Nutrition

FOR

DUMMIES®

4TH EDITION

Nutrition For Dummies, 4th Edition

Cheat Sheet

Measurements Used in Nutrition

Abbreviation	Measurement	Equivalent	Abbreviation	Measurement	Equivalent
g	gram	1,000 milligrams	lb	pound	0.45 kilograms
		1,000,000 micrograms			16 ounces
mg	milligram	$\frac{1}{1,000}$ gram	l	liter	1,000 milliliters
mcg	microgram	$\frac{1}{1,000,000}$ gram			10 deciliters
kg	kilogram	1,000 grams	dl	deciliter	$\frac{1}{10}$ liter
		2.2 pounds	ml	milliliter	$\frac{1}{1,000}$ liter

When You May Need Extra Vitamins

Special circumstances require extra vitamins, and some of those circumstances are listed here. Read Chapter 10 before adding any vitamin supplements to your diet.

✔ When you're pregnant, you need extra amounts of vitamins C, D, E, B12, riboflavin, folate, and protein.

✔ When you're breast-feeding your baby, you need extra vitamin A, E, thiamin, riboflavin, and folate. You also need extra vitamin D, vitamin C, and niacin.

✔ What? You still smoke? Then you need more vitamin C than nonsmokers.

✔ Are you a woman approaching menopause? You need calcium and extra vitamin D.

✔ Is your diet strictly vegetarian — meaning no food of animal origin, not even milk and eggs? You need extra vitamin D and B12.

✔ Are you a couch potato who plans to start working out? Take it slow, and take an extra dose of vitamin E.

✔ Do you have very light or very dark skin? You should take vitamin D supplements.

When You May Need Extra Minerals

Here are some examples of when you should consider taking mineral supplements. Read Chapter 11 before adding these minerals to your diet.

✔ If you're a man, taking a daily supplement of 200 micrograms of selenium may cut your risk of prostate cancer by two-thirds.

✔ If you're a woman, you probably lose 1.4 milligrams of iron during each menstrual period. To remedy this, some doctors prescribe a daily iron supplement.

✔ If you're pregnant, studies suggest (but don't prove) that you may need extra copper to protect nerve cells in the fetal brain.

✔ If you're breast-feeding your baby, you need extra calcium, phosphorus, magnesium, iron, zinc, and selenium.

✔ If you're a woman approaching menopause, or if you're an older man, extra calcium is recommended.

✔ If you're a strict vegetarian, iron supplements should be standard fare. Calcium may also be necessary.

The 19 Essential Vitamins and Minerals

✔ Vitamin A	✔ Vitamin E	✔ Vitamin C	✔ Iron	✔ Niacin	✔ Selenium
✔ Vitamin B12	✔ Calcium	✔ Magnesium	✔ Riboflavin (vitamin B2)	✔ Iodine	✔ Folate
✔ Vitamin D	✔ Vitamin K	✔ Thiamin (vitamin B1)	✔ Vitamin B6		
✔ Choline	✔ Phosphorous		✔ Zinc		

For Dummies: Bestselling Book Series for Beginners

Nutrition For Dummies,® 4th Edition

Cheat Sheet

Key Elements Used in Nutrition Words

Element	Meaning
amyl-	starch
an-	without
anti-	against
-ase	an enzyme
di-	two
-emia	found in the blood
gastro-	referring to the stomach

Element	Meaning
gly-	referring to sugars
hydr-, hydro-	water (*also:* hydrogen)
hyper-	above normal
hypo-	below normal
lact-, lacti-, lacto-	milk

Element	Meaning
lip-, lipo-	fat
macro-	large
micro-	very small
mono-	one
-ose	sugar
tri-	three

How to Keep Food Safe as Well as Nutritious

- Wash your hands before (and after) touching food.
- Wash all fruits and vegetables before you use them.
- Follow the directions on the food package for storing and preparing food safely.
- Handle all raw meat, fish, and poultry as though it were contaminated (sometimes, it is!).
- Cook foods thoroughly.
- Keep hot foods hot, cold foods cold.
- Never eat or drink anything containing raw eggs.
- Use a separate cutting board for raw meat, fish, and poultry.
- Never taste any questionable food "just to be sure it's all right." When in doubt, throw it out.

Easy Ways to Cut Calories

- Use low-fat or no-fat dairy products
- Use sugar substitutes instead of sugar
- Skim the fat off all soups and stews
- Choose low-fat desserts
- Serve poultry without skin
- Avoid high-fat, oily salad dressings
- Make open-face sandwiches with just one slice of bread
- Eliminate high-fat ingredients in any dish
- Don't butter the veggies
- Rinse the fat off chopped meat with hot water

Fast Online Help with Nutrition Puzzles

Here's a quick and handy list of recommended Web sites to visit when you need even more nutrition information.

- American Council on Science and Health (ASCH): www.acsh.org
- American Dietetic Association: www.eatright.org
- The American Cancer Society: www.cancer.org
- The American Heart Association: www.americanheart.org
- Center for Science in the Public Interest (CSPI): www.cspinet.org
- The Food Allergy and Anaphylaxis Network: www.foodallergy.org
- International Food Information Council (IFIC): ific.org
- U.S. Department of Agriculture Nutrient Database: www.nal.usda.gov/fnic/foodcomp/search
- U.S. Food and Drug Administration: www.fda.gov
- USDA Food and Nutrition Information Center (FNIC): www.nal.usda.gov/fnic

For Dummies: Bestselling Book Series for Beginners

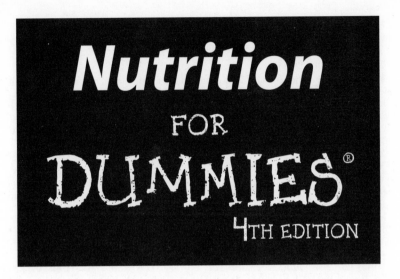

Nutrition FOR DUMMIES® 4TH EDITION

by Carol Ann Rinzler

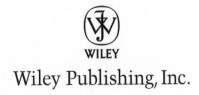

WILEY

Wiley Publishing, Inc.

Nutrition For Dummies,® 4th Edition

Published by
Wiley Publishing, Inc.
111 River St.
Hoboken, NJ 07030-5774
www.wiley.com

WILEY

About the Author

Carol Ann Rinzler is a noted authority on health and nutrition and holds an MA from Columbia University. She has written a nutrition column for the *New York Daily News* and is the author of more than 20 health-related books, including *Controlling Cholesterol For Dummies*, *Weight Loss Kit For Dummies*, and the highly acclaimed *Estrogen and Breast Cancer: A Warning to Women*. Rinzler lives in New York with her husband, wine writer Perry Luntz, and their amiable cat, Kat.

Dedication

This book is dedicated to my husband, Perry Luntz, a fellow writer who, as always, stayed patient as a saint and even-tempered beyond belief while I was racing pell-mell (and not always pleasantly) to deadline.

Author's Acknowledgments

This new edition of *Nutrition For Dummies* has given me the opportunity to work with yet another group of thoroughly pleasant professionals at the Dummies group of Wiley Publishing. Acquisitions Editor Michael Lewis enthusiastically welcomed the new edition and kept the project moving smoothly. Senior Project Editor Natalie Harris was incredibly soothing to the author, not to mention totally in command of the hundreds, maybe even thousands, of details it takes to update a nutrition book. I appreciate Danielle Voirol, maybe more than she knows; medical and science writers understand very well that without skillful, knowledgeable copy editors, we would be walking over factual cliffs every day of our writing lives. Finally, I am grateful to Alfred Bushway, PhD, for once again reading and commenting on the manuscript. Thanks, guys.

Publisher's Acknowledgments

We're proud of this book; please send us your comments through our Dummies online registration form located at www.dummies.com/register/.

Some of the people who helped bring this book to market include the following:

Acquisitions, Editorial, and Media Development

Project Editor: Natalie Faye Harris

(Previous Edition: Alissa Schwipps)

Acquisitions Editor: Mike Lewis

(Previous Edition: Natasha Graf)

Copy Editor: Danielle Voirol

(Previous Edition: Neil Johnson)

Editorial Program Coordinator: Hanna K. Scott

Technical Editor: Alfred Bushway, PhD

Editorial Manager: Christine Beck

Editorial Assistants: Erin Calligan, Nadine Bell, David Lutton

Cover Photo: © Ron Chapple/Thinkstock/ PictureQuest

Cartoons: Rich Tennant (www.the5thwave.com)

Composition Services

Project Coordinator: Tera Knapp

Layout and Graphics: Carl Byers, Andrea Dahl, Brooke Graczyk, Joyce Haughey, Stephanie D. Jumper, Barbara Moore, Barry Offringa, Jill Proll

Proofreaders: Leeann Harney, Jessica Kramer, Dwight Ramsey, Techbooks

Indexer: Techbooks

Publishing and Editorial for Consumer Dummies

Diane Graves Steele, Vice President and Publisher, Consumer Dummies

Joyce Pepple, Acquisitions Director, Consumer Dummies

Kristin A. Cocks, Product Development Director, Consumer Dummies

Michael Spring, Vice President and Publisher, Travel

Kelly Regan, Editorial Director, Travel

Publishing for Technology Dummies

Andy Cummings, Vice President and Publisher, Dummies Technology/General User

Composition Services

Gerry Fahey, Vice President of Production Services

Debbie Stailey, Director of Composition Services

Contents at a Glance

Table of Contents

Introduction

· ·

*O*nce upon a time people simply sat down to dinner, eating to fill up an
empty stomach or just for the pleasure of it. Nobody said, "Wow, that
cream soup is loaded with calories," or asked whether the bread was a high-
fiber loaf or fretted about the chicken being served with the skin still on. No
longer. Today, the dinner table can be a battleground between health and
pleasure. You plan your meals with the precision of a major general moving
his troops into the front lines, and for most people, the fight to eat what's
good for you rather than what tastes good has become a lifelong struggle.

This book is designed to end the war between your need for good nutrition
and your equally compelling need for tasty meals. In fact (listen up, here!),
what's good for you can also be good to eat — and vice versa.

About This Book

Nutrition For Dummies, 4th Edition, doesn't aim to send you back to the class-
room, sit you down, and make you take notes about what to put on the table
every day from now until you're 104 years old. You're reading a reference
book, so you don't have to memorize anything — when you want more info,
just jump in anywhere to look it up.

Instead, this book means to give you the information you need to make wise
food choices — which always means choices that please the palate and soul,
as well as the body. Some of what you'll read here is really, *really* basic:
definitions of vitamins, minerals, proteins, fats, carbohydrates, and — can
you believe this? — plain old water. You'll also read tips about how to put
together a nutritious shopping list and how to use food to make meals so
good you can't wait to eat them.

For those who know absolutely nothing about nutrition except that it deals
with food, this book is a starting point. For those who know more than a little
about nutrition, this book is a refresher course to bring you up to speed on
what has happened since the last time you checked out a calorie chart.

For those who want to know *absolutely everything,* this 4th edition of Nutrition for Dummies book is UP TO DATE, with hot new info from the 2005 revisions of the Dietary Guidelines for Americans, new recommended daily allowances for all the nutrients a healthy body needs, plus all the twisty "this is good for you" and "this is really, really rotten" bits and pieces of food info that nutrition scientists have come up with since, well, the last edition.

Conventions Used in This Book

The following conventions are used throughout the text to make things consistent and easy to understand:

- ✔ All Web addresses appear in `monofont`.

- ✔ New terms appear in *italic* and are closely followed by an easy-to-understand definition.

- ✔ **Bold** is used to highlight the action parts of numbered steps, as well as key words in bulleted lists.

- ✔ Nutrition experts commonly use metric terms such as gram (g), milligram (mg), and microgram (mcg) to describe quantities of protein, fat, carbohydrates, vitamins, minerals, and other nutrients. Feel free to use the Cheat Sheet at the front of this book whenever you forget what each means.

What You Don't Have to Read

What? Not read something printed in a book? Well, yeah. Some small parts of this book are fun or informative but not necessarily vital to your understanding of nutrition. For example:

- ✔ **Text in sidebars:** The sidebars are the shaded boxes that appear here and there. They share personal stories and observations but aren't necessary reading.

- ✔ **Anything with a Technical Stuff icon attached:** This information is interesting but not critical to your understanding of nutrition.

- ✔ **The stuff on the copyright page:** No kidding. You'll find nothing here of interest unless you're inexplicably enamored by legal language and Library of Congress numbers.

Foolish Assumptions

Every book is written with a particular reader in mind, and this one is no different. As I wrote this book, I made the following basic assumptions about who you are and why you plunked down your hard-earned cash for an entire volume about nutrition:

- ✔ You didn't study nutrition in high school or college and now you've discovered that you have a better shot a staying healthy if you know how to put together well-balanced, nutritious meals.

- ✔ You're confused by conflicting advice on vitamins and minerals, protein, fats and carbs. In other words, you need a reliable road map through the nutrient maze.

- ✔ You want basic information, but you don't want to become an expert in nutrition or spend hours digging your way through medical textbooks and journals.

How This Book Is Organized

The following is a brief summary of each part in *Nutrition For Dummies,* 4th Edition. You can use this guide as a fast way to check out what you want to read first. One really nice thing about this book is that you don't have to start with Chapter 1 and read straight through to the end. *Au contraire,* as the French like to say when they mean "on the contrary." You can dive in absolutely anywhere and still come up with tons of tasty information about how food helps your body work.

Part I: The Basic Facts about Nutrition

Chapter 1 defines nutrition and its effects on your body. This chapter also tells you how to read a nutrition study and how to judge the value of nutrition information in newspapers, magazines, and on TV. Chapter 2 is a really clear guide to how your digestive system works to transform food and beverages into the nutrients you need to sustain a healthy body. Chapter 3 concentrates on calories, the energy factor in food and beverages. Chapter 4 tells you how much of each nutrient you need to stay in tiptop form. Chapter 5 details some of the rules on dietary supplements — the pills, powders, and potions that add nutritional punch to your regular diet.

Part II: What You Get from Food

Chapter 6 gives you the facts about protein: where you get it and what it does in your body. Chapter 7 does the same job for dietary fat, while Chapter 8 explains carbohydrates: sugars, starches, and that indigestible but totally vital substance in carbohydrate foods — ta-da! — dietary fiber. Chapter 9 outlines the risks and, yes, some newly proven benefits of alcohol beverages.

Chapter 10 is about vitamins, the substances in food that trigger so many vital chemical reactions in your body. Chapter 11 is about minerals, substances that often work in tandem with vitamins. Chapter 12 explains phytochemicals, newly important substances in food. Chapter 13 is about water, the essential liquid that comprises as much as 70 percent of your body weight. This chapter also describes the functions of electrolytes, special minerals that maintain your fluid balance (the correct amount of water inside and outside your body cells).

Part III: Healthy Eating

Chapter 14 is about *hunger* (the need for food) and *appetite* (the desire for food). Balancing these two eating factors makes maintaining a healthful weight possible for you. Chapter 15 on the other hand, is about food preference: why you like some foods and really, really hate others. (Broccoli, anyone?) Chapter 16 tells you how to assemble a healthful diet. It's based on the Dietary Guidelines for Americans created by the U.S. Departments of Agriculture and Health and Human Services, plus some recent updates from the National Academy of Sciences' Institute of Medicine, so you know it's good for you. Chapter 17 explains how to use nutritional guidelines to plan nutritious, appetizing meals at home. Chapter 18 shows you how to take the guidelines out to dinner so that you can judge the value of foods in all kinds of restaurants, from the posh white-tablecloth ones to fast-food havens.

Part IV: Food Processing

Chapter 19 asks and answers this simple question: What is food processing? Chapter 20 shows you how cooking affects the way food looks and tastes, as well as its nutritional value. Chapter 21 does the same for freezing, canning, drying, and irradiating techniques. Chapter 22 gives you the lowdown on chemicals used to keep food fresh.

Part V: Food and Medicine

Chapter 23 explains why some food gives some people hives and presents strategies for identifying and avoiding the food to which you may be allergic. Chapter 24 is about how eating or drinking certain foods and beverages may affect your mood — a hot topic these days with nutrition researchers. Chapter 25 tells you how foods may interact with medical drugs — an important subject for anyone who ever has taken, now takes, or ever plans to take medicine. Chapter 26 tells you how some foods may actually act as preventive medicine or relieve the symptoms of certain illnesses ranging from the horrible-but-not-really-serious common cold to the Big Two: heart disease and cancer.

Part VI: The Part of Tens

Could there even be a *For Dummies* book without The Part of Tens? Not a chance. This part (Chapters 27, 28, and 29) provides ten great nutritional Web site addresses, lists ten common foods with near-magical status, and last — but definitely not least — lays out ten easy ways to cut calories from food.

Icons Used in This Book

Icons are a handy *For Dummies* way to catch your attention as you slide your eyes down the page. The icons come in several varieties, each with its own special meaning:

Nutrition is full of stuff that "everybody knows." This masked marvel clues you in to the real facts when (as often happens) everybody's wrong!

This little guy looks smart because he's marking the place where you find definitions of the words used by nutrition experts.

The Official Word icon says, "Look here for scientific studies, statistics, definitions, and recommendations used to create standard nutrition policy."

This time, the same smart fella is pointing to clear, concise explanations of technical terms and processes — details that are interesting but not necessarily critical to your understanding of a topic. In other words, skip them if you want, but try a few first.

Bull's-eye! This is time- and stress-saving information that you can use to improve your diet and health.

This is a watch-out-for-the-curves icon, alerting you to nutrition pitfalls such as (oops!) leaving the skin on the chicken — turning a low-fat food into one that is high in fat and cholesterol. This icon also warns you about physical dangers such as supplements to avoid because they may do more damage than good to your health.

Where to Go from Here

Ah, here's the best part. *For Dummies* books are not linear (a fancy way of saying they proceed from A to B to C . . . and so on). In fact, you can dive right in anywhere, say at L, M, or N, and still make sense of what you're reading because each chapter delivers a complete message.

For example, if carbohydrates are your passion, go right to Chapter 8. If you want to know how to pick and choose from a menu when you're eating out, skip to Chapter 18. If you've always been fascinated by food processing, your choice is Chapter 19. You can use the Table of Contents to find broad categories of information or the Index to look up more specific things.

If you're not sure where you want to go, why not just begin at the beginning, Part I? It gives you all the basic info you need to understand nutrition and points to places where you can find more detailed information.

Part I
The Basic Facts about Nutrition

The 5th Wave   By Rich Tennant

"Yes, we told them about the pectin and flavonoids, but they seem a little slow to catch on. Maybe if we just left them alone with the snake a while..."

In this part . . .

To use food wisely, you need a firm grasp of the basics. In this part, I define nutrition and give you a detailed explanation of digestion (how your body turns food into nutrients). I also explain why calories are useful and set forth a no-nonsense starter guide to your daily requirements of vitamins, minerals, and other good stuff.

Chapter 1

What's Nutrition, Anyway?

*W*elcome aboard! You're about to begin your very own *Fantastic Voyage.* (You know. That's the 1966 movie in which Raquel Welch and a couple of guys were shrunk down to the size of a molecule to sail through the body of a politician shot by an assassin who had . . . hey, maybe you should just check out the next showing on your favorite cable movie channel.)

In any event, as you read, chapter by chapter, you can follow a route that carries food (meaning food and beverages) from your plate to your mouth to your digestive tract and into every tissue and cell. Along the way, you'll have the opportunity to see how your organs and systems work. You'll observe firsthand why some foods and beverages are essential to your health. And you'll discover how to manage your diet so you can get the biggest bang (nutrients) for your buck (calories). Bon voyage!

Nutrition Equals Life

Technically speaking, *nutrition* is the science of how the body uses food. In fact, nutrition is life. All living things, including you, need food and water to live. Beyond that, you need good food, meaning food with the proper nutrients, to live well. If you don't eat and drink, you'll die. Period. If you don't eat and drink nutritious food and beverages:

  ✔ Your bones may bend or break (not enough calcium).

  ✔ Your gums may bleed (not enough vitamin C).

  ✔ Your blood may not carry oxygen to every cell (not enough iron).

Essential nutrients for Fido, Fluffy, and your pet petunia

Vitamin C isn't the only nutrient that's essential for one species but not for others. Many organic compounds (substances similar to vitamins) and elements (minerals) are essential for your green or furry friends but not for you, either because you can synthesize them from the food you eat or because they're so widely available in the human diet and you require such small amounts that you can get what you need without hardly trying.

Two good examples are the organic compounds choline and myoinositol. *Choline* is an essential nutrient for several species of animals, including dogs, cats, rats, and guinea pigs. Although choline has now been declared essential for human beings (more about that in Chapter 10), human bodies produce choline on their own, and you can get choline from eggs, liver, soybeans, cauliflower, and lettuce. *Myoinositol* is

an essential nutrient for gerbils and rats, but human beings synthesize it naturally and use it in many body processes, such as transmitting signals between cells.

Here's a handy list of nutrients that are essential for animals and/or plants but not for you:

Organic Compounds	*Elements*
Carnitine	Arsenic
Myoinositol	Cadmium
Taurine	Lead
	Nickel
	Silicon
	Tin
	Vanadium

And on, and on, and on. Understanding how good nutrition protects you against these dire consequences requires a familiarity with the language and concepts of nutrition. Knowing some basic chemistry is helpful (don't panic: Chemistry can be a cinch when you read about it in plain English). A smattering of sociology and psychology is also useful, because although nutrition is mostly about how food revs up and sustains your body, it's also about the cultural traditions and individual differences that explain how you choose your favorite foods (see Chapter 15).

To sum it up: Nutrition is about why you eat what you eat and how the food you get affects your body and your health.

First principles: Energy and nutrients

Nutrition's primary task is figuring out which foods and beverages (in what quantities) provide the energy and building material you need to construct and maintain every organ and system. To do this, nutrition concentrates on food's two basic attributes: energy and nutrients.

Energy from food

Energy is the ability to do work. Virtually every bite of food gives you energy, even when it doesn't give you nutrients. The amount of energy in food is measured in *calories,* the amount of heat produced when food is burned (metabolized) in your body cells. You can read all about calories in Chapter 3. But right now, all you need to know is that food is the fuel on which your body runs. Without enough food, you don't have enough energy.

Nutrients in food

Nutrients are chemical substances your body uses to build, maintain, and repair tissues. They also empower cells to send messages back and forth to conduct essential chemical reactions, such as the ones that make it possible for you to

- Breathe
- Move
- Eliminate waste
- Think
- See
- Hear
- Smell
- Taste

. . . and do everything else natural to a living body.

Food provides two distinct groups of nutrients:

- **Macronutrients (macro = big):** Protein, fat, carbohydrates, and water
- **Micronutrients (micro = small):** Vitamins and minerals

What's the difference between these two groups? The amount you need each day. Your daily requirements for macronutrients generally exceed 1 gram. (For comparison's sake, 28 grams are in an ounce.) For example, a man needs about 63 grams of protein a day (slightly more than two ounces), and a woman needs 50 grams (slightly less than two ounces).

Your daily requirements for micronutrients are much smaller. For example, the Recommended Dietary Allowance (RDA) for vitamin C is measured in milligrams ($\frac{1}{1,000}$ of a gram), while the RDAs for vitamin D, vitamin B12, and folate are even smaller and are measured in micrograms ($\frac{1}{1,000,000}$ of a gram). You can find out much more about the RDAs, including how they vary for people of different ages, in Chapter 4.

What's an essential nutrient?

A reasonable person may assume that an essential nutrient is one you need to sustain a healthy body. But who says a reasonable person thinks like a nutritionist? In nutritionspeak, an *essential nutrient* is a very special thing:

✔ **An essential nutrient cannot be manufactured in the body.** You have to get essential nutrients from food or from a nutritional supplement.

✔ **An essential nutrient is linked to a specific deficiency disease.** For example, people who go without protein for extended periods of time develop the protein-deficiency disease *kwashiorkor*. People who don't get enough vitamin C develop the vitamin C–deficiency disease *scurvy*. A diet rich in the essential nutrient cures the deficiency disease, but you need the proper nutrient. In other words, you can't cure a protein deficiency with extra amounts of vitamin C.

Not all nutrients are essential for all species of animals. For example, vitamin C is an essential nutrient for human beings but not for dogs. A dog's body makes the vitamin C it needs. Check out the list of nutrients on a can or bag of dog food. See? No C. The dog already has the C it — sorry, he or she — requires.

Essential nutrients for human beings include many well-known vitamins and minerals, several *amino acids* (the so-called building blocks of proteins), and at least two fatty acids. For more about these essential nutrients, see Chapters 6, 7, 10, and 11.

Protecting the nutrients in your food

Identifying nutrients is one thing. Making sure you get them into your body is another. Here, the essential idea is to keep nutritious food nutritious by preserving and protecting its components.

Some people see the term *food processing* as a nutritional dirty word. Or words. They're wrong. Without food processing and preservatives, you and I would still be forced to gather (or kill) our food each morning and down it fast before it spoiled. For more about which processing and preservative techniques produce the safest, most nutritious — and yes, delicious — dinners, check out Chapters 19, 20, 21 and 22.

Considering how vital food preservation can be, you may want to think about when you last heard a rousing cheer for the anonymous cook who first noticed that salting or pickling food could extend food's shelf life. Or for the guys who invented the refrigeration and freezing techniques that slow food's natural tendency to degrade (translation: spoil). Or for Louis Pasteur, the man who made it ab-so-lute-ly clear that heating food to boiling kills bugs that might otherwise cause food poisoning. Hardly ever, that's when. So give them a hand, right here. Cool.

Other interesting substances in food

The latest flash in the nutrition sky is caused by phytochemicals. *Phyto* is the Greek word for plants, so *phytochemicals* are simply — yes, you've got it — chemicals from plants. Although the 13-letter group name may be new to you, you're already familiar with some phytochemicals. Vitamins are phytochemicals. Pigments such as beta carotene, the deep yellow coloring in fruits and vegetables that your body can convert to a form of vitamin A, are phytochemicals.

And then there are *phytoestrogens,* hormone-like chemicals that grabbed the spotlight when it was suggested that a diet high in phytoestrogens, such as the isoflavones found in soybeans, may lower the risk of heart disease and reduce the incidence of reproductive cancers (cancers of the breast, ovary, uterus, and prostate). More recent studies suggest that phytoestrogens may have some problems of their own, so to find out more about phytochemicals, including phytoestrogens, check out Chapter 12.

You are what you eat

Oh boy, I bet you've heard this one before. But it bears repeating, because the human body really is built from the nutrients it gets from food: water, protein, fat, carbohydrates, vitamins, and minerals. On average, when you step on the scale

- ✔ About 60 percent of your weight is water.
- ✔ About 20 percent of your weight is fat.
- ✔ About 20 percent of your weight is a combination of mostly protein (especially in your muscles) plus carbohydrates, minerals, and vitamins.

An easy way to remember your body's percentage of water, fat, and protein and other nutrients is to think of it as the "60-20-20 Rule."

What's a body made of?

Sugar and spice and everything nice . . . Oops. What I meant to say was the human body is made of water and fat and protein and carbohydrates and vitamins and minerals.

On average, when you step on the scale, approximately 60 percent of your weight is water, 20 percent is body fat (slightly less for a man), and 20 percent is a combination of mostly protein, plus carbohydrates, minerals, vitamins, and other naturally occurring biochemicals.

Based on these percentages, you can reasonably expect that an average 140-pound person's body weight consists of about

✔ 84 pounds of water

✔ 28 pounds of body fat

✔ 28 pounds of a combination of protein (up to 25 pounds), minerals (up to 7 pounds), carbohydrates (up to 1.4 pounds), and vitamins (a trace).

Yep, you're right: Those last figures do total more than 28 pounds. That's because "up to"

(as in "up to 25 pounds of protein") means that the amounts may vary from person to person.

For example, a young person's body has proportionately more muscle and less fat than an older person's, while a woman's body has proportionately less muscle and more fat than a man's. As a result, more of a man's weight comes from protein and calcium, while more of a woman's body comes from fat. Protein-packed muscles and mineral-packed bones are denser tissue than fat.

Weigh a man and a woman of roughly the same height and size, and he's likely to tip the scale higher every time.

The National Research Council, *Recommended Dietary Allowances* (Washington D.C.: National Academy Press, 1989); Eleanor Noss Whitney, Corinne Balog Cataldo, and Sharon Rady Rolfes, *Understanding Normal and Clinical Nutrition* (Minneapolis/St. Paul: West Publishing Company, 1994)

Your nutritional status

Nutritional status is a phrase that describes the state of your health as related to your diet. For example, people who are starving do not get the nutrients or calories they need for optimum health. These people are said to be *malnourished* (mal = bad), which means their nutritional status is, to put it gently, definitely not good. Malnutrition may arise from

✔ **A diet that doesn't provide enough food.** This situation can occur in times of famine or through voluntary starvation because of an eating disorder or because something in your life disturbs your appetite. For example, older people may be at risk of malnutrition because of tooth loss or age-related loss of appetite or because they live alone and sometimes just forget to eat.

✔ **A diet that, while otherwise adequate, is deficient in a specific nutri-ent.** This kind of nutritional inadequacy can lead to — surprise! — a defi-ciency disease, such as beriberi, the disease caused by a lack of vitamin B1 (thiamine).

✔ **A metabolic disorder or medical condition that prevents your body from absorbing specific nutrients, such as carbohydrates or protein.** One common example is diabetes, the inability to produce enough insulin, the hormone your body uses to metabolize (digest) carbohy-drates. Another is celiac disease, a condition that makes it impossible for the body to digest gluten, a protein in wheat. Need more info on either diabetes or celiac disease? Check out *Diabetes For Dummies, 2nd Edition,* and *Living Gluten-Free for Dummies.* Of course.

Doctors and registered dieticians have many tools with which to rate your nutritional status. For example, they can

✔ Review your medical history to see whether you have any conditions (such as dentures) that may make eating certain foods difficult or that interfere with your ability to absorb nutrients.

✔ Perform a physical examination to look for obvious signs of nutritional deficiency, such as dull hair and eyes (a lack of vitamins?), poor posture (not enough calcium to protect the spinal bones?), or extreme thinness (not enough food? An underlying disease?).

✔ Order laboratory blood and urine tests that may identify early signs of malnutrition, such as the lack of red blood cells that characterizes anemia caused by an iron deficiency.

At every stage of life, the aim of a good diet is to maintain a healthy nutri-tional status.

Fitting food into the medicine chest

Food is medicine for the body and the soul. Good meals make good friends, and modern research validates the virtues of not only Granny's chicken soup but also heart-healthy sulfur compounds in garlic and onions, anti-cholesterol dietary fiber in grains and beans, bone-building calcium in milk and greens, and mood elevators in coffee, tea, and chocolate.

Of course, foods pose some risks as well: food allergies, food intolerances, food and drug interactions, and the occasional harmful substances such as the dreaded *saturated fats* and *trans fats* (quick — Chapter 7!). In other words, constructing a healthful diet can mean tailoring food choices to your own special body. Not to worry: You can do it. Especially after reading through Part V. Would a *For Dummies* book leave you unarmed? Not a chance!

Finding Nutrition Facts

Getting reliable information about nutrition can be a daunting challenge. For the most part, your nutrition information is likely to come from TV and radio talk shows or news, your daily newspaper, your favorite magazine, a variety of nutrition-oriented books, and the Internet. How can you tell whether what you hear or read is really right?

Nutritional people

The people who make nutrition news may be scientists, reporters, or simply someone who wandered in with a new theory (Artichokes prevent cancer! Never eat cherries and cheese at the same meal! Vitamin C gives you hives!), the more bizarre the better. But several groups of people are most likely to give you news you can use with confidence. For example:

✔ **Nutrition scientists:** These are people with graduate degrees (usually in chemistry, biology, biochemistry, or physics) engaged in research dealing primarily with the effects of food on animals and human beings.

✔ **Nutrition researchers:** Researchers may be either nutrition scientists or professionals in another field, such as medicine or sociology, whose research (study or studies) concentrates on the effects of food.

✔ **Nutritionists:** These are people who concentrate on the study of nutrition. In some states, a person who uses the title "nutritionist" must have a graduate degree in basic science courses related to nutrition.

✔ **Dietitians:** These people have undergraduate degrees in food and nutrition science or the management of food programs. A person with the letters R.D. after his or her name has completed a dietetic internship and passed an American Dietetic Association licensing exam.

✔ **Nutrition reporters and writers:** These are people who specialize in giving you information about the medical and/or scientific aspects of food. Like reporters who concentrate on politics or sports, nutrition reporters gain their expertise through years of covering their beat. Most have the science background required to translate technical information into language nonscientists can understand; some have been trained as dietitians, nutritionists, or nutrition scientists.

Consumer alert: Regardless of the source, nutrition news should always pass what you may call *The Reasonableness Test*. In other words, if a story or report or study sounds ridiculous, it probably is.

Want some guidelines for evaluating nutrition studies? Read on.

Can you trust this study?

You open your morning newspaper or turn on the evening news and read or hear that a group of researchers at an impeccably prestigious scientific organization has published a study showing that yet another thing you've always taken for granted is hazardous to your health. For example, the study says drinking coffee stresses your heart, adding salt to food raises blood pressure, or fatty foods increase your risk of cancer or heart disease.

So you throw out the offending food or drink or rearrange your daily routine to avoid the once-acceptable, now-dangerous food, beverage, or additive. And then what happens? Two weeks, two months, or two years down the road, a second, equally prestigious group of scientists publishes a study conclusively proving that the first group got it wrong: In fact, this study shows coffee has no effect on the risk of heart disease — and may even improve athletic performance; salt does not cause hypertension except in certain sensitive individuals; only *some* fatty foods are risky.

Who's right? Nobody seems to know. That leaves you, a layperson, on your own to come up with the answer. Never fear — you may not be a nutritionist, but that doesn't mean you can't apply a few common-sense rules to any study you read about, rules that say: "Yes, this may be true," or "No, this may not be."

Does this study include human beings?

True, animal studies can alert researchers to potential problems, but working with animals alone cannot give you conclusive proof.

Different species react differently to various chemicals and diseases. For example, although cows and horses can digest grass and hay, human being can't. And while outright poisons such as cyanide clearly traumatize any living body, many foods or drugs that harm a laboratory rat won't harm you. And vice versa. For example, mouse and rat embryos suffer no ill effects when their mothers are given thalidomide, the sedative that's known to cause deformed fetal limbs when given to pregnant monkeys — and human beings — at the point in pregnancy when limbs are developing. (And here's an astounding turn: Modern research shows that thalidomide is beneficial for treating or preventing *human* skin problems related to Hansen's disease [leprosy], cancer, and/or autoimmune conditions, such as rheumatoid arthritis, in which the body mistakenly attacks its own tissues.)

Are enough people in this study?

Hey, researchers' saying, "Well, I did give this to a couple of people," is simply not enough. The study must include sufficient numbers and a variety of individuals, too. If you don't have enough people in the study — several hundred to many thousand — to establish a pattern, there's always the possibility that an effect occurred by chance.

If you don't include different types of people, which generally means young and old men and women of different racial and ethnic groups, your results may not apply across the board. For example, the original studies linking high blood cholesterol levels to an increased risk of heart disease and linking small doses of aspirin to a reduced risk of a second heart attack involved only men. It wasn't until follow-up studies were conducted with women that researchers were able to say with any certainty that high cholesterol is dangerous and aspirin is protective for women as well — but not in quite the same way: In January 2006, the *Journal of the American Medical Association* reported that men taking low dose aspirin tend to lower their risk of heart attack. For women, the aspirin reduces the risk of stroke. Vive la difference!

Is there anything in the design or method of this study that may affect the accuracy of its conclusions?

Some testing methods are more likely to lead to biased or inaccurate conclusions. For example, a retrospective study (which asks people to tell what they did in the past) is always considered less accurate than a prospective study (one that follows people while they're actually doing what the researchers are studying), because memory isn't always accurate. People tend to forget details or, without meaning to, alter them to fit the researchers' questions.

Are the study's conclusions reasonable?

When a study comes up with a conclusion that seems illogical to you, chances are the researchers feel the same way. For example, in 1990, the long-running Nurses' Study at the Harvard School of Public Health reported that a high-fat diet raised the risk of colon cancer. But the data showed a link only to diets high in beef. No link was found to diets high in dairy fat. In short, this study was begging for a second study to confirm (or deny) its results.

And while we wait for that second and, naturally, third study, you can bet we're keeping an open mind. The nature of life is that things *do* change, sometimes in surprising ways. Consider dioxin, a toxic contaminant found in some fish. Consider Olestra, the calorie-free fat substitute that makes some tummies rumble. As you read this page, dioxin's still a bad actor, but in 2005 researchers at the University of Cincinnati and the University of Western Australia announced that eating foods containing Olestra may speed your body's elimination of — you guessed it — dioxin. A-maz-ing.

Chapter 2

Digestion: The 24-Hour Food Factory

● ●

In This Chapter

▶ Getting acquainted with your digestive organs

▶ Following the food through your body

▶ Absorbing nutrients and passing them along to your body

● ●

*W*hen you see (or smell) something appetizing, your digestive organs leap into action. Your mouth waters. Your stomach contracts. Intestinal glands begin to secrete the chemicals that turn food into the nutrients that build new tissues and provide the energy you need to keep zipping through the days, months, and years.

This chapter introduces you to your digestive system and explains exactly how your body digests the many different kinds of foods you eat, all the while extracting the nutrients you need to keep on truckin'.

Introducing the Digestive System

Your digestive system may never win a Tony, Oscar, or Emmy, but it certainly deserves your applause for its ability to turn complex food into basic nutrients. Doing this requires not a cast of thousands but a group of digestive organs, each designed specifically to perform one role in the two-part process. Read on.

The digestive organs

Although exceedingly well-organized, your digestive system is basically one long tube that starts at your mouth, continues down through your throat to your stomach, and then goes on to your small and large intestines and past the rectum to end at your anus.

In between, with the help of the liver, pancreas, and gallbladder, the usable (digestible) parts of everything that you eat are converted to simple compounds that your body can easily absorb to burn for energy or to build new tissue. The indigestible residue is bundled off and eliminated as waste.

Figure 2-1 shows the body parts and organs that comprise your digestive system.

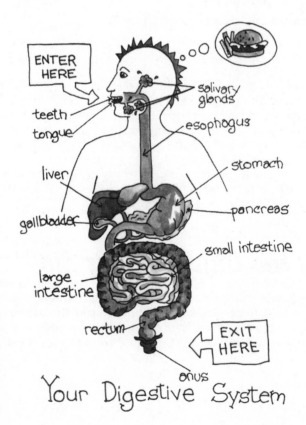

Figure 2-1:
Your
digestive
system in all
its glory.

ENTER HERE

salivary glands

teeth

tongue

esophagus

liver

stomach

gallbladder

pancreas

large intestine

small intestine

rectum

EXIT HERE

anus

Your Digestive System

Digestion: A two-part process

Digestion is a two-part process — half mechanical, half chemical:

- *Mechanical digestion* takes place in your mouth and your stomach. Your teeth break food into small pieces that you can swallow without choking. In your stomach, a churning action continues to break food into smaller particles.

- *Chemical digestion* occurs at every point in the digestive tract where enzymes and other substances, such as *hydrochloric acid* (from stomach glands) and *bile* (from the liver), dissolve food, releasing the nutrients inside.

Understanding How Your Body Digests Food

Each organ in the digestive system plays a specific role in the digestive drama. But the first act occurs in two places that are never listed as part of the digestive tract: your eyes and nose.

The eyes and nose

When you see appetizing food, you experience a conditioned response. (For the lowdown on how your digestive system can be conditioned to respond to food, see Chapter 14; for information on your food preferences, see Chapter 15). In other words, your thoughts — "Wow! That looks good!" — stimulate your brain to tell your digestive organs to get ready for action.

What happens in your nose is purely physical. The tantalizing aroma of good food is transmitted by molecules that fly from the surface of the food to settle on the membrane lining of your nostrils; these molecules stimulate the receptor cells on the olfactory nerve fibers that stretch from your nose back to your brain. When the receptor cells communicate with your brain — "Listen up, there's good stuff here!" — your brain sends encouraging messages to your mouth and digestive tract.

In both cases — eyes and nose — the results are the same: "Start the saliva flowing," they say. "Warm up the stomach glands. Alert the small intestine." In other words, the sight and scent of food has made your mouth water and your stomach contract in anticipatory hunger pangs.

But wait! Suppose you hate what you see or smell? For some people, even the thought of liver is enough to make them want to barf — or simply leave the room. At that point, your body takes up arms to protect you: You experience a *rejection reaction* — a reaction similar to that exhibited by babies given something that tastes bitter or sour. Your mouth purses and your nose wrinkles as if to keep the food (and its odor) as far away as possible. Your throat tightens, and your stomach *turns* — muscles contracting not in anticipatory pangs but in movements preparatory for vomiting up the unwanted food. Not a pleasant moment.

But assume you like what's on your plate. Go ahead. Take a bite.

The mouth

Lift your fork to your mouth, and your teeth and salivary glands swing into action. Your teeth chew, grinding the food, breaking it into small, manageable pieces. As a result:

- ✔ You can swallow without choking.
- ✔ You break down the indigestible wrapper of fibers surrounding the edible parts of some foods (fruits, vegetables, whole grains) so that your digestive enzymes can get to the nutrients inside.

At the same time, salivary glands under your tongue and in the back of your mouth secrete the watery liquid called *saliva,* which performs two important functions:

- ✔ Moistening and compacting food so that your tongue can push it to the back of your mouth and you can swallow, sending the food down the slide of your *gullet* (esophagus) into your stomach.
- ✔ Providing *amylases,* enzymes that start the digestion of complex carbohydrates (starches), breaking the starch molecules into simple sugars (Check out Chapter 8 for more on carbs.)

No protein digestion occurs in your mouth, though saliva does contain very small amounts of lingual lipases, fat-busting enzymes secreted by cells at the base of the tongue; however, the amount is so small that the fat digestion that occurs in the mouth is insignificant.

The stomach

If you were to lay your digestive tract out on a table, most of it would look like a simple, rather narrow tube. The exception is your stomach, a pouchy part just below your *gullet* (esophagus).

Turning starches into sugars

Salivary enzymes (like amylases) don't lay a finger on proteins and leave fats pretty much alone, but they do begin to digest complex carbohydrates, breaking the long, chainlike molecules of starches into individual units of sugars; this simple experiment enables you to taste first-hand the effects of amylases on carbohydrates.

1. **Put a small piece of plain, unsalted cracker on your tongue.**

   No cheese, no chopped liver — just the cracker, please.

2. **Close your mouth and let the cracker sit on your tongue for a few minutes.**

   Do you taste a sudden, slight sweetness? That's the salivary enzymes breaking a long, complex starch molecule into its component parts (sugars).

3. **Okay, you can swallow now.**

   The rest of the digestion of the starch takes place farther down, in your small intestine.

Like most of the digestive tube, your stomach is circled with strong muscles whose rhythmic contractions — called *peristalsis* — move food smartly along and turn your stomach into a sort of food processor that mechanically breaks pieces of food into ever smaller particles. While this is going on, glands in the stomach wall are secreting *stomach juices* — a potent blend of enzymes, hydrochloric acid, and mucus.

One stomach enzyme — *gastric alcohol dehydrogenase* — digests small amounts of alcohol, an unusual nutrient that can be absorbed directly into your bloodstream even before it's been digested. For more about alcohol digestion, including why men can drink more than women without becoming tipsy, see Chapter 9.

Other enzymes, plus stomach juices, begin the digestion of proteins and fats, separating them into their basic components — amino acids and fatty acids.

Stop! If the words amino acids and fatty acids are completely new to you and if you are suddenly consumed by the desire to know more about them this instant, stick a pencil in the book to hold your place and flip ahead to Chapters 6 and 7, where I discuss them in detail.

Stop again!! For the most part, digestion of carbohydrates comes to a screeching — though temporary — halt in the stomach because the stomach juices are so acidic that they deactivate *amylases,* the enzymes that break complex carbohydrates apart into simple sugars. However, stomach acid can break some carbohydrate bonds, so a bit of carb digestion does take place.

Back to the action. Eventually, your churning stomach blends its contents into a thick soupy mass called *chyme* (from *cheymos,* the Greek word for juice). When a small amount of chyme spills past the stomach into the small intestine, the digestion of carbohydrates resumes in earnest, and your body begins to extract nutrients from food.

The small intestine

Open your hand and put it flat against your belly button, with your thumb pointing up to your waist and your pinkie pointing down.

Your hand is now covering most of the relatively small space into which your 20-foot-long small (20 feet? small?) intestine is neatly coiled. When the soupy, partially-digested chyme spills from your stomach into this part of the digestive tube, a whole new set of gastric juices are released. These include:

✔ *Pancreatic and intestinal enzymes* that finish the digestion of proteins into amino acids

✔ *Bile,* a greenish liquid (made in the liver and stored in the gallbladder) that enables fats to mix with water

✔ *Alkaline pancreatic juices* that make the chyme less acidic so that amylases (the enzymes that break down carbohydrates) can go back to work separating complex carbohydrates into simple sugars

✔ *Intestinal alcohol dehydrogenase,* which digests alcohol not previously absorbed into your bloodstream

While these chemicals are working, contractions of the small intestine continue to move the food mass down through the tube so that your body can absorb sugars, amino acids, fatty acids, vitamins, and minerals into cells in the intestinal wall.

The lining of the small intestine is a series of folds covered with projections that have been described as "finger-like" or "small nipples." The technical name for these small fingers/nipples is *villi.* Each villus is covered with smaller projections called *microvilli,* and every villus and microvillus is programmed to accept a specific nutrient — and no other.

Nutrients are absorbed not in their order of arrival in the intestine but according to how fast they're broken down into their basic parts:

✔ Carbohydrates — which separate quickly into single sugar units — are absorbed first.

✔ Proteins (as amino acids) go next.

✔ Fats — which take longest to break apart into their constituent fatty acids — are last. That's why a high-fat meal keeps you feeling fuller longer than a meal such as chow mein or plain tossed salad, which are mostly low-fat carbohydrates.

✔ Vitamins that dissolve in water are absorbed earlier than vitamins that dissolve in fat.

Peephole: The first man to watch a living human gut at work

William Beaumont, M.D., was a surgeon in the United States Army in the early 19th century. His name survives in the annals of medicine because of an excellent adventure that began on June 6, 1822. Alexis St. Martin, an 18-year-old French Canadian fur trader, was wounded by a musket ball that discharged accidentally, tearing through his back and out his stomach, leaving a wound that healed but didn't close.

St. Martin's injury seems not to have affected what must have been a truly sunny disposition: Two years later, when all efforts to close the hole in his gut had failed, he granted Beaumont permission to use the wound as the world's first window on a working human digestive system. (To keep food and liquid from spilling out of the small opening, Beaumont kept it covered with a cotton bandage.)

Beaumont's method was simplicity itself. At noon on August 1, 1825, he tied small pieces of food (cooked meat, raw meat, cabbage, bread) to a silk string, removed the bandage, and inserted the food into the hole in St. Martin's stomach.

An hour later, he pulled the food out. The cabbage and bread were half digested; the meat, untouched. After another hour, he pulled the string out again. This time, only the raw meat remained untouched, and St. Martin, who now

had a headache and a queasy stomach, called it quits for the day. But in more than 230 later trials, Beaumont — with the help of his remarkably compliant patient — discovered that although carbohydrates (cabbage and bread) were digested rather quickly, it took up to eight hours for the stomach juices to break down proteins and fats (the beef). Beaumont attributed this to the fact that the cabbage had been cut into small pieces and the bread was porous. Modern nutritionists know that carbohydrates are simply digested faster than proteins and that digesting fats (including those in beef) takes longest of all.

By withdrawing gastric fluid from St. Martin's stomach, keeping it at 100° F (the temperature recorded on a thermometer stuck into the stomach), and adding a piece of meat, Beaumont was able to clock exactly how long the meat took to fall apart: 10 hours.

Beaumont and St. Martin separated in 1833 when the patient, now a sergeant in the United States Army, was posted elsewhere, leaving the doctor to write "Experiments and Observations on the Gastric Juice and the Physiology of Digestion." The treatise is now considered a landmark in the understanding of the human digestive system.

After you've digested your food and absorbed its nutrients through your small intestine:

- Amino acids, sugars, vitamin C, the B vitamins, iron, calcium, and magnesium are carried through the bloodstream to your liver, where they are processed and sent out to the rest of the body.

- Fatty acids, cholesterol, and vitamins A, D, E, and K go into the lymphatic system and then into the blood. They, too, end up in the liver, are processed, and are shipped out to other body cells.

Inside the cells, nutrients are *metabolized,* or burned for heat and energy or used to build new tissues. The metabolic process that gives you energy is called *catabolism* (from *katabole,* the Greek word for casting down). The metabolic process that uses nutrients to build new tissues is called *anabolism* (from *anabole,* the Greek word for raising up).

How the body uses nutrients for energy and new tissues is, alas, a subject for another chapter. In fact, this subject is enough to fill seven different chapters, each devoted to a specific kind of nutrient. For information about metabolizing proteins, turn to Chapter 6. I discuss fats in Chapter 7, carbohydrates in Chapter 8, alcohol in Chapter 9, vitamins in Chapter 10, minerals in Chapter 11, and water in Chapter 13.

The large intestine

After every useful, digestible ingredient other than water has been wrung out of your food, the rest — indigestible waste such as fiber — moves into the top of your large intestine, the area known as your *colon.* The colon's primary job is to absorb water from this mixture and then to squeeze the remaining matter into the compact bundle known as feces.

Feces (whose brown color comes from leftover bile pigments) are made of indigestible material from food, plus cells that have sloughed off the intestinal lining and bacteria — quite a lot of bacteria. In fact, about 30 percent of the entire weight of the feces is bacteria. No, these bacteria aren't a sign you're sick. On the contrary, they prove that you're healthy and well. These bacteria are good guys, microorganisms that live in permanent colonies in your colon, where they:

- Manufacture vitamin B12, which is absorbed through the colon wall

- Produce vitamin K, also absorbed through the colon wall

- Break down amino acids and produce nitrogen (which gives feces a characteristic odor)

- Feast on indigestible complex carbohydrates (fiber), excreting the gas that sometimes makes you physically uncomfortable — or a social pariah

Chew! Chew! All aboard the Nutrient Express!

Think of your small intestine as a busy train station whose apparent chaos of arrivals and departures is actually an efficient, well-ordered system. (Please forgive the terrible pun in the title of this sidebar. My husband — who inherited a gift for this sort of thing from his mother — made me do it.)

As I was saying, the small intestine resembles a three-level, miniature Grand Central Terminal:

✔ Level 1 is the *duodenum* (at the top, right after your stomach).

✔ Level 2 is the *jejunum* (in the middle).

✔ Level 3 is the *ileum* (the last part before the colon).

This three-station tube hums away as nutrients arrive and depart, with millions of "trains" (the nutrients) running on millions of "tracks" (the microvilli) designed to accommodate only one kind of train — and no other.

The system absorbs and ships out nutrients accounting for more than 90 percent of all the protein, fat, and carbohydrates that you consume, plus smaller percentages of vitamins and minerals. The train schedule looks something like this:

Level 1	Duodenum	Iron, calcium, magnesium
Level 2	Jejunum	Simple sugars (the end products of carbohydrate digestion) and water-soluble vitamins (vitamin C and the B vitamins, other than vitamin B12)
Level 3	Ileum	Amino acids (the end product of protein digestion), fat-soluble vitamins (vitamins A, D, E, and K), fatty acids (the end products of fat digestion), cholesterol, vitamin B12, sodium, potassium, and alcohol

When the bacteria have finished, the feces — perhaps the small remains of yesterday's copious feast — pass down through your rectum and out through your anus. But not necessarily right away: Digestion of any one meal may take longer than a day to complete.

After that, digestion's done!

Chapter 3

Calories: The Energizers

Automobiles burn gasoline to get the energy they need to move. Your body burns *(metabolizes)* food to produce energy in the form of heat. This heat warms your body and (as energy) powers every move you make.

Nutritionists measure the amount of heat produced by metabolizing food in units called kilocalories. A *kilocalorie* is the amount of energy it takes to raise the temperature of 1 kilogram of water 1 degree on a Centigrade (Celsius) thermometer at sea level.

In common use, nutritionists substitute the word *calorie* for *kilocalorie*. This information isn't scientifically accurate: Strictly speaking, a calorie is really $\frac{1}{1000}$ of a kilocalorie. But the word calorie is easier to say and easier to remember, so that's the term you see whenever you read about the energy in food. And few nutrition-related words have caused as much confusion and concern as the lowly calorie. Read on to find out what calories mean to you and your nutrition.

Counting the Calories in Food

When you read that a serving of food — say, one banana — has 105 calories, that means metabolizing the banana produces 105 calories of heat that your body can use for work.

You may wonder which kinds of food have the most calories. Here's how the calories measure up in 1 gram of the following foods:

✔ **Protein:** 4 calories

✔ **Carbohydrates:** 4 calories

✔ **Alcohol:** 7 calories

✔ **Fat:** 9 calories

In other words, ounce for ounce, proteins and carbohydrates give you fewer than half as many calories as fat. That's why — again, ounce for ounce — high-fat foods, such as cream cheese, are high in calories, while low-fat foods, such as bagels (minus the cream cheese, of course), are not.

Sometimes foods that seem to be equally low-calorie really aren't. You have to watch all the angles, paying attention to fat in addition to protein and carbohydrates. Here's a good example: A chicken breast and a hamburger are both high-protein foods. Both should have the same number of calories per ounce. But if you serve the chicken without its skin, it contains very little fat, while the hamburger is (sorry about this) full of it. A 3-ounce serving of skinless chicken provides 140 calories, while a 3-ounce burger yields 230 to 245 calories, depending on the cut of the meat.

Empty calories

All food provides calories. All calories provide energy. But not all calories come with a full complement of extra benefits such as amino acids, fatty acids, fiber, vitamins, and minerals. Some foods are said to give you *empty calories.* This term has nothing to do with the calorie's energy potential or with calories having a hole in the middle. It describes a calorie with no extra benefits.

The best-known empty-calorie foods are table sugar and *ethanol* (the kind of alcohol found in beer, wine, and spirits). On their own, sugar and ethanol give you energy — but no nutrients. (See Chapter 8 for more about sugar and Chapter 9 for more about alcohol.)

People who abuse alcohol aren't always thin, but the fact that they often substitute alcohol for food can lead to nutritional deficiencies, most commonly a deficiency of thiamin (vitamin B1), resulting in loss of appetite, an upset stomach, depression, and an inability to concentrate. (For more on vitamin deficiency problems, check out Chapter 10.)

Measuring the number of calories

Nutrition scientists measure the number of calories in food by actually burning the food in a *bomb calorimeter,* which is a box with two chambers, one inside the other. The researchers weigh a sample of the food, put the sample on a dish, and put the dish into the inner chamber of the calorimeter. They fill the inner chamber with oxygen and then seal it so the oxygen can't escape. The outer chamber is filled with a measured amount of cold water, and the oxygen in the first chamber (inside the chamber with the water) is ignited with an electric spark. When the food burns, an observer records the rise in the temperature of the water in the outer chamber. If the temperature of the water goes up 1 degree per kilogram, the food has 1 calorie; 2 degrees, 2 calories; and 235 degrees, 235 calories — or one 8-ounce chocolate malt!

Bomb Calorimeter

Of course, it's only fair to point out that sugar and alcohol are ingredients often found in foods that do provide other nutrients. For example, sugar is found in bread, and alcohol is found in beer — two very different foods that both have calcium, phosphorus, iron, potassium, sodium, and B vitamins.

In the United States, some people are malnourished because they can't afford enough food to get the nutrients they need. The school lunch program started by President Franklin Delano Roosevelt in 1935 and expanded by almost every president, Republican and Democrat, since then has been a largely successful attempt to prevent malnutrition among poor schoolchildren.

But many Americans who can afford enough food nevertheless are malnourished because they simply don't know how to choose a diet that gives them nutrients as well as calories. For these people, eating too many foods with empty calories can cause significant health problems, such as having weak bones; being underweight (yes, being too thin can be a problem); getting bleeding gums, skin rashes, and other nasties; and developing mental disorders, including depression and preventable retardation.

Every calorie counts

People who say that "calories don't count" or that "some calories count less than others" are usually trying to convince you to follow a diet that concentrates on one kind of food to the exclusion of most others. One common example that seems to arise like a phoenix in every generation of dieters is the *high-protein diet.*

The high-protein diet says to cut back or even entirely eliminate carbohydrate foods on the assumption that because your muscle tissue is mostly protein, the protein foods you eat will go straight from your stomach to your muscles, while everything else turns to fat. In other words, this diet says that you can stuff yourself with protein foods until your eyes bug out, because no matter how many calories you get, they'll all be protein calories and they'll all end up in your muscles, not on your hips. Boy, wouldn't it be nice if that were true? The problem is, it isn't. Here's the absolute truth: All calories, regardless of where they come from, give you energy. If you take in more energy (calories) than you spend each day, you'll gain weight. If you take in less than you use up, you'll lose weight. This nutrition rule is an equal opportunity, one-size-fits-all proposition that applies to everyone.

How Many Calories Do You Need?

Think of your energy requirements as a bank account. You make deposits when you consume calories. You make withdrawals when your body spends energy on work. Nutritionists divide the amount of energy you withdraw each day into two parts:

✔ The energy you need when your body is at rest

✔ The energy you need to do your daily "work"

To keep your energy account in balance, you need to take in enough each day to cover your withdrawals. As a general rule, infants and adolescents burn more energy per pound than adults do, because they're continually making large amounts of new tissue. Similarly, an average man burns more energy than an average woman because his body is larger and has more muscle, thus leading to the totally unfair but totally true proposition that a man who weighs, say, 150 pounds can consume about 10 percent more calories than a woman who weighs 150 pounds and still not gain weight. For the numbers, check out the next section and Table 3-1.

Resting energy expenditure (REE)

Even when you're at rest, your body is busy. Your heart beats. Your lungs expand and contract. Your intestines digest food. Your liver processes nutrients. Your glands secrete hormones. Your muscles flex, usually gently. Cells send electrical impulses back and forth among themselves, and your brain continually signals to every part of your body.

The energy that your resting body uses to do all this stuff is called (surprise! surprise!) *resting energy expenditure,* abbreviated REE. The REE, also known as the *basal metabolism,* accounts for a whopping 60 to 70 percent of all the energy you need each day.

To find your resting energy expenditure (REE), you must first figure out your weight in kilograms (kg). One kilogram equals 2.2 pounds. So to get your weight in kilograms, divide the number in pounds by 2.2. For example, if you weigh 150 pounds, that's equal to 68.2 kg (150 ÷ 2.2). Plug that into the appropriate equation in Table 3-1 — and bingo! You have your REE.

Table 3-1	How Many Calories Do You Need When You're Resting?
Sex and Age	**Equation to Figure Out Your REE**
Males	
18–30 years	$(15.3 \times \text{weight in kg}) + 679$
31–60 years	$(11.6 \times \text{weight in kg}) + 879$
Older than 60 years	$(13.5 \times \text{weight in kg}) + 487$
Females	
18–30 years	$(14.7 \times \text{weight in kg}) + 496$
31–60 years	$(8.7 \times \text{weight in kg}) + 829$
Older than 60 years	$(10.5 \times \text{weight in kg}) + 596$

The National Research Council, Recommended Dietary Allowances (Washington, D.C.: National Academy Press, 1989)

Sex, glands, and chocolate cake

A *gland* is an organ that secretes *hormones,* which are chemical substances that can change the function — and sometimes the structure — of other body parts. For example, your pancreas secretes *insulin,* a hormone that enables you to digest and metabolize carbohydrates. At puberty, your sex glands secrete either the female hormones estrogen and progesterone or the male hormone testosterone; these hormones trigger the development of secondary sex characteristics, such as the body and facial hair that make us look like either men or women.

Hormones can also affect your REE, how much energy you use when your body's at rest. Your pituitary gland, a small structure in the center of your brain, stimulates your thyroid gland (which sits at the front of your throat) to secrete hormones that influence the rate at which your tissues burn nutrients to produce energy.

When your thyroid gland doesn't secrete enough hormones (a condition known as *hypothyroidism*), you burn food more slowly and your REE drops. When your thyroid secretes excess amounts of hormones (a condition known as *hyperthyroidism*), you burn food faster and your REE is higher.

When you're frightened or excited, your adrenal glands (two small glands, one on top of each kidney) release *adrenaline,* the hormone that serves as your body's call to battle stations. Your heartbeat increases. You breathe faster. Your muscles clench. And you burn food faster, converting it as fast as possible to the energy you need for the reaction commonly known as *fight or flight.* But these effects are temporary. The effects of the sex glands, on the other hand, last as long as you live. Read on.

How your hormones affect your energy needs

If you're a woman, you know that your appetite rises and falls in tune with your menstrual cycle. In fact, this fluctuation parallels what's happening to your REE, which goes up just before or at the time of ovulation. Your appetite is highest when menstrual bleeding starts and then falls sharply. Yes, you really are hungrier (and need more energy) just before you get your period.

Being a man (and making lots of testosterone) makes satisfying your nutritional needs on a normal American diet easier. Your male bones are naturally denser, so you're less dependent on dietary or supplemental calcium to prevent *osteoporosis* (severe loss of bone tissue) late in life. You don't lose blood through menstruation, so you need only two-thirds as much iron. Best of all, you can consume about 10 percent more calories than a woman of the same weight without adding pounds.

Teenage boys' developing wide shoulders and biceps while teenage girls get hips is no accident. Testosterone, the male hormone, promotes the growth of muscle and bone. Estrogen gives you fatty tissue. As a result, the average male body has proportionally more muscle; the average female body, proportionally more fat.

Muscle is active tissue. It expands and contracts. It works. And when a muscle works, it uses more energy than fat (which insulates the body and provides a source of stored energy but does not move an inch on its own). What this muscle versus fat battle means is that the average man's REE is about 10 percent higher than the average woman's. In practical terms, that means a 140-pound man can hold his weight steady while eating about 10 percent more than a 140-pound woman who is the same age and performs the same amount of physical work.

No amount of dieting changes this unfair situation. A woman who exercises strenuously may reduce her body fat so dramatically that she no longer menstruates — an occupational hazard for some professional athletes. But she'll still have proportionately more body fat than an adult man of the same weight. If she eats what he does, and they perform the same amount of physical work, she still requires fewer calories than he to hold her weight steady.

And here's a really rotten possibility. Muscle weighs more than fat. This interesting fact is one that many people who take up exercise to lose weight discover by accident. One month into the barbells and step-up-step-down routine, their clothes fit better, but the scale points slightly higher because they've traded fat for muscle — and you know what that means: Sometimes you can't win for losing. (Sorry, but I just couldn't resist.)

Energy for work

Your second largest chunk of energy is the energy you withdraw to spend on physical work. That's everything from brushing your teeth in the morning to hoeing a row of petunias in the garden or working out in the gym.

Your total energy requirement (the number of calories you need each day) is your REE plus enough calories to cover the amount of work you do.

Does thinking about this use up energy? Yes, but not as much as you'd like to imagine. To solve a crossword puzzle — or write a chapter of this book — the average brain uses about 1 calorie every four minutes. That's only one-third the amount needed to keep a 60-watt bulb burning for the same length of time.

Table 3-2 defines the energy level of various activities ranging from the least energetic (sleep) to the most (playing football, digging ditches). Table 3-3 shows how many calories you use in an hour's worth of different kinds of work.

Table 3-2	How Active Are You When You're Active?
Activity Level	*Activity*
Resting	Sleeping, reclining
Very light	Seated and standing activities, painting, driving, laboratory work, typing, sewing, ironing, cooking, playing cards, and playing a musical instrument
Light	Walking on a level surface at 2.5 to 3 mph, garage work, electrical trades, carpentry, restaurant trades, housecleaning, child care, golfing, sailing, and table tennis
Moderate	Walking 3.5 to 4 mph, weeding and hoeing, carrying a load, cycling, skiing, tennis, and dancing
Heavy	Walking with a load uphill, tree felling, heavy manual digging, basketball, climbing, football, and soccer
Exceptionally heavy	Professional athletic training

The National Research Council, Recommended Dietary Allowances (Washington, D.C.: National Academy Press, 1989)

Table 3-3	How Many Calories Do You Need to Do the Work You Do?
Activity Level	*Calories Needed for This Work for One Hour*
Very light	80–100
Light	110–160
Moderate	170–240
Heavy	250–350
Exceptionally heavy	350+

"Food and Your Weight," House and Garden Bulletin, No. 74 (Washington, D.C.: U.S. Department of Agriculture)

Enjoying the extras

Are you a sensible foodie? If you're supposed to have no more than 2,000 calories a day, can you pack all the vitamins, minerals, protein, heart-healthy fats, and carbs you need into 1,800 calories? Do that, and the folks who wrote the *Dietary Guidelines for Americans 2005* (more about that in Chapter 16) say, reward yourself. Use the "leftover" 200 calories — called *discretionary calories* — for anything that makes your mouth water. Naturally, some expert spoilsports disagree. They say that giving you an inch (those leftover calories) means you'll take a mile (three pieces of chocolate cake). Prove them wrong and celebrate your smarts. Yum!

How Much Should You Weigh?

Through the years, a number of charts have purported to lay out *standard* or *healthy weights* for adult Americans, but some set the figures so low that you can hardly get there without severely restricting your diet — or being born again with a different body, preferably with light bones and no curves.

Studying weight charts

Table 3-4 is one moderate, eminently usable set of weight recommendations that originally appeared in the 1990 edition of *Dietary Guidelines for Americans* published by the U.S. Department of Agriculture and the U.S. Department of Health and Human Services. The weights in this chart are listed in ranges for people (men and women) of specific heights. Naturally, height is measured without shoes, and weight is measured without clothes. (For more — much more — on the *Dietary Guidelines,* see Chapter 16.)

Because most people gain some weight as they grow older, Table 3-4 does a really sensible thing by dividing the ranges into two broad categories, one for men and women ages 19 to 34, the other for men and women ages 35 and older.

People with a small frame and proportionately more fat tissue than muscle tissue (muscle is heavier than fat) are likely to weigh in at the low end. People with a large frame and proportionately more muscle than fat are likely to weigh in at the high end. As a general (but by no means invariable) rule, that means that women — who have smaller frames and less muscle — weigh less than men of the same height and age.

Fittest and fattest U.S. cities

June is bustin' out all over. How about you? For several years, the guys at *Men's Fitness* magazine have rated the top 25 fattest and fittest cities in the United States. Of course, *Men's Fitness* is published in Southern California, where long legs, slim hips, tight abs, and a taste for sprouts are handed out at birth. As a result, the magazine's pundits may not know that in other places like, oh, New York, Chicago, Milwaukee, you-pick-it, Americans come in all shapes and sizes. And they may have missed the fact that running for a bus or climbing subway stairs constitutes a daily workout in metro areas. Or that compared to high-fat, goat-cheese pizza, a West Coast fave, city bagels are health food.

Nonetheless, the magazine's lists are a warning for the weighty. I'll tell you right off the bat that in 2005, the 25 fittest cities (starting with the best) were Seattle, Honolulu, Colorado Springs, San Francisco, Denver, Portland (Oregon), Tucson, San Diego, Albuquerque, Boston, Virginia Beach (Virginia), Minneapolis, Fresno, Milwaukee, Omaha, San Jose (California), Jacksonville, Austin, Oakland, Los Angeles, Arlington (Texas), Washington, D.C., Cleveland, and Nashville-Davidson. Yay!

The 25 fattest (starting with the worst) were Houston, Philadelphia, Detroit, Memphis, Chicago, Dallas, New Orleans, New York, Las Vegas, San Antonio, El Paso, Phoenix, Indianapolis, Fort Worth, Mesa (Arizona), Columbus (Ohio), Wichita (Kansas), Miami (Florida), Long Beach (California), Oklahoma City, Tulsa, Atlanta, Charlotte (North Carolina), and Baltimore. Shape up, guys. *Men's Fitness* is watching you!

I feel honor bound to tell you that the 2000 and 2005 editions of the *Dietary Guidelines* leave out the higher weight allowances for older people, which means that the healthy weights for everyone, young or old, are the ones listed in the column for 19- to 34-year-olds. I'm going to go out on a limb here to say that I prefer the 1990 recommendations because they're

- ✔ Achievable without constant dieting
- ✔ Realistic about how your body changes as you get older
- ✔ Less likely to make you totally crazy about your weight

. . . which is a pretty good description of how nutritional guidelines need to work, don't you think?

Another way to rate your weight: Calculating your BMI

As you run your finger down the chart in Table 3-4, remember that the numbers are guidelines — no more, no less.

Table 3-4	How Much Should You Weigh?	
Height	*Weight (Pounds) for 19- to 34-Year-Olds*	*Weight (Pounds) for 35-Year-Olds and Older*
5'	97–128	108–138
5'1"	101–132	111–143
5'2"	104–137	115–148
5'3"	107–141	119–152
5'4"	111–146	122–157
5'5"	114–150	126–162
5'6"	118–155	130–167
5'7"	121–160	134–172
5'8"	125–164	138–178
5'9"	129–169	142–183
5'10"	132–174	146–188
5'11"	136–179	151–194
6'	140–184	155–199
6'1"	144–189	159–205
6'2"	148–195	164–210
6'3"	152–200	168–216
6'4"	156–205	173–222
6'5"	160–211	177–228
6'6"	164–216	182–234

Nutrition and Your Health: Dietary Guidelines for Americans, 3rd ed. (Washington D.C.: U.S. Department of Agriculture, U.S. Department of Health and Human Services, 1990)

Squeezing people into neat little boxes is a reassuring exercise, but in real life, human beings constantly confound the rules. We all know chubby people who live long and happy lives and trim and skinny ones who leave us sooner than they should. However, people who are overweight have a higher risk of developing conditions such as arthritis, diabetes, and heart disease, so you need a way to find out whether your current weight puts you at risk.

What do they mean when they say that you're fat?

Obesity is a specific medical condition in which the body accumulates an overabundance of fatty tissue. One way American nutritionists determine who's obese is by comparing a person's weight with the figures on the weight/height charts (see Table 3-4):

✔ If your weight is 20 to 40 percent higher than the chart recommends, you're mildly obese.

✔ If your weight is 40 to 99 percent higher, you're moderately obese.

✔ If your weight is more than double the weight on the chart, you're severely obese.

One good guide is the *Body Mass Index (BMI),* a number that measures the relationship between your weight and your height and offers some predictive estimate of your risk of weight-related disease.

The Body Mass Index (BMI) provides a second way to determine who's tipping the scales. In the United States, a BMI below 18.5 is currently considered underweight, 18.5–24.9 is normal, 25.0–29.9 is overweight, and 30.0 and higher is obese. Other countries have slightly different standards. For example, in Australia, a BMI below 19 is underweight, 20–25 is normal, 26–30 is overweight, and 31+ is obese. In Canada, a BMI below 18.5 is underweight, 18.5–24.9 is normal, 25–29.9 is overweight, 30–34.9 is Class 1 obese, 35–39.9 is Class 2 obese, and 40+ is Class 3 obese. In Great Britain, a BMI below 20 is underweight, 20–25 is normal, 25–30 is overweight, and 30+ is obese.

To calculate your BMI, perform the following steps:

1. **Divide your weight (in pounds) by your height (in inches) squared.**

2. **Multiply the result of Step 1 by 705.**

For example, if you are 5'3" (63 inches) tall and weigh 138 pounds, the equations for your BMI look like this:

$$\text{BMI} = \frac{138}{63 \times 63 \text{ inches}} \times 705 = 24.5$$

Currently, the healthiest BMI seems to be 21.0. A BMI higher than 28 (168 pounds for a 5'5" woman; 195 pounds for a 5'10" man) appears to double the risk of diabetes, heart disease, and death.

How reliable are the numbers? Considering confounding variables

Weight charts and tables and numbers and stats are so plentiful that you may think they're totally reliable in predicting who's healthy and who's not. So here's a surprise: They aren't.

The problem is that real people and their differences keep sneaking into the equation. For example, the value of the Body Mass Index in predicting your risk of illness or death appears to be tied to your age. If you're in your 30s, a lower BMI is clearly linked to better health. If you're in your 70s or older, no convincing evidence points to how much you weigh playing a significant role in determining how healthy you are or how much longer you'll live. In between, from age 30 to age 74, the relationship between your BMI and your health is, well, in-between — more important early on, less important later in life.

In other words, the simple evidence of your own eyes is true. Although Americans sometimes seem totally obsessed with the need to lose weight, the fact is that many larger people, even people who are clearly obese, do live long, happy, and healthy lives. To figure out why, many nutrition scientists now are focusing not only on weight or weight/height (the BMI) but on the importance of *confounding variables,* which is sciencespeak for "something else is going on here."

Here are three potential confounding variables in the obesity/health equation:

- Maybe people who are overweight are more prone to illness because they exercise less, in which case stepping up the workouts may reduce the perceived risk of being overweight.

- People who are overweight may be more likely to be sick because they eat lots of foods containing high-calorie ingredients, such as saturated fat, that can trigger adverse health effects; in this case, the remedy may simply be a change in diet.

- Maybe people who are overweight have a genetic predisposition to a serious disease. If that's true, you'd have to ask whether losing 20 pounds really reduces their risk of disease to the level of a person who is naturally 20 pounds lighter. Perhaps not: In a few studies, people who successfully lost weight actually had a higher rate of death.

Adding to the confusion is the fact that an obsessive attempt to lose weight may itself be hazardous to your health (see Chapter 14). Every year, Americans spend $30 billion to $50 billion (yes, you read that right) on diet clubs, special foods, and over-the-counter remedies aimed at weight loss. Often the diets, the pills, and the foods don't work, which can leave dieters feeling worse than they did before they started.

The chance that the diet fails is only half the bad news. Here's the rest: Some foods that effectively lower calorie intake and some drugs that effectively reduce appetite have potentially serious side effects. For example, some fat substitutes prevent your body from absorbing important nutrients (see Chapter 19), and some prescription diet drugs, such as the combination once known as Phen-Fen, are linked to serious, even fatal, diseases.

Facing the numbers when they don't fit your body

Right about here, you probably feel the strong need for a really big chocolate bar (not such a bad idea now that nutritionists have discovered that dark chocolate is rich in disease-fighting antioxidants). But it also makes sense to consider the alternative: realistic rules that enable you to control your weight safely and effectively. Check out the following:

- ✔ **Rule No. 1: Not everybody starts out with the same set of genes — or fits into the same pair of jeans.** Some people are naturally larger and heavier than others. If that's you, and all your vital stats satisfy your doctor, don't waste time trying to fit someone else's idea of perfection. Relax and enjoy your own body.

- ✔ **Rule No. 2: If you're overweight and your doctor agrees with your decision to diet, you don't have to set world records to improve your health.** Even a moderate drop in poundage can be highly beneficial. According to *The New England Journal of Medicine* (www.nejm.org on the Net), losing just 10 to 15 percent of your body weight can lower high blood sugar, high cholesterol, and high blood pressure, reducing your risks of diabetes, heart disease, and stroke.

- ✔ **Rule No. 3: The only number you really need to remember is 3,500, the number of calories it takes to gain or lose one pound of body fat.** In other words, one pound of body fat equals 3,500 calories. So if you simply

  - • Cut your calorie consumption from 2,000 calories a day to 1,700 and continue to do the same amount of physical work, you'll lose one pound of fat in just 12 days.

- Go the other way, increasing from 1,700 to 2,000 calories a day without increasing the amount of work you do, 12 days later you'll be one pound heavier.

✔ **Rule No. 4: Moderation is the best path to weight control.** Moderate calorie deprivation on a sensible diet produces healthful, moderate weight loss; this diet includes a wide variety of different foods containing sufficient amounts of essential nutrients. Abusing this rule and cutting calories to the bone can turn you literally into skin and bones, depriving you of the nutrients you need to live a normal healthy life. For more on the potentially devastating effects of starvation, voluntary and otherwise, check out Chapter 14.

✔ **Rule No. 5: Be more active.** Doing exercise allows you to take in more calories and still lose weight. In addition, exercise reduces the risk of many health problems, such as heart disease. Sounds like a recipe for success.

How many calories do you really need?

Figuring out ex-act-ly how many calories to consume each day can be a, well, consuming task. Luckily, the *Dietary Guidelines for Americans 2005* lays out a list of the average daily calorie allowance for healthy adults with a healthful BMI — 21.5 for women and 22.5 for men — based on the amount of activity a person performs each day. Table 3-5 shows numbers. Note that in this context, *sedentary* means a lifestyle with only the light physical activity associated with daily living; *moderately active* means a lifestyle that adds physical activity equal to a daily 1.5–3 mile walks at a speed of 3–4 miles per hour; *active* means adding physical activity equal to walking 3 miles a day at the 3–4 mph clip.

Table 3-5	Matching Daily Calories with Daily Lifestyle		
Gender/Age*	*Calories If Sedentary*	*Calories If Moderately Active*	*Calories If Active*
Female			
19-30 years	2,000	2,000–2,200	2,400
31-50	1,800	2,000	2,200
51+	1,600	1,800	2,000–2,200

(continued)

Table 3-5 *(continued)*

Gender/Age*	Calories If Sedentary	Calories If Moderately Active	Calories If Active
Male			
19-30	2,400	2,600–2,800	3,000
31-50	2,200	2,400–2,600	2,800–3,000
50+	2,000	2,200–2,400	2,400–2,600

* As a rule, men have proportionately more active tissue (muscle) than women do, so an average man's calorie requirements are about 10 percent higher than an average woman's.
Dietary Guidelines for Americans, 6th ed. (Washington D.C.: U.S. Department of Agriculture, U.S. Department of Health and Human Services, 2005)

The last word on calories

Calories are not your enemy. On the contrary, they give you the energy you need to live a healthy life.

The trick is managing your calories and not letting them manage you. After you know that fats are more fattening than proteins and carbohydrates and that your body burns food to make energy, you can strategize your energy intake to match your energy expenditure, and vice versa. Here's how: Turn straight to Chapter 16 to find out about a healthful diet and Chapter 17 to find out about planning nutritious meals.

Chapter 4

How Much Nutrition Do You Need?

A healthful diet provides sufficient amounts of all the nutrients that your body needs. The question is, how much is enough?

Today, three sets of recommendations provide the answers, and each comes with its own virtues and deficiencies. The first, and most familiar, is the *RDA* (short for *Recommended Dietary Allowance*). The second, originally known as the Estimated Safe and Adequate Daily Dietary Intakes (ESADDIs), now shortened to *Adequate Intake* or simply *AI,* describes recommended amounts of nutrients for which no RDAs exist. The third is the *DRI (Dietary Reference Intake),* an umbrella term that includes RDAs plus several innovative categories of nutrient recommendations.

Confused? Not to worry. This chapter spells it all out.

RDAs: Guidelines for Good Nutrition

The Recommended Dietary Allowances (RDAs) were created in 1941 by the Food and Nutrition Board, a subsidiary of the National Research Council, which is part of the National Academy of Sciences in Washington, D.C.

RDAs originally were designed to make planning several days' meals in advance easy for you. The *D* in RDA stands for dietary, not daily, because the RDAs are an average. You may get more of a nutrient one day and less the next, but the idea is to hit an average over several days.

For example, the current RDA for vitamin C is 75 mg for a woman and 90 mg for a man (age 18 and older). One 8-ounce glass of fresh orange juice has 120 mg vitamin C, so a woman can have an 8-ounce glass of orange juice on Monday and Tuesday, skip Wednesday, and still meet the RDA for the three days. A man may have to toss in something else — maybe a stalk of broccoli — to be able to do the same thing. No big deal.

The amounts recommended by the RDAs provide a margin of safety for healthy people, but they're not therapeutic. In other words, RDA servings won't cure a nutrient deficiency, but they can prevent one from occurring.

The essentials

RDAs offer recommendations for protein and 18 essential vitamins and minerals, which include:

- Vitamin A
- Vitamin D
- Vitamin E
- Vitamin K
- Vitamin C
- Thiamin (vitamin B1)
- Riboflavin (vitamin B2)
- Niacin
- Vitamin B6

- Folate
- Vitamin B12
- Phosphorus
- Magnesium
- Iron
- Zinc
- Copper
- Iodine
- Selenium

The newest essential nutrient, choline, won its wings in 2002, but no RDAs have yet been established. Calcium also has an Adequate Intake (AI) rather than an RDA.

Recommendations for carbohydrates, fats, dietary fiber, and alcohol

What nutrients are missing from the RDA list of essentials? Carbohydrates, fiber, fat, and alcohol. The reason is simple: If your diet provides enough

protein, vitamins, and minerals, it's almost certain to provide enough carbohydrates and probably more than enough fat. Although no specific RDAs
exist for carbohydrates and fat, guidelines definitely exist for them and for
dietary fiber and alcohol.

In 1980, the U.S. Public Health Service and the U.S. Department of Agriculture
joined forces to produce the first edition of *Dietary Guidelines for Americans*
(see Chapter 16). This report has been modified many times. The latest set of
recommendations, issued in the spring of 2005, sets parameters for what you
can consider reasonable amounts of calories, carbohydrates, dietary fiber,
fats, protein, and alcohol. According to these guidelines, as a general rule,
you need to

✔ Balance your calorie intake with energy output in the form of regular
   exercise. Check out Chapter 3 for specifics on how many calories a
   person of your weight, height, and level of activity (couch potato?
   marathon runner?) needs to consume each day.

✔ Eat enough carbohydrates (primarily the complex ones from fruits, vegetables, and whole grains) to account for 45 to 65 percent of your total
   daily calories. That's 900 to 1,300 calories on a 2,000-calorie diet.

✔ Take in an appropriate amount of dietary fiber, currently described as 14
   grams dietary fiber for every 1,000 calories.

✔ Get no more than 20 to 35 percent of your daily calories from dietary fat.
   Therefore, if your daily diet includes about 2,000 calories, only 400 to
   700 calories should come from fat.

   Less than 10 percent of your daily calories should come from saturated
   fatty acids, and your daily diet should have less than 300 mg cholesterol.
   Eat as little trans fat as possible. The Nutrition Facts label on foods now
   shows a gram amount for trans fats, but there's no upper limit because
   any amount is considered, well, less than okey-dokey. (For the skinny on
   saturated, unsaturated, and trans fats, plus cholesterol, check out
   Chapter 7).

✔ If you choose to drink alcoholic beverages, do so in moderation, meaning one drink a day for a woman and two for a man.

Different people, different needs

Because different bodies require different amounts of nutrients, RDAs currently address as many as 22 specific categories of human beings: boys and
girls, men and women, from infancy through middle age. The RDAs recently
were expanded to include recommendations for groups of people ages 50 to

70 and 70 and older. Eventually, recommendations will be made for people older than 85. These expanded groupings are a really good idea. In 1990, the U.S. Census counted 31.1 million Americans who are older than 65. By 2050, the U.S. Government expects more than 60 million to be alive and kickin'. You wouldn't want these baby boomers to miss their RDAs, now would you?

But who you are affects the recommendations. If age is important, so is gender. For example, because women of childbearing age lose iron when they menstruate, their RDA for iron is higher than the RDA for men. On the other hand, because men who are sexually active lose zinc through their ejaculations, the zinc RDA for men is higher than the zinc RDA for women.

Finally, gender affects body composition, which influences RDAs. Consider protein: The RDA for protein is set in terms of grams of protein per kilogram (2.2 pounds) of body weight. Because the average man weighs more than the average woman, his RDA for protein is higher than hers. The RDA for an adult male, age 19 or older, is 56 grams; for a woman, it's 46 grams.

AIs: The Nutritional Numbers Formerly Known as ESADDIs

In addition to the RDAs, the Food and Nutrition Board created Estimated Safe and Adequate Daily Dietary Intakes (ESADDI), now renamed *Adequate Intake (AI),* for eight nutrients considered necessary for good health, even though nobody really knows exactly how much your body needs. Not to worry: Sooner or later some smart nutrition researcher will come up with a hard number and move the nutrient to the RDA list. Or not. In the meantime, new reports have established AIs for various age groups for the following nutrients:

- ✔ Pantothenic acid
- ✔ Biotin
- ✔ Choline
- ✔ Calcium

- ✔ Molybdenum
- ✔ Manganese
- ✔ Fluoride
- ✔ Chromium

DRI: A Newer Nutrition Guide

In 1993, the Food and Nutrition Board's Dietary Reference Intakes committee established several panels of experts to review the RDAs and other recommendations for major nutrients (vitamins, minerals, and other food components) in light of new research and nutrition information.

The first order of business was to establish a new standard for nutrient recommendations called the *Dietary Reference Intake (DRI).* DRI is an umbrella term that embraces several categories of nutritional measurements for vitamins, minerals, and other nutrients. It includes the:

- **Estimated Average Requirement (EAR):** the amount that meets the nutritional needs of half the people in any one group (such as teenage girls or people older than 70). Nutritionists use the EAR to figure out whether an entire population's normal diet provides adequate amounts of nutrients.

- **Recommended Dietary Allowance (RDA):** The RDA, now based on information provided by the EAR, is still a daily average for individuals, the amount of any one nutrient known to protect against deficiency.

- **Adequate Intake (AI):** The AI is a new measurement, providing recommendations for nutrients for which no RDA is set. (***Note:*** AI replaces ESADDI.)

- **Tolerable Upper Intake Level (UL):** The UL is the highest amount of a nutrient you can consume each day without risking an adverse effect.

The DRI panel's first report, listing new recommendations for calcium, phosphorus, magnesium, and fluoride, appeared in 1997. Its most notable change was upping the recommended amount of calcium from 800 mg to 1,000 mg for adults ages 31 to 50 as well as post-menopausal women taking estrogen supplements; for post menopausal women not taking estrogen, the recommendation is 1,500 mg.

The second DRI Panel report appeared in 1998. The report included new recommendations for thiamin, riboflavin, niacin, vitamin B6, folate, vitamin B12, pantothenic acid, biotin, and choline. The most important revision was increasing the folate recommendation to 400 mcg a day based on evidence showing that folate reduces a woman's risk of giving birth to a baby with spinal cord defects and lowers the risk of heart disease for men and women. (See the sidebar "Reviewing terms to describe nutrient recommendations" in this chapter or the Cheat Sheet at the front of the book to brush up on your metric abbreviations.)

As a result of the 1989 DRI Panel report, the FDA ordered food manufacturers to add folate to flour, rice, and other grain products. (Multivitamin products already contain 400 mcg of folate.) In May 1999, data released by the Framingham Heart Study, which has followed heart health among residents of a Boston suburb for nearly half a century, showed a dramatic increase in blood levels of folate. Before the fortification of foods, 22 percent of the study participants had folate deficiencies; after the fortification, the number fell to 2 percent.

A DRI report with revised recommendations for vitamin C, vitamin E, the mineral selenium, beta-carotene, and other antioxidant vitamins was published in 2000. In 2001, new DRIs were released for vitamin A, vitamin K, arsenic, boron, chromium, copper, iodine, iron, manganese, molybdenum, nickel, silicon, vanadium, and zinc. And in 2004, the Institute of Medicine (IOM) released new recommendations for sodium, potassium, chloride, and water, plus a special report on recommendations for two groups of older adults (ages 50 to 70 and 71 and over). Put these findings all together, and they spell out the recommendations you find in this chapter.

Table 4-1 shows the most recent RDAs for vitamins for healthy adults; Table 4-2 shows RDAs for minerals for healthy adults. Where no RDA is given, an AI is indicated by an asterisk (*) by the column heading. The complete reports on which this table is based are available online. Go to `www.iom.edu/ Object.File/Master/21/372/0.pdf`. Prefer hard copy? IOM plans to consolidate the reports into one book to be published late in 2006. (If you want an idea of what kinds of foods provide these vitamins, check out Chapter 10.)

Hankering for more details? Notice something missing? Right — no recommended allowances for protein, fat, carbohydrates and, of course, water. You'll find those (respectively) in Chapters 6, 7, 8, and 13.

Reviewing terms used to describe nutrient recommendations

Nutrient listings use the metric system. RDAs for protein are listed in grams. The RDA and AIs for vitamins and minerals are shown in milligrams (mg) and micrograms (mcg). A milligram is $\frac{1}{1000}$ of a gram; a microgram is $\frac{1}{1000}$ of a milligram.

Vitamin A, vitamin D, and vitamin E are special cases. For instance, one form of vitamin A is *preformed vitamin A*, a form of the nutrient that your body can use right away. Preformed vitamin A, known as *retinol*, is found in food from animals — liver, milk, and eggs. Carotenoids (red or yellow pigments in plants) also provide vitamin A. But to get vitamin A from carotenoids, your body has to convert the pigments to chemicals similar to retinol. Because retinol is a ready-made nutrient, the RDA for vitamin A is listed in units called retinol equivalents (RE). One mcg (microgram) RE is approximately equal to 3.33 international units (IU, the former unit of measurement for vitamin A).

Vitamin D consists of three compounds: vitamin D1, vitamin D2, and vitamin D3. Cholecalciferol, the chemical name for vitamin D3, is the most active of the three, so the RDA for vitamin D is measured in equivalents of cholecalciferol.

Your body gets vitamin E from two classes of chemicals in food: tocopherols and tocotrienols. The compound with the greatest vitamin E activity is a tocopherol: *alpha*-tocopherol. The RDA for vitamin E is measured in milligrams of *alpha*-tocopherol equivalents (a-TE).

Table 4-1		**Vitamin RDAs for Healthy Adults**			
g	= Gram		RE	= retinol equivalent	
mg	= milligram		a-TE	= alpha-tocopherol equivalent	
mcg	= microgram		NE	= niacin equivalent	

Age (Years)	Vitamin A (RE/IU)†	Vitamin D (mcg/IU)‡*	Vitamin E (a-TE)	Vitamin K (mcg)*	Vitamin C (mg)
Males					
19–30	900/2,970	5/200	15	120	90
31–50	900/2,970	5/200	15	120	90
51–70	900/2,970	10/400	15	120	90
Older than 70	900/2,970	15/600	15	120	90
Females					
19–30	700/2,310	5/200	15	90	75
31–50	700/2,310	5/200	15	90	75
51–70	700/2,310	10/400	15	90	75
Older than 70	700/2,310	15/600	15	90	75
Pregnant (age-based)	750–770/ 2,475–2,541	5/200	15	75–90	70
Nursing (age-based)	1,200–1,300/ 3,960–4,290	5/200	19	76–90	95

* Adequate Intake (AI)
† The "official" RDA for vitamin A is still 1,000 RE/5,000 IU for a male, 800 RE/4,000 IU for a female who isn't pregnant or nursing; the lower numbers listed on this chart are the currently recommended levels for adults.
‡ The current recommendations are the amounts required to prevent vitamin D deficiency disease; recent studies suggest that the optimal levels for overall health may actually be higher, in the range of 800–1,000 IU a day.

Table 4-1 (continued)

Age (years)	Thiamin (Vitamin B1) (mg)	Riboflavin (Vitamin B2) (mg)	Niacin (NE)	Pantothenic acid (mg)*	Vitamin B6 (mg)	Folate (mcg)	Vitamin B12 (mcg)	Biotin (mcg)*
Males								
19–30	1.2	1.3	16	5	1.3	400	2.4	30
31–50	1.2	1.3	16	5	1.3	400	2.4	30
50–70	1.2	1.3	16	5	1.7	400	2.4	30
Older than 70	1.2	1.1	16	5	1.7	400	2.4	30
Females								
19–30	1.1	1.1	14	5	1.3	400	2.4	30
31–50	1.1	1.1	14	5	1.3	400	2.4	30
51–70	1.1	1.1	14	5	1.5	400	2.4	30
Older than 70	1.1	1.1	14	5	1.5	400	2.4	30
Pregnant	1.4	1.1	18	6	1.9	600	2.6	30
Nursing	1.4	1.1	17	7	2.0	500	2.8	35

* Adequate Intake (AI)

Table 4-2		**Mineral RDAs for Healthy Adults**				
Age (years)	Calcium (mg)*	Phosphorus (mg)	Magnesium (mg)	Iron (mg)	Zinc (mg)	Copper (mcg)
Males						
19–30	1,000	700	400	8	11	900
31–50	1,000	700	420	8	11	900
51–70	1,200	700	420	8	11	900
Older than 70	1,200	700	420	8	11	900
Females						
19–30	1,000	700	310	18	8	900
31–50	1,000	700	320	18	8	900
51–70	1,000/1,500**	700	320	8	8	900
Older than 70	1,000/1,500**	700	320	8	8	900
Pregnant	1,000–1,300	700–1,250	350–400	27	11–12	1,000
Nursing	1,000–1,300	700–1,250	310–350	9–10	12–13	1,300

* Adequate Intake (AI)
** The lower recommendation is for postmenopausal women taking estrogen supplements; the higher figure is for postmenopausal women not taking estrogen supplements.

Age (years)	Iodine (mcg)	Selenium (mcg)	Molybdenum (mcg)	Manganese (mg)*	Fluoride (mg)*	Chromium (mcg)*	Choline (mg)*
Males							
19–30	150	55	45	2.3	4	36	550
31–50	150	55	45	2.3	4	36	550
51–70	150	55	45	2.3	4	30	550
Older than 70	150	55	45	2.3	4	30	550
Females							
19–30	150	55	45	1.8	3	25	425
31–50	150	55	45	1.8	3	25	425

Age (years)	Iodine (mcg)	Selenium (mcg)	Molybdenum (mcg)	Manganese (mg)*	Fluoride (mg)*	Chromium (mcg)*	Choline (mg)*
51–70	150	55	45	1.8	3	20	425
Older than 70	150	55	45	1.8	3	20	425
Pregnant	220	60	50	2.0	1.5–4.0	29–30	450
Nursing	290	70	50	2.6	1.5–4.0	44–45	550

*Adequate Intake (AI)

Adapted with permission from Recommended Dietary Allowances (Washington D.C.: National Academy Press, 1989), and DRI panel reports, 1997-2004

No Sale Ever Is Final

The slogan "No Sale Ever Is Final," printed on the sales slips at one of my favorite clothing stores, definitely applies to nutritional numbers. RDAs, AIs, and DRIs should always be regarded as works in progress, subject to revision at the first sign of a new study. In other words, in an ever-changing world, here's one thing of which you can be *absolutely* certain: The numbers in this chapter will change. Sorry about that.

Chapter 5

A Supplemental Story

The Food and Drug Administration (FDA) estimates that every year, Americans buy millions of bottles and boxes of dietary supplements, a $19 billion business that includes everything from plain old vitamin C to — yuck! — desiccated (dried) liver. You can stir up a good food fight in any group of nutrition experts simply by asking whether all these supplements are (a) necessary, (b) economical, or (c) safe. But when the argument's over, you still may not have a satisfactory *official* answer, so this brief chapter aims to provide the information you need to make your own sensible choices.

Introducing Dietary Supplements

The vitamin pill you may pop each morning is a dietary supplement. So are the calcium antacids many American women consider standard nutrition. Echinacea, the herb reputed to short-circuit your winter cold, is, and so is the vanilla-flavored meal-in-a-can liquid your granny chug-a-lugs every afternoon just before setting off on her daily mile power walk. The FDA classifies each of these as a dietary supplement because they meet the agency's definition: any pill, tablet, capsule, powder, or liquid you take by mouth that contains a dietary ingredient.

Of course, that raises another question: What's a dietary ingredient? Answer:

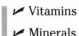

- ✔ Vitamins
- ✔ Minerals

✔ Herbs

✔ Amino acids (the "building blocks of protein" described in Chapter 6)

✔ Enzymes

✔ Organ tissue, such as desiccated (dried) liver

✔ Some hormones, such as melatonin, which is promoted as a sleep aid

✔ Metabolites (substances produced when nutrients are digested)

✔ Extracts

Dietary supplements may be single-ingredient products, such as vitamin E capsules, or they may be combination products, such as the nutrient-packed protein powders favored by some athletes.

Examining Why People Use Dietary Supplements

In a country where food is plentiful and affordable, you have to wonder why so many people opt to scarf down pills instead of just plain food.

Many people consider vitamin and mineral supplements a quick and easy way to get nutrients without so much shopping and kitchen time and without all the pesky fat and sugars in food. Others take supplements as nutritional insurance (for more on recommended dietary allowances of vitamins and minerals, see Chapter 4). And some even use supplements as substitutes for medical drugs. In general, nutrition experts, including the American Dietetic Association, the National Academy of Sciences, and the National Research Council, prefer that you invest your time and money whipping up meals and snacks that supply the nutrients you need in a balanced, tasty diet. Nonetheless, every expert worth his or her vitamin C admits that in certain circumstances, supplements can be a definite plus.

In 2002, the American Medical Association (AMA), which for decades had turned thumbs down on vitamin supplements, changed its collective mind after a review of 26 years' worth of scientific studies relating vitamin levels to the risk of chronic illness. Robert H. Fletcher and Kathleen M. Fairfield, the Harvard-based authors of the study, which was published in the *Journal of the American Medical Association (JAMA),* said, yes, true vitamin-deficiency diseases such as scurvy and beriberi are rare in Western countries. But *suboptimal vitamin levels* — sciencespeak for slightly less than you need — are a real problem. If "slightly less than you need" sounds slightly less than important, consider this:

✔ Suboptimal intake of folate and two other B vitamins (B6 and B12) raises your risk of heart disease, colon cancer, breast cancer, and birth defects.

✔ Suboptimal vitamin D intake means a higher risk of rickets and osteoporosis.

✔ Suboptimal levels of antioxidant vitamins A, E, and C are linked to a particular form of heart disease and some forms of cancer.

Hence the new AMA rule: "It's prudent for all adults to take vitamin supplements."

But just as that bit of info was settling in, a new study (you can read more about this in Chapter 10) said, "Hold it! There's too much Vitamin A in that pill!" That was followed by more new research on too much vitamin E. As you read this, vitamin manufacturers are tumbling over each other in the race to get new, lower formulations to market.

When food isn't enough

Illness, age, diet preferences, and some gender-related conditions may put you in a spot where you can't get all the nutrients you need from food alone.

Digestive illnesses, unfriendly drugs, injury, and chronic illness

Certain metabolic disorders and diseases of the digestive organs (liver, gallbladder, pancreas, and intestines) interfere with the normal digestion of food and the absorption of nutrients. Some medicines may also interfere with normal digestion, meaning you need supplements to make up the difference. People who suffer from certain chronic diseases, who have suffered a major injury (such as a serious burn), or who have just been through surgery may need more nutrients than they can get from food. In these cases, a doctor may prescribe supplements to provide the hard-to-get vitamins, minerals, and other nutrients.

Checking with your doctor or pharmacist before opting for a supplement you hope will have medical effects (make you stronger, smooth your skin, ease your anxiety) is a smart idea. The bad old days when doctors were total ignoramuses about nutrition may not be gone forever, but they're fading fast. Besides, your doctor is the person most familiar with your health, knows what medications you're taking, and can warn you of potential side effects.

Vegetarianism

Vitamin B12 is found only in food from animals, such as meat, milk, and eggs. (Some seaweed does have B12, but the suspicion is that the vitamin comes from microorganisms living in the plant.) Without these foods, *vegans* — vegetarians who don't eat any foods of animal origin — almost certainly have to get their vitamin B12 from supplements or fortified foods.

Using supplements as insurance

Healthy people who eat a nutritious diet still may want to use supplements to make sure they're getting adequate nutrition. Plenty of recent research supports their choice.

Protecting against disease

Taking supplements may reduce the likelihood of some types of cancer and other diseases. After analyzing data from a survey of 871 men and women, epidemiologists at Seattle's Fred Hutchinson Cancer Center found that people taking a daily multivitamin for more than ten years were 50 percent less likely to develop colon cancer. In addition, selenium supplements seem to reduce the risk of prostate cancer, and vitamin C seems to lower the risk of cataracts.

Supplementing aging appetites

As you grow older, your appetite may decline and your sense of taste and smell may falter. If food no longer tastes as good as it once did, if you have to eat alone all the time and don't enjoy cooking for one, or if dentures make chewing difficult, you may not be taking in all the foods that you need to get the nutrients you require. Dietary supplements to the rescue!

If you're so rushed that you literally never get to eat a full, balanced meal, you may benefit from supplements regardless of your age.

Meeting a woman's special needs

And what about women? At various stages of their reproductive lives, they, too, benefit from supplements-as-insurance:

✔ **Before menopause:** Women, who lose iron each month through menstrual bleeding, rarely get sufficient amounts of iron from a typical American diet providing fewer than 2,000 calories a day. For them, and for women who are often on a diet to lose weight, iron supplements may be the only practical answer.

Iron is a mineral element, so it may be called "iron" or "elemental iron" on the label. Iron pills contain a compound of elemental iron ("ferrous" or "ferric," from *ferrum,* the Latin word for iron), plus an ingredient such as a sulfur derivative or lactic acid to enable your body to use the iron. On the label, the combination reads "ferrous sulfate" or "ferrous lactate." Different iron compounds dissolve at different rates in your stomach, yielding different amounts of elemental iron, so supplement labels usually list the iron this way: Ferrous sulfate 325 mg/Elemental iron 65 mg. Translation? This pill has 325 milligrams of ferrous sulfate, yielding 65 milligrams plain old iron. Sometimes the label omits the first part and simply says: Iron 65 mg.

If your doctor says, "Take one 325-milligram pill a day," she means 325 milligrams iron compound, not plain elemental iron.

✔ **During pregnancy and lactation:** Women who are pregnant or nursing often need supplements to provide the nutrients they need to build new maternal and fetal tissue or to produce nutritious breast milk. In addition, supplements of the B vitamin folate now are known to decrease a woman's risk of giving birth to a child with a neural tube defect (a defect of the spinal cord and column).

Never self-prescribe supplements while you're pregnant. Large amounts of some nutrients may actually be hazardous for your baby. For example, taking megadoses of vitamin A while you're pregnant can increase the risk of birth defects.

✔ **Through adulthood:** True, women older than 19 can get the calcium they require (1,000 milligrams/day) from four 8-ounce glasses of nonfat skim milk a day, three 8-ounce containers of yogurt made with nonfat milk, 22 ounces of canned salmon (with the soft edible bones; no, you definitely should not eat the hard bones in fresh salmon!), or any combination of the above. However, expecting women to do this nutritional balancing act every single day may be unrealistic. The simple alternative is calcium supplements.

Supplement Safety: An Iffy Proposition

The Food and Drug Administration (FDA) regulates food and drugs (no surprise there). Before the agency allows a new food or a new drug on the market, the manufacturer must submit proof that the product is safe. Drug manufacturers must also meet a second test, showing that their new medicine is *efficacious*, a fancy way of saying that the drug and the dosage in which it's sold will cure or relieve the condition for which it's prescribed.

Nobody says the drug-regulation system's perfect. Reality dictates that manufacturers test a drug only on a limited number of people for a limited period of time. So you can bet that some new drugs will trigger unexpected, serious, maybe even life-threatening side effects when used by thousands of people or taken for longer than the testing period. For proof, look no further than Phen-Fen, a diet drug combination that appeared to control weight safely during premarket testing but turned lethal after it reached pharmacy shelves.

Sweet trouble

Nobody wants to choke down a yucky supplement, but pills that look or taste like candy may be hazardous to a child's health. Some nutrients are troublesome — or even deadly — in high doses (see Chapters 10 and 11), especially for kids. For example, the Food and Drug Administration warns the lethal dose for young children may be as low as 3 grams (3,000 milligrams)

elemental iron, the amount in 49 tablets with 65 milligrams iron apiece. If you have youngsters in your house, protect them by buying neutral-tasting supplements and keeping all pills, nutrient and otherwise, in a safe cabinet, preferably high off the floor and locked tight to resist tiny prying fingers.

But at least the FDA can require that premarket safety and/or effectiveness info be displayed on foods and drugs. Unfortunately, the agency has no such power when it comes to dietary supplements.

In 1994, Congress passed and President Clinton signed into law the Dietary Supplement Health and Education Act, which limits the FDA's control over dietary supplements. Under this law, The FDA can't

✔ Require premarket tests to prove that supplements are safe and effective

✔ Limit the dosage in any dietary supplement

✔ Halt or restrict sales of a dietary supplement unless evidence shows that the product has caused illness or injury *when used according to the directions on the package;* in other words, if you experience a problem after taking slightly more or less of a supplement than directed on the label, the FDA can't help you

As a result, the FDA has found it virtually impossible to take products off drugstore shelves even after reports of illness and injury. For example, supplements containing the herb *ephedra* are reputed to enhance weight loss and sports performance. More than 600 reports of illness and at least 100 deaths have been linked to the use of ephedra supplements. The herb is banned by professional football and college athletics in the U.S. and by the Olympics. However, the FDA didn't act until February 2003, following the death of Baltimore Orioles pitcher Steve Bechler, who reportedly had been using ephedra products to control his weight.

Bechler's untimely death rang warning bells across the country, including in Washington, D.C., where the FDA ruled that henceforth every bottle of ephedra must carry strong warnings that the popular herb can cause potentially lethal heart attacks or strokes. In the sports world, ephedra was immediately forbidden in minor league but not major league baseball. The FDA banned all ephedra products, but the ban was partially reversed in April 2005, when a federal judge ruled that products containing low doses of ephedra were safe and could remain on the market. Some in Congress are pressing for a law that would enable FDA to ban any supplements considered even potentially hazardous to your precious health. Stay tuned.

By the way, ephedra isn't the only herbal supplement that can make you *really* uncomfortable. Table 5-1 lists some equally problematic herbal products that you need to approach with caution — or avoid altogether. In many cases, even small amounts are hazardous.

Table 5-1	Some Potentially Hazardous Herbals
Herb	*Known Side Effects and Reactions*
Blue cohosh	Nausea, vomiting, dizziness, smooth muscle (such as the uterus) contractions
Chaparral	Liver damage, liver failure
Comfrey	Possible liver damage
Kombuchu tea	Potentially fatal liver damage, intestinal upset
Lobelia (Indian tobacco)	Potentially fatal convulsions, coma
Pennyroyal	Potentially fatal liver damage, convulsions, coma
Senna	Severe gastric irritation, diarrhea
Stephania (also known as magnolia)	Kidney damage (sometimes severe enough to require dialysis or transplant)
Valerian	Severe withdrawal symptoms

"Vitamin and nutritional supplements," Mayo Clinic Health Letter (supplement), June 1997; Nancy Beth Jackson, "Doctors' warning: Beware of herbs' side effects," The New York Times, November 18, 1998; Jane Brody, "Taking a gamble on herbs as medicine," The New York Times, February 9, 1999; Carol Ann Rinzler, The Complete Book of Herbs, Spices, and Condiments (New York: Facts on File, 1990)

Choosing the Most Effective Supplements

Okay, you've read about the virtues and drawbacks of supplements. You've decided which supplements you think may do you some good. Now it's crunch time, and all you really want to know is how to choose the safest, most effective products. The guidelines in this section can help.

Choosing a well-known brand

Even though the FDA can't require manufacturers to submit safety and effectiveness data, a respected name on the label offers some assurance of a quality product. It also promises a fresh product; well-known brands generally sell out more quickly. The initials *USP* (U.S. Pharmacopoeia, a reputable testing organization) are another quality statement, and so are the words "release assured" or "proven release," which mean the supplement is easily absorbed by your body.

Checking the ingredient list

Check the supplement label. In the early 1990s, the FDA introduced the consumer-friendly nutrition food label with its mini-nutrition guide to nutrient content, complete ingredient listings, and dependable information about how eating certain foods may affect your risk of chronic illnesses, such as heart disease and cancer. (For more about the nutrition labels, see Chapter 17.)

The FDA's new supplement labels must list all ingredients. The label for vitamin and mineral products must give you the quantity per nutrient per serving plus the *%DV* (percentage daily value), the percentage of the RDA (Recommended Dietary Allowance). The listings for other dietary supplements, such as botanicals (herbs) and phytochemicals (see Chapter 12), must show the quantity per serving plus the part of the plant from which the ingredient is drawn (root, leaves, and so on). A manufacturer's own proprietary blend of two or more botanicals must list the weight of the total blend.

Figure 5-1 shows an example of the new supplement labels.

Looking for the expiration date

Over time, all dietary supplements become less potent. Always choose the product with the longest useful shelf life. Pass on the ones that will expire before you can use all the pills, such as the 100-pill bottle with an expiration date 30 days from now.

Checking the storage requirements

Even when you buy a product with the correct expiration date, it may be less effective if you don't keep it in the right place. Some supplements must be refrigerated; the rest you need to store, like any food product, in a cool, dry place. Avoid putting dietary supplements in a cabinet above the stove or refrigerator — true, the fridge is cold inside, but the motor pulsing away outside emits heat.

Nutrition Labeling for Dietary Supplements

(Effective March 1999)

Statement of identity.

GINSENG
A DIETARY SUPPLEMENT

Net quantity of contents.

60 CAPSULES

Structure-function claim.

"When you need to perform your best, take ginseng."

This statement has not been evaluated by the Food and Drug Administration. This product is not intended to diagnose, treat, cure, or prevent any disese.

Directions.

DIRECTIONS FOR USE: Take one capsule daily.

Supplement Facts panel.

Supplement Facts

Serving Size 1 Capsule

Amount Per Capsule

Oriental Ginseng, powdered (root)   250 mcg*

*Daily Value not established.

Other ingredients in descending order of predominance and by common name or proprietary blend.

Other ingredients: Gelatin, water, and glycerin.
ABC Company
Anywhere, MD 00001

Figure 5-1: Supplement labels are now consumer-friendly.

Name and place of business of manufacturer, packer, or distributor. This is the address to write for more product information.

Nutrients for the 21st-century body

Hate taking pills? Bored with trying to get all the foods required to meet your nutrients needs? A vitamin company in New South Wales (New Zealand) has your back. Or should I say, your bottom? AussieBum "Essence" underwear is made with material impregnated with "micro-encapsulated organic substances" that stay functional for up to 15 washings, releasing antioxidant "dermo-protective oils" onto your skin. And I just found them on, yes, eBay! You can't make this stuff up.

Choosing a sensible dose

Unless your doctor prescribes a dietary supplement as medicine, you don't need products marked "therapeutic," "extra-strength," or any variation thereof. Pick one that gives you no more than the RDA for any ingredient.

Avoiding hype

When the label promises something that's too good to be true — "Buy me! You'll live forever" — you know it's too good to be true. The FDA doesn't permit supplement marketers to claim that their products cure or prevent disease (that would make them medicines that require premarket testing). But the agency does allow claims that affect function, such as "maintains your cholesterol" (the no-no medical claim would be "lowers your cholesterol").

Another potential hype zone is the one labeled "natural," as in "natural vitamins are better." If you took Chem 101 in college, you know that the ascorbic acid (vitamin C) in oranges has exactly the same chemical composition as the ascorbic acid some nutritional chemist cooks up in her lab. But the ascorbic acid in a "natural" vitamin pill may come without additives such as coloring agents or fillers used in "regular" vitamin pills. In other words, if you aren't sensitive to the coloring agents or fillers in plain old pills, don't spend the extra dollars for "natural." If you are sensitive, do. What could be simpler? (For more on "natural" versus "synthetic" food ingredients, see Chapter 22.)

Good Reasons for Getting Nutrients from Food Rather Than Supplements

Despite this chapter's focus on the wonders of supplements, I feel obligated to play devil's advocate and report to you the arguments in favor of healthy people getting all or most of their nutrients from food rather than supplements.

Cost

If you're willing to plan and prepare nutritious meals, you can almost always get your nutrients less expensively from fresh fruits, vegetables, whole grains, dairy products, meat, fish, and poultry. Besides, food usually tastes better than supplements.

Unexpected bonuses

Food is a package deal containing vitamins, minerals, protein, fat, carbohydrates, and fiber, plus a cornucopia of as-yet-unidentified substances called phytochemicals (phyto = plant, chemicals = well, chemicals) that may be vital to your continuing good health. Think of lycopene, the red pigment in tomatoes that recently was found to reduce the risk of prostate cancer. Think of genistein and daidzein, the estrogen-like substances in soybeans that appear to reduce your risk of heart disease. Who knows what else is hiding in your apples, peaches, pears, and plums? Do you want to be the only one on your block who misses out on these goodies? Of course not. For more about the benefits of phytochemicals, see Chapter 12.

Safety

Several common nutrients may be toxic when you scarf them down in *megadose servings* (amounts several times larger than the RDAs). Not only are large doses of vitamin A linked to birth defects, but they may also cause symptoms similar to a brain tumor. Niacin megadoses may cause liver damage. Megadoses of vitamin B6 may cause (temporary) damage to nerves in arms, legs, fingers, and toes. All these effects are more likely to occur with supplements. Pills slip down easily, but regardless of how hungry you are, you probably won't eat enough food to reach toxic levels of nutrients. (To read more about the hazards of megadoses, see Chapters 10 and 11.)

The best statement about the role of supplements in good nutrition may be a paraphrase of Abraham Lincoln's famous remark about politicians and voters: "You may fool all the people some of the time; you can even fool some of the people all the time; but you can't fool all of the people all the time." If Honest Abe were with us now and were a sensible nutritionist rather than President, he might amend his words: "Supplements are valuable for all people some of the time and for some people all the time, but they're probably not necessary for all people all the time."

Part II
What You Get from Food

The 5th Wave
By Rich Tennant

"I'm not actually buying this stuff; I'm just using it to hide the fruit, legumes and greens until we get checked out."

In this part . . .

*H*ere's the lowdown on things you've heard about practically forever: protein, fat, carbohydrates, alcohol, vitamins, minerals, and water, with the absolutely newest numbers available on how much of what nutrients you need to keep your body humming happily.

This is a *For Dummies* book, so you don't have to read straight through from protein to water to see how things work. You can skip from chapter to chapter, back and forth, side to side. Any way you take it, this part is bound to clue you in to the value of the nutrients in food.

Chapter 6

Powerful Protein

· ·

In This Chapter

▶ Determining what protein is

▶ Finding the proteins in your body

▶ Getting the best quality protein from food

▶ Gauging how much protein you need

· ·

*P*rotein is an essential nutrient whose name comes from the Greek word *protos,* which means "first." To visualize a molecule of protein, close your eyes and see a very long chain, rather like a chain of sausage links. The links in the chains are *amino acids,* commonly known as the building blocks of protein. In addition to carbon, hydrogen, and oxygen atoms, amino acids contain a nitrogen (amino) group. The *amino group* is essential for synthesizing (assembling) specialized proteins in your body.

In this chapter, you can find out more — maybe even more than you ever wanted to know — about this molecule, how your body uses the proteins you take in as food, and how the body makes some special proteins you need for a healthy life.

Looking Inside and Out: Where Your Body Puts Protein

The human body is chock-full of proteins. Proteins are present in the outer and inner membranes of every living cell. Here's where else protein makes an appearance:

✔ Your hair, your nails, and the outer layers of your skin are made of the protein keratin. Keratin is a *scleroprotein,* or a protein resistant to digestive enzymes. So if you bite your nails, you can't digest them.

✔ Muscle tissue contains myosin, actin, myoglobin, and a number of other proteins.

✔ Bone has plenty of protein. The outer part of bone is hardened with minerals such as calcium, but the basic, rubbery inner structure is protein; and bone marrow, the soft material inside the bone, also contains protein.

✔ Red blood cells contain *hemoglobin,* a protein compound that carries oxygen throughout the body. *Plasma,* the clear fluid in blood, contains fat and protein particles known as *lipoproteins,* which ferry cholesterol around and out of the body.

Putting Protein to Work: How Your Body Uses Protein

Your body uses proteins to build new cells, maintain tissues, and synthesize new proteins that make it possible for you to perform basic bodily functions.

About half the dietary protein that you consume each day goes into making *enzymes,* the specialized worker proteins that do specific jobs such as digesting food and assembling or dividing molecules to make new cells and chemical substances. To perform these functions, enzymes often need specific vitamins and minerals.

Your ability to see, think, hear, and move — in fact, to do just about everything that you consider part of a healthy life — requires your nerve cells to send messages back and forth to each other and to other specialized kinds of cells, such as muscle cells. Sending these messages requires chemicals called *neurotransmitters.* Making neurotransmitters requires — guess what — proteins.

Finally, proteins play an important part in the creation of every new cell and every new individual. Your chromosomes consist of *nucleoproteins,* which are substances made of amino acids and nucleic acids. See the "DNA/RNA" sidebar in this chapter for more information about nucleoproteins.

Packing Back the Protein: What Happens to the Proteins You Eat

The cells in your digestive tract can absorb only single amino acids or very small chains of two or three amino acids called *peptides.* So proteins from food are broken into their component amino acids by digestive enzymes — which are, of course, specialized proteins. Then other enzymes in your body cells build new proteins by reassembling the amino acids into specific compounds that your body needs to function. This process is called *protein synthesis.* During protein synthesis

✔ Amino acids hook up with fats to form *lipoproteins,* the molecules that ferry cholesterol around and out of the body. Or amino acids may join up with carbohydrates to form the *glycoproteins* found in the mucus secreted by the digestive tract.

✔ Proteins combine with phosphoric acid to produce *phosphoproteins,* such as casein, a protein in milk.

✔ Nucleic acids combine with proteins to create *nucleoproteins,* which are essential components of the cell nucleus and of cytoplasm, the living material inside each cell.

The carbon, hydrogen, and oxygen that are left over after protein synthesis is complete are converted to glucose and used for energy (see Chapter 7). The nitrogen residue (ammonia) isn't used for energy. It's processed by the liver, which converts the ammonia to urea. Most of the urea produced in the liver is excreted through the kidneys in urine; very small amounts are sloughed off in skin, hair, and nails.

Every day, you *turn over* (reuse) more proteins than you get from the food you eat, so you need a continuous supply to maintain your protein status. If your diet does not contain sufficient amounts of proteins, you start digesting the proteins in your body, including the proteins in your muscles and — in extreme cases — your heart muscle.

DNA/RNA

Nucleoproteins are chemicals in the nucleus of every living cell. They're made of proteins linked to *nucleic acids* — complex compounds that contain phosphoric acid, a sugar molecule, and nitrogen-containing molecules made from amino acids.

Nucleic acids (molecules found in the chromosomes and other structures in the center of your cells) carry the genetic codes — genes that help determine what you look like, your general intelligence, and who you are. They contain one of two sugars, either *ribose* or *deoxyribose.* The nucleic acid containing ribose is called *ribonucleic acid* (RNA). The nucleic acid containing deoxyribose is called *deoxyribonucleic acid* (DNA).

DNA, a long molecule with two strands twisting about each other (the *double helix*), carries and transmits the genetic inheritance in your chromosomes. In other words, DNA supplies instructions that determine how your body cells are formed and how they behave. RNA, a single-strand molecule, is created in the cell nucleus according to the pattern determined by the DNA. Then RNA carries the DNA's instructions to the rest of the cell.

Knowing about DNA is important because it's the most distinctly "you" thing about your body. Chances that another person on Earth has exactly the same DNA as you are really small. That's why DNA analysis is used increasingly in identifying criminals or exonerating the innocent. Some people are even proposing that parents store a sample of their children's DNA so that they'll have a conclusive way of identifying a missing child, even years later.

Examining Protein Types: Not All Proteins Are Created Equal

All proteins are made of building blocks called amino acids, but not all proteins contain all the amino acids you require. This section helps you figure out how you can get the most useful proteins from your varied diet.

Essential and nonessential proteins

To make all the proteins that your body needs, you require 22 different amino acids. Ten are considered *essential,* which means you can't synthesize them in your body and must obtain them from food (two of these, arginine and histidine, are essential only for children). Several more are *nonessential:* If you don't get them in food, you can manufacture them yourself from fats, carbohydrates, and other amino acids. Three — glutamine, ornithine, and taurine — are somewhere in between essential and nonessential for human beings: They're essential only under certain conditions, such as with injury or disease.

Essential Amino Acids	*Nonessential Amino Acids*
Arginine*	Alanine
Histidine*	Asparagine
Isoleucine	Aspartic acid
Leucine	Citrulline
Lysine	Cysteine
Methionine	Glutamic acid
Phenlyalanine	Glycine
Threonine	Hydroxyglutamic acid
Tryptophan	Norleucine
Valine	Proline
	Serine
	Tyrosine

* Essential for children; nonessential for adults

High-quality and low-quality proteins

Because an animal's body is similar to yours, its proteins contain similar combinations of amino acids. That's why nutritionists call proteins from foods of animal origin — meat, fish, poultry, eggs, and dairy products — *high-quality proteins*. Your body absorbs these proteins more efficiently; they can be used without much waste to synthesize other proteins. The proteins from plants — grains, fruit, vegetables, legumes (beans), nuts, and seeds — often have limited amounts of some amino acids, which means their nutritional content is not as high as animal proteins.

Super soy: The special protein food

Nutrition fact No. 1: Food from animals has complete proteins. **Nutrition fact No. 2:** Vegetables, fruits, and grains have incomplete proteins. **Nutrition fact No. 3:** Nobody told the soybean.

Unlike other vegetables, including other beans, soybeans have complete proteins with sufficient amounts of all the amino acids essential to human health. In fact, food experts rank soy proteins on par with egg whites and casein (the protein in milk), the two proteins easiest for your body to absorb and use (see Table 6-1).

Some nutritionists think soy proteins are even better than the proteins in eggs and milk, because the proteins in soy come with no cholesterol and very little of the saturated fat known to clog your arteries and raise your risk of heart attack. Better yet, more than 20 recent studies suggest that adding soy foods to your diet can actually lower your cholesterol levels.

One-half cup of cooked soybeans has 14 grams of protein; 4 ounces of tofu has 13. Either serving gives you approximately twice the protein you get from one large egg or one 8-ounce glass of skim milk, or two-thirds the protein in 3 ounces of lean ground beef. Eight ounces of fat-free soy milk has 7 milligrams protein — a mere 1 milligram less than a similar serving of skim milk — and no cholesterol. Soybeans are also jam-packed with dietary fiber, which helps move food through your digestive tract.

In fact, soybeans are such a good source of food fiber that I feel obligated to add a cautionary note here. One day after I'd read through a bunch of studies about soy's effect on cholesterol levels, I decided to lower my cholesterol level right away. So I had a soy burger for lunch, a half cup of soybeans and no-fat cheese for an afternoon snack, and another half cup with tomato sauce at dinner. Delicacy prohibits me from explaining in detail how irritated and upset all that fiber made my digestive tract, but I'm sure you get the picture.

If you choose to use soybeans (or any other dry beans for that matter), take it slow — a little today, a little more tomorrow, and a little bit more the day after that.

The basic standard against which you measure the value of proteins in food is the egg. Nutrition scientists have arbitrarily given the egg a *biological value* of 100 percent, meaning that, gram for gram, it's the food with the best supply of complete proteins. Other foods that have proportionately more protein may not be as valuable as the egg because they lack sufficient amounts of one or more essential amino acids.

For example, eggs are 11 percent protein, and dry beans are 22 percent protein. However, the proteins in beans don't provide sufficient amounts of *all* the essential amino acids, so they (the beans) are not as nutritionally complete as proteins from animal foods. The prime exception is the soybean, a legume that's packed with abundant amounts of all of the amino acids essential for adults. Soybeans are an excellent source of proteins for vegetarians, especially *vegans,* which are vegetarians who avoid all products of animal origin, including milk and eggs.

The term used to describe the value of the proteins in any one food is *amino acid score.* Because the egg contains all the essential amino acids, it scores 100. Table 6-1 shows the protein quality of representative foods relative to the egg.

Table 6-1	Scoring the Amino Acids in Food	
Food	*Protein Content (Grams)*	*Amino Acid Score (Compared to the Egg)*
Egg	33	100
Fish	61	100
Beef	29	100
Milk (cow's whole)	23	100
Soybeans	29	100
Dry beans	22	75
Rice	7	62–66
Corn	7	47
Wheat	13	50
Wheat (white flour)	12	36

Nutritive Value of Foods (Washington, D.C.: U.S. Department of Agriculture, 1991); George M. Briggs and Doris Howes Calloway, Nutrition and Physical Fitness, 11th ed. (New York: Holt, Rinehart and Winston, 1984)

Homocysteine and your heart

Homocysteine is an *intermediate,* a chemical released when you metabolize (digest) protein. Unlike other amino acids, which are vital to your health, homocysteine can be hazardous to your heart, raising your risk of heart disease by attacking cells in the lining of your arteries by making them reproduce more quickly (the extra cells may block your coronary arteries) or by causing your blood to clot (ditto).

Years and years ago, before cholesterol moved to center stage, some smart heart researchers labeled homocysteine the major nutritional culprit in heart disease. Today, they've been vindicated. The American Heart Association cites high homocysteine levels as an independent probable (but not major) risk factor for heart disease, perhaps explaining why some people with low cholesterol have heart attacks.

But wait! The good news is that information from several studies, including the Harvard/ Brigham and Women's Hospital Nurses' Health Study in Boston, suggest that a diet rich in the B vitamin folate lowers blood levels of homocysteine. Most fruits and vegetables have plentiful amounts of folate. Stocking up on them may protect your heart.

Complete proteins and incomplete proteins

Another way to describe the quality of proteins is to say that they're either complete or incomplete. A *complete protein* is one that contains ample amounts of all essential amino acids; an *incomplete protein* does not. A protein low in one specific amino acid is called a *limiting protein* because it can build only as much tissue as the smallest amount of the necessary amino acid. You can improve the protein quality in a food containing incomplete/ limiting proteins by eating it along with one that contains sufficient amounts of the limited amino acids. Matching foods to create complete proteins is called *complementarity.*

For example, rice is low in the essential amino acid lysine, and beans are low in the essential amino acid methionine. By eating rice with beans, you improve (or complete) the proteins in both. Another example is pasta and cheese. Pasta is low in the essential amino acids lysine and isoleucine; milk products have abundant amounts of these two amino acids. Shaking Parmesan cheese onto pasta creates a higher-quality protein dish. In each case, the foods have complementary amino acids. Other examples of complementary protein dishes are peanut butter with bread, and milk with cereal. Many such combinations are a natural and customary part of the diet in parts of the world where animal proteins are scarce or very expensive. Here are some categories of foods with incomplete proteins:

- ✔ **Grain foods:** Barley, bread, bulgur wheat, cornmeal, kasha, and pancakes

- ✔ **Legumes:** Black beans, black-eyed peas, fava beans, kidney beans, lima beans, lentils, peanut butter, peanuts, peas, split peas, and white beans

- ✔ **Nuts and seeds:** Almonds, Brazil nuts, cashews, pecans, walnuts, pumpkin seeds, sesame seeds (tahini), and sunflower seeds

In order for the foods to complement each other, you must eat them together. In other words, rice and beans at one meal, not rice for lunch and beans for dinner. Table 6-2 shows how to combine foods to improve the quality of their proteins.

Table 6-2	How to Combine Foods to Complement Proteins	
This Food	*Complements This Food*	*Examples*
Whole grains	Legumes (beans)	Rice and beans
Dairy products	Whole grains	Cheese sandwich, pasta with cheese, pancakes (wheat and milk/egg batter)
Legumes (beans)	Nuts and/or seeds	Chili soup (beans) with caraway seeds
Dairy products	Legumes (beans)	Chili beans with cheese
Dairy products	Nuts and seeds	Yogurt with chopped nut garnish

The lowdown on gelatin and your fingernails

Everyone knows that gelatin is protein that strengthens fingernails. Too bad everyone's wrong. Gelatin is produced by treating animal bones with acid, a process that destroys the essential amino acid tryptophan. Surprise: Bananas are high in tryptophan. Slicing bananas onto your gelatin increases the quality of the protein. Adding milk makes it even better, but that still may not heal your splitting nails. The fastest way to a cure is a visit to the dermatologist, who can tell you whether the problem is an allergy to nail polish, too much time spent washing dishes, a medical problem such as a fungal infection, or just plain peeling nails. Then the dermatologist may prescribe a different nail polish (or none at all), protective gloves, a fungicide (a drug that wipes out fungi), or a lotion product that strengthens the natural glue that holds the layers of your nails together.

Deciding How Much Protein You Need

The National Academy of Sciences Food and Nutrition Board, which sets the requirements (for example, RDAs) for vitamins and minerals, also sets goals for daily protein consumption. As with other nutrients, the board has different recommendations for different groups of people: young or older, men or women.

Calculating the correct amount

As a general rule, the National Academy of Sciences says healthy people need to get 10 to 35 percent of their daily calories from protein. More specifically, the Academy has set a Dietary Reference Intake (DRI) of 45 grams protein per day for a healthy woman and 52 grams per day for a healthy man. (Check out Chapter 4 for a complete explanation of the DRI.)

These amounts are easily obtained from two to three 3-ounce servings of lean meat, fish, or poultry (21 grams each). Vegetarians can get their protein from 2 eggs (12–16 grams), 2 slices of prepacked fat-free cheese (10 grams), 4 slices of bread (3 grams each), and one cup of yogurt (10 grams).

As you grow older, you synthesize new proteins less efficiently, so your muscle mass (protein tissue) diminishes while your fat content stays the same or rises. This change is why some folks erroneously believe that muscle "turns to fat" in old age. Of course, you still use protein to build new tissue, including hair, skin, and nails, which continue to grow until you cross over into The Great Beyond. By the way, the idea that nails continue to grow after death — a staple of shock movies and horror comics — arises from the fact that after death, tissue around the nails shrinks, making a corpse's nails simply look longer. Who else would let you in on these secrets?

Dodging protein deficiency

The first sign of protein deficiency is likely to be weak muscles — the body tissue most reliant on protein. For example, children who do not get enough protein have shrunken, weak muscles. They may also have thin hair, their skin may be covered with sores, and blood tests may show that the level of albumin in their blood is below normal. *Albumin* is a protein that helps maintain the body's fluid balance, keeping a proper amount of liquid in and around body cells.

A protein deficiency may also show up in your blood. Red blood cells live for only 120 days. Protein is needed to produce new ones. People who do not get enough protein may become *anemic,* having fewer red blood cells than they need. Protein deficiency may also show up as fluid retention (the big belly on a starving child), hair loss, and muscle wasting caused by the body's attempt to protect itself by digesting the proteins in its own muscle tissue. That's why victims of starvation are, literally, skin and bones.

Given the high protein content of a normal American diet (which generally provides far more protein than you actually require), protein deficiency is rare in the United States except as a consequence of eating disorders such as *anorexia nervosa* (refusal to eat) and *bulimia* (regurgitation after meals).

Boosting your protein intake: Special considerations

Anyone who's building new tissue quickly needs extra protein. For example, the Dietary Reference Intake (DRI) for protein for women who are pregnant or nursing is 71 grams per day. Injuries also raise your protein requirements. An injured body releases above-normal amounts of protein-destroying hormones from the pituitary and adrenal glands. You need extra protein to protect existing tissues, and after severe blood loss, you need extra protein to make new hemoglobin for red blood cells. Cuts, burns, or surgical procedures mean that you need extra protein to make new skin and muscle cells. Fractures mean extra protein is needed to make new bone. The need for protein is so important when you've been badly injured that if you can't take protein by mouth, you'll be given an intravenous solution of amino acids with glucose (sugar) or emulsified fat.

Do athletes need more proteins than the rest of us? Recent research suggests that the answer may be yes, but athletes easily meet their requirements by increasing the amount of food in their normal diet.

Avoiding protein overload

Yes, you can get too much protein. Several medical conditions make it difficult for people to digest and process proteins properly. As a result, waste products build up in different parts of the body.

People with liver disease or kidney disease either don't process protein efficiently into urea or don't excrete it efficiently through urine. The result may be uric acid kidney stones or *uremic poisoning* (an excess amount of uric acid in the blood). The pain associated with *gout* (a form of arthritis that affects nine men for every one woman) is caused by uric acid crystals collecting in the spaces around joints. Doctors may recommend a low-protein diet as part of the treatment in these situations.

Chapter 7

The Lowdown on Fat and Cholesterol

*T*he chemical family name for fats and related compounds such as cholesterol is *lipids* (from *lipos,* the Greek word for fat). Liquid fats are called *oils;* solid fats are called, well, *fat.* With the exception of *cholesterol* (a fatty substance that has no calories and provides no energy), fats are high-energy nutrients. Gram for gram, fats have more than twice as much energy potential (calories) as protein and carbohydrates (affectionately referred to as *carbs*): 9 calories per fat gram versus 4 calories per gram for proteins and carbs. (For more calorie facts, see Chapter 3.)

In this chapter, I cut the fat away from the subject of fats and zero in on the essential facts you need to put together a diet with just enough fat (yes, you do need fat) to provide the bounce that every diet requires. And then I deal with that ultimate baddie — cholesterol. Surprise! You need some of that, too. Onward.

Finding the Facts about Fat Stuff

Fats are sources of energy that add flavor to food — the sizzle on the steak, you can say. However, as anyone who's spent the last 30 years on planet Earth knows, fats may also be hazardous to your health. The trick is separating the good from the bad. Trust me. It can be done. And this section explains how.

Understanding how your body uses fat

Here's a sentence that you probably never thought you'd read: A healthy body needs fat. Your body uses *dietary fat* (the fat that you get from food) to make tissue and manufacture biochemicals, such as hormones. Some of the body fat made from food fat is *visible.* Even though your skin covers it, you can *see* the fat in the *adipose* (fatty) *tissue* in female breasts, hips, thighs, buttocks, and belly or male abdomen and shoulders.

This visible body fat

- Provides a source of stored energy
- Gives shape to your body
- Cushions your skin (imagine sitting in a chair for a while to read this book without your buttocks to pillow your bones)
- Acts as an insulation blanket that reduces heat loss

Other body fat is invisible. You can't see this body fat because it's tucked away in and around your internal organs. This hidden fat is

- Part of every cell membrane (the outer skin that holds each cell together)
- A component of *myelin,* the fatty material that sheathes nerve cells and makes it possible for them to fire the electrical messages that enable you to think, see, speak, move, and perform the multitude of tasks natural to a living body; brain tissue also is rich in fat
- A shock absorber that protects your organs (as much as possible) if you fall or are injured
- A constituent of hormones and other biochemicals, such as vitamin D and bile

Pulling energy from fat

Although fat has more energy (calories) per gram than proteins and carbohydrates, your body has a more difficult time pulling the energy out of fatty foods. Imagine a chain of long balloons — the kind people twist into shapes that resemble dachshunds, flowers, and other amusing things. When you drop one of these balloons into water, it floats. That's exactly what happens when you swallow fat-rich foods. The fat floats on top of the watery food-and-liquid mixture in your stomach, which limits the effect that *lipases* — fat-busting digestive enzymes in the mix below — can have on it. Because fat is digested more slowly than proteins and carbohydrates, you feel fuller (a condition called *satiety*) longer after eating high-fat food.

Into the intestines

When the fat moves down your digestive tract into your small intestine, an intestinal hormone called *cholestokinin* beeps your gallbladder, signaling for the release of bile. *Bile* is an emulsifier, a substance that enables fat to mix with water so that lipases can start breaking the fat into glycerol and fatty acids. These smaller fragments may be stored in special cells (fat cells) in adipose tissue, or they may be absorbed into cells in the intestinal wall, where one of the following happens:

- ✔ They're combined with oxygen (or burned) to produce heat/energy, water, and the waste product carbon dioxide.
- ✔ They're used to make lipoproteins that haul fats, including cholesterol, through your bloodstream.

Into the body

Glucose, the molecule you get by digesting carbohydrates, is the body's basic source of energy. Burning glucose is easier and more efficient than burning fat, so your body always goes for carbohydrates first. But if you've used up all your available glucose — maybe you're stranded in a cabin in the Arctic, you haven't eaten for a week, a blizzard's howling outside, and the corner deli 500 miles down the road doesn't deliver — then it's time to start in on your body fat.

The first step is for an enzyme in your fat cells to break up stored triglycerides (the form of fat in adipose tissue). The enzyme action releases glycerol and fatty acids, which travel through your blood to body cells, where they combine with oxygen to produce heat/energy, plus water — lots of water — and the waste product carbon dioxide. As anyone who has used a high-protein/high-fat/low-carb weight-loss diet such as the Atkins regimen can tell you, in addition to all that water, burning fat without glucose produces a second waste product called ketones. In extreme cases, high concentrations of ketones (a condition known as *ketosis*) alter the acid/alkaline balance (or pH) of your blood and may trip you into a coma. Left untreated, ketosis can lead to death. Medically, this condition is most common among people with diabetes. For people on a low-carb diet, the more likely sign of ketosis is stinky urine or breath that smells like acetone (nail polish remover).

Focusing on the fats in food

Food contains three kinds of fats: triglycerides, phospholipids, and sterols. Here's how they differ:

- ✔ **Triglycerides:** You use these fats to make adipose tissue and burn for energy.
- ✔ **Phospholipids:** Phospholipids are hybrids — part lipid, part phosphate (a molecule made with the mineral phosphorus) — that act as tiny rowboats,

ferrying hormones and fat-soluble vitamins A, D, E, and K through your blood and back and forth in the watery fluid that flows across cell membranes. (By the way, the official name for fluid around cells is *extracellular fluid*. See why I just called it watery fluid?)

✔ **Sterols (steroid alcohols):** These are fat and alcohol compounds with no calories. Vitamin D is a sterol. So is the sex hormone testosterone. And so is cholesterol, the base on which your body builds hormones and vitamins.

Getting the right amount of fat

Getting the right amount of fat in your diet is a delicate balancing act. Too much, and you increase your risk of obesity, diabetes, heart disease, and some forms of cancer. (The risk of colon cancer seems to be tied more clearly to a diet high in fat from meat rather than fat from dairy products.) Too little fat, and infants don't thrive, children don't grow, and everyone, regardless of age, is unable to absorb and use fat-soluble vitamins that smooth the skin, protect vision, bolster the immune system, and keep reproductive organs functioning.

In the fall of 2002, the National Academies' Institute of Medicine (IOM) recommended that no more than 20 to 45 percent of daily calories should come from fat. On a 2,000-calorie daily diet, that's 400 to 900 calories from fats a day. The Dietary Guidelines for Americans 2005 (see Chapter 16) lowers that to 20 to 30 percent of total calories. Translation: 400 to 600 of the calories on a 2,000-calorie/day regimen.

Because your body doesn't need to get saturated fats, cholesterol, or trans fats from food, neither IOM nor the *Dietary Guidelines for Americans 2005* have set levels for these nutrients, except to say, "Keep them as low as possible, please."

This advice about fat intake is primarily for adults. Although many organizations, such as the American Academy of Pediatrics, the American Heart Association, and the National Heart, Lung, and Blood Institute, recommend restricting fat intake for older children, they stress that infants and toddlers require fatty acids for proper physical growth and mental development, and that's why Mother Nature made human breast milk (see Chapter 28) so high in fatty acids. Never limit the fat in your baby's diet without checking first with your pediatrician.

Essential fatty acids

An *essential fatty acid* is one that your body needs but cannot assemble from other fats. You have to get it whole, from food. Linoleic acid, found in vegetable oils, is an essential fatty acid. Two others — linolenic acid and arachidonic acid — occupy a somewhat ambiguous position. You can't make them from scratch, but you can make them if you have enough linoleic acid on hand, so food scientists can work up a good fight about whether linolenic and arachidonic acids are actually "essential." In practical terms, who cares? Linoleic acid is so widely available in food, you're unlikely to experience a deficiency of any of the three — linoleic, linolenic, or arachidonic acids — as long as 2 percent of the calories you get each day come from fat.

In 2002, the Institute of Medicine (IOM) published the first daily recommendations for two essential fatty acids, *alpha*-linolenic acid and linolenic acid. The former is an omega-3 fatty acid (more about that later on in this chapter) that's found in fish oils, milk, and some veggie oils. The latter is an omega-6 fatty acid (ditto), found in safflower and corn oil. IOM recommends that

- ✔ Women get 12 grams linolenic acid and 1.1 grams *alpha*-linolenic acid per day

- ✔ Men get 17 grams linolenic acid and 1.6 grams *alpha*-linolenic acid per day

Finding fat in all kinds of foods

As a general rule:

- ✔ Fruits and vegetables have only traces of fat, primarily unsaturated fatty acids.

- ✔ Grains have small amounts of fat, up to 3 percent of their total weight.

- ✔ Dairy products vary. Cream is a high-fat food. Regular milks and cheeses are moderately high in fat. Skim milk and skim milk products are low-fat foods. Most of the fat in any dairy product is saturated fatty acids.

- ✔ Meat is moderately high in fat, and most of its fats are saturated fatty acids.

- ✔ Poultry (chicken and turkey), without the skin, is relatively low in fat.

- ✔ Fish may be high or low in fat, primarily unsaturated fatty acids that — lucky for the fish — remain liquid even when the fish is swimming in cold water. (Saturated fats harden when cooled.)

- ✔ Vegetable oils, butter, and lard are high-fat foods. Most of the fatty acids in vegetable oils are unsaturated; most of the fatty acids in lard and butter are saturated.

- ✔ Processed foods, such as cakes, breads, canned or frozen meat, and vegetable dishes, are generally higher in fat than plain grains, meats, fruits, and vegetables.

Here's a simple guide to finding which foods are high (or low) in fat. Oils are virtually 100 percent fat. Butter and lard are close behind. After that, the fat level drops, from 70 percent for some nuts down to 2 percent for most bread. The rule to take away from these numbers? A diet high in grains and plants always is lower in fat than a diet high in meat and oils.

Defining fatty acids and their relationship to dietary fat

Fatty acids are the building blocks of fats. Chemically speaking, a *fatty acid* is a chain of carbon atoms with hydrogen atoms attached and a *carbon-oxygen-oxygen-hydrogen group* (the unit that makes it an acid) at one end.

All the fats in food are combinations of fatty acids. Nutritionists characterize fatty acids as saturated, monounsaturated, or polyunsaturated, depending on how many hydrogen atoms are attached to the carbon atoms in the chain. The more hydrogen atoms, the more saturated the fatty acid. Depending on which fatty acids predominate, a food fat is likewise characterized as saturated, monounsaturated, or polyunsaturated.

- A *saturated fat,* such as butter, has mostly saturated fatty acids. Saturated fats are solid at room temperature and get harder when chilled.

- A *monounsaturated fat,* such as olive oil, has mostly monounsaturated fatty acids. Monounsaturated fats are liquid at room temperature; they get thicker when chilled.

- A *polyunsaturated fat,* such as corn oil, has mostly polyunsaturated fatty acids. Polyunsaturated fats are liquid at room temperature; they stay liquid when chilled.

So why is margarine, which is made from unsaturated fats such as corn and soybean oil, a solid? Because it's been artificially saturated by food chemists who add hydrogen atoms to some of its unsaturated fatty acids. This process, known as *hydrogenation,* turns an oil, such as corn oil, into a solid fat that can be used in products such as margarines without leaking out all over the table. A fatty acid with extra hydrogen atoms is called a *hydrogenated fatty acid.* Another name for hydrogenated fatty acid is trans fatty acid. *Trans fatty acids* are not healthy for your heart. Because of those darned extra hydrogen atoms, they are, well, more saturated, and they act like — what else? — saturated fats, clogging arteries and raising the levels of cholesterol in your blood. To make it easier for you to control your trans fat intake, the Food and Drug Administration now requires a new line on the Nutritional Facts label that tells you exactly how many grams of trans fats are in any product you buy.

In the meantime, as I explain in *Controlling Cholesterol For Dummies* (a whole doggone book — published by Wiley — on how to whip your cholesterol profile into shape), the same smart food chemists who invented hydrogenation have now come up with trans fat–free margarines and spreads, including some that are made with plant sterols and stanols.

Plant *sterols* are natural compounds found in oils in grains, fruits, and vegetables, including soybeans, while *stanols* are compounds created by adding hydrogen atoms to sterols from wood pulp and other plant sources. Sterols and stanols work like little sponges, sopping up cholesterol in your intestines before it can make its way into your bloodstream. As a result, your total cholesterol levels and your levels of low-density lipoproteins (otherwise known as LDLs or "bad cholesterol") go down. In some studies, one to two 1-tablespoon servings a day of sterols and stanols can lower levels of bad cholesterol by 10 to 17 percent, with results showing up in as little as two weeks. Wow!

A nutritional fish story

When Sir William Gilbert, lyricist to songsmith Sir Arthur Sullivan, wrote, "Here's a pretty kettle of fish!" he may well have been talking about the latest skinny on seafood.

The good news from a 2002 Harvard survey of more than 43,000 male health professionals shows that the ones who eat 3 to 5 ounces of fish just once a month have a 40 percent lower risk of *ischemic stroke,* a stroke caused by a blood clot in a cranial artery. The Harvard study did not include women, but a report on women and stroke published in the *Journal of the American Medical Association* in 2000 says that women who eat about 4 ounces of fish — think one small can of tuna — two to four times a week appear to cut their risk of stroke by a similar 40 percent.

These benefits are, in large part, because of the presence of *omega-3 fatty acids,* which are unsaturated fatty acids found most commonly in fatty fish such as salmon and sardines. The primary omega-3 is *alpha*-linolenic acid, which your body converts to hormonelike substances called eicosanoids. The *eicosanoids* — eicosapentaenoic acid (EPA) and docosahexaenoic acid (DHA) — reduce inflammation,

perhaps by inhibiting an enzyme called COX-2, which is linked to inflammatory diseases such as rheumatoid arthritis (RA). The Arthritis Foundation says omega-3s relieve RA joint inflammation, swelling, and pain.

Omega-3s also are heart-friendly. The fats make the tiny blood particles called platelets less sticky, reducing the possibility that they'll clump together to form blood clots that might obstruct a blood vessel and trigger a heart attack. Omega-3s also knock down levels of bad cholesterol so effectively that the American Heart Association recommends eating fish at least twice a week. Besides, fish also is a good source of *taurine,* an amino acid the journal *Circulation* notes helps maintain the elasticity of blood vessels, which means that the vessels may dilate to permit blood or — horrors! — a blot clot to flow through.

Did I mention that omega-3s are bone builders? Fish oils enable your body to create *calciferol,* a naturally occurring form of vitamin D, the nutrient that enables your body to absorb bone-building calcium — which may be why omega-3s appear to help hold minerals in bone — and increase the formation of new bone.

(continued)

(continued)

A pretty kettle of fish, indeed.

You can find respectable amounts of omega-3s in

- Anchovies
- Haddock
- Herring
- Mackerel
- Salmon
- Sardines
- Scallops
- Tuna (albacore)
- Broccoli
- Kale
- Spinach
- Canola oil
- Walnut oil
- Flaxseed oil

Consumer Alert No. 1

Before you shout, "Waiter! Bring me the salmon, mackerel, herring, or whatever," here's the other side of the coin. Earlier research suggests that frequent servings of fish may increase the risk of a stroke caused by bleeding in the brain. This situation is common among Native Alaskans who eat plenty of fish and have a higher than normal incidence of hemorrhagic, or bleeding, strokes. True, the Harvard study found no significant link between fish consumption and bleeding strokes, but researchers say more studies are needed to nail down the relationship — or lack thereof.

Consumer Alert No. 2

Not all omegas are equally beneficial. Omega-6 fatty acids — polyunsaturated fats found in beef, pork, and several vegetable oils, including corn, sunflower, cottonseed, soybean, peanut, and sesame oils — are chemical cousins of omega-3s, but the omega-6s lack the benefits of the omega-3s.

Consumer Alert No. 3

Wait! Don't go just yet. Despite all the benefits fish bring to a healthful diet, my technical editor, University of Maine Food Science Professor Alfred Bushway, wants me to remind you that some fish, particularly those caught in the wild (rather than raised on a fish farm), may be contaminated with metals such as mercury, which has made its way into the water as industrial pollution and may be hazardous for women who are or may be pregnant. Check the food bulletins in your local newspaper or check the FDA's hotline (listed on its Web site, which you can find in Chapter 27) for the most up-to-date data.

Now it's really a pretty kettle of fish!

Table 7-1 shows the kinds of fatty acids found in some common dietary fats and oils. Fats are characterized according to their predominant fatty acids. For example, as you can plainly see in the table, nearly 25 percent of the fatty acids in corn oil are monounsaturated fatty acids. Nevertheless, because corn oil has more polyunsaturated fatty acid, corn oil is considered a polyunsaturated fatty acid. Note for math majors: Some of the totals in Table 7-1 don't add up to 100 percent because these fats and oils also contain other kinds of fatty acids in amounts so small that they don't affect the basic character of the fat.

Exploring the chemical structure of fatty acids

If you don't have a clue about the chemical structure of fatty acids, reading this explanation may be worth your while. The concepts are simple, and the information you find here applies to all kinds of molecules, not just fatty acids.

Molecules are groups of atoms hooked together by chemical bonds. Different atoms form different numbers of bonds with other atoms. For example, a hydrogen atom can form one bond with one other atom; an oxygen atom can form two bonds with other atoms; and a carbon atom can form four bonds to other atoms.

To actually see how this works, visualize a carbon atom as one of those round pieces in a child's Erector set or Tinkertoy kit. Your carbon atom (C) has — figuratively speaking, of course — four holes: one on top, one on the bottom, and one on each side. If you stick a peg into each hole and attach a small piece of wood representing a hydrogen atom (H) to the pegs on the top, the bottom, and the left, you have a structure that looks like this:

Methyl group

This unit, called a *methyl group,* is the first piece in any fatty acid. To build the rest of the fatty acid, you add carbon atoms and hydrogen atoms to form a chain. At the end, you tack on a group with one carbon atom, two oxygen atoms, and a hydrogen atom. This group is called an *acid group,* the part that makes the chain of carbon and hydrogen atoms a fatty acid.

Saturated Fatty Acid

The preceding molecule is a *saturated fatty acid* because it has a hydrogen atom at every available carbon link in the chain. A *monounsaturated fatty acid* drops two hydrogen atoms and forms one double bond (two lines instead of one) between two carbon atoms. A *polyunsaturated fatty acid* drops more hydrogen atoms and forms several (poly) double bonds between several carbon atoms. Every hydrogen atom still forms one bond, and every carbon atom still forms four bonds, but they do so in a slightly different way. These sketches are not pictures of real fatty acids, which have many more carbons in the chain and have their double bonds in different places, but they can give you an idea of what fatty acids look like up close.

Instead of this:

(a saturated fatty acid)

You get this:

(a monosaturated fatty acid)

or

(a polyunsaturated fatty acid)

And that's the whole deal!

Table 7-1	What Fatty Acids Are in That Fat or Oil?			
Fat or Oil	*Saturated Fatty Acid (%)*	*Monounsaturated Fatty Acid (%)*	*Polyunsaturated Fatty Acid (%)*	*Kind of Fat or Oil*
Canola oil	7	53	22	Mono-unsaturated
Corn oil	13	24	59	Poly-unsaturated
Olive oil	14	74	9	Mono-unsaturated
Palm oil	52	38	10	Saturated
Peanut oil	17	46	32	Mono-unsaturated
Safflower oil	9	12	74	Poly-unsaturated
Soybean oil	15	23	51	Poly-unsaturated
Soybean-cottonseed oil	18	29	48	Poly-unsaturated
Butter	62	30	5	Saturated
Lard	39	45	11	Saturated*

* Because more than one-third of its fats are saturated, nutritionists label lard a saturated fat. Nutritive Value of Foods (Washington, D.C.: U.S. Department of Agriculture); Food and Life (New York: American Council on Science and Health)

Considering Cholesterol and You

I mention earlier in this chapter that your body actually *needs* fat, and here's another sentence that may blow your (nutritional) mind: Every healthy body *needs* cholesterol. Look carefully and you find cholesterol in and around your cells, in your fatty tissue, in your organs, and in your glands. What's it doing there? Plenty of useful things. For example, cholesterol

✔ Protects the integrity of cell membranes

✔ Helps enable nerve cells to send messages back and forth

✔ Is a building block for vitamin D (a sterol), made when sunlight hits the fat just under your skin (for more about vitamin D, see Chapter 10)

✔ Enables your gallbladder to make *bile acids,* digestive chemicals that, in turn, enable you to absorb fats and fat-soluble nutrients such as vitamin A, vitamin D, vitamin E, and vitamin K

✔ Is a base on which you build steroid hormones such as estrogen and testosterone

Cholesterol and heart disease

Doctors measure your cholesterol level by taking a sample of blood and counting the milligrams of cholesterol in 1 deciliter (1/10 liter) of blood. When you get your annual report from the doctor, your total cholesterol level looks something like this: 225 mg/dl. Translation: You have 225 milligrams of cholesterol in every tenth of a liter of blood. Why does this matter? Because cholesterol makes its way into blood vessels, sticks to the walls, and forms deposits that eventually block the flow of blood. The more cholesterol you have floating in your blood, the more cholesterol is likely to cross into your arteries, where it may increase your risk of heart attack or stroke.

As a general rule, the National Cholesterol Education Program (NCEP) says that for adults, a cholesterol level higher than 250 mg/dl is a high risk factor for heart disease; between 200 mg/dl and 250 mg/dl is considered a moderate risk factor; below 200 mg/dl is considered a low risk factor.

Cholesterol levels alone are not the entire story. Many people with high cholesterol levels live to a ripe old age, but others with low total cholesterol levels develop heart disease. Worse yet, recent research indicates that low cholesterol levels may increase the risk of stroke. In other words, cholesterol is only one of several risk factors for heart disease. Here are some more:

✔ An unfavorable ratio of lipoproteins (see the following section)

✔ Smoking

✔ Obesity

✔ Age (being older is riskier)

✔ Sex (being male is riskier)

✔ A family history of heart disease

To estimate your own risk of heart disease/heart attack, check out the NCEP heart attack risk calculator at hin.nhlbi.nih.gov/atpiii/calculator.asp.

Cholesterol season

Even if you allow yourself to indulge in (a few) high-cholesterol ice cream cones and burgers every day of the year, your cholesterol level may still be naturally lower in the summer than in winter.

The basis for this intriguing culinary conclusion is the 2004 University of Massachusetts SEASONS (Seasonal Variation in Blood Lipids) Study of 517 healthy men and women ages 20 to 70. The volunteers started out with an average cholesterol level of 213 mg/dl (women) to 222 mg/dl (men). A series of five blood tests during the one-year study showed an average drop of 4 points in the summer for men and 5.4 points for women. People with high cholesterol (above 240 mg/dl) did better, dropping as much as 18 points in the summer.

U. Mass cardiologists say one explanation for the summer downswing may be the normal increase in human blood volume in hot weather. Cholesterol levels reflect the total amount of cholesterol in your bloodstream. With more blood in the stream, the amount of cholesterol per deciliter declines, producing a lower total cholesterol reading. A second possibility is that people tend to eat less and be more active in summer. They lose weight, and weight loss equals lower cholesterol.

The first bit of wisdom from this study is obvious: Being physically active reduces your cholesterol level. The second is that environment matters. In other words, if you're planning to start a new cholesterol-buster diet, you may just do better to start during the cool weather, when your efforts may lower your total cholesterol as much as 12 points over a reasonable period of time, say, six months. Then when your doctor runs a follow-up test the following summer, you'll get the added benefit of the seasonal slip to make you feel really, really good about how well you're doing. And there's this: For more on controlling your cholesterol, zip out and get yourself a copy of (what else?) *Controlling Cholesterol For Dummies*. By me.

Living with lipoproteins

A *lipoprotein* is a fat (lipo = fat, remember?) and protein particle that carries cholesterol through your blood. Your body makes four types of lipoproteins: chylomicrons, very low-density lipoproteins (VLDLs), low-density lipoproteins (LDLs), and high-density lipoproteins (HDLs). As a general rule, LDLs take cholesterol into blood vessels; HDLs carry it out of the body.

A lipoprotein is born as a *chylomicron,* made in your intestinal cells from protein and triglycerides (fats). After 12 hours of traveling through your blood and around your body, a chylomicron has lost virtually all of its fats. By the time the chylomicron makes its way to your liver, the only thing left is protein.

The liver, a veritable fat and cholesterol factory, collects fatty acid fragments from your blood and uses them to make cholesterol and new fatty acids. Time out! How much cholesterol you get from food may affect your liver's daily output: Eat more cholesterol, and your liver may make less. If you eat less cholesterol, your liver may make more. And so it goes.

Churning out harmful lipoproteins

Okay, after your liver has made cholesterol and fatty acids, it packages them with protein as very low-density lipoproteins (VLDLs), which have more protein and are denser than their precursors, the chylomicrons. As VLDLs travel through your bloodstream, they lose triglycerides, pick up cholesterol, and turn into low-density lipoproteins (LDLs). LDLs supply cholesterol to your body cells, which use it to make new cell membranes and manufacture sterol compounds such as hormones. That's the good news.

The bad news is that both VLDLs and LDLs are soft and squishy enough to pass through blood vessel walls. The larger and squishier they are, the more likely they are to slide into your arteries, which means that VLDLs are more hazardous to your health than plain old LDLs. These fluffy, fatty lipoproteins carry cholesterol into blood vessels, where it can cling to the inside wall, forming deposits, or *plaques*. These plaques may eventually block an artery, prevent blood from flowing through, and trigger a heart attack or stroke. Whew! Got all that?

VLDLs and LDLs are sometimes called "bad cholesterol," but this characterization is a misnomer. They aren't cholesterol; they're just the rafts on which cholesterol sails into your arteries. Traveling through the body, LDLs continue to lose cholesterol. In the end, they lose so much fat that they become mostly protein — turning them into high-density lipoproteins, the particles sometimes called "good cholesterol." Once again, this label is inaccurate. HDLs aren't cholesterol: They're simply protein and fat particles too dense and compact to pass through blood vessel walls, so they carry cholesterol out of the body rather than into arteries.

That's why a high level of HDLs may reduce your risk of heart attack regardless of your total cholesterol levels. Conversely, a high level of LDLs may raise your risk of heart attack, even if your overall cholesterol level is low. Hey, on second thought, maybe that does qualify them as "good" and "bad" cholesterol.

Setting limits on the bad guys

At one point, back in the dawn of the Cholesterol Age, like, say, five years ago, the "safe" upper limit for LDLs was assumed to be around 160 mg/dl. Now, the National Heart, Lung, and Blood Institute, American College of Cardiology, and the American Heart Association have all put their stamps of approval on the National Cholesterol Education Program's (NCEP) recommendations for new, lower levels of LDLs based on the presence of the risk factors I list under "Cholesterol and heart disease." You know — diabetes, high blood pressure, obesity . . . those risk factors.

For healthy people with two or more risk factors, the new goal is to push LDLs below 130 mg/dl. For high-risk patients with heart disease or blood vessel problems and more than two risk factors, it's LDLs below 100 mg/dl. For very high-risk patients who are hospitalized with heart disease or have heart disease plus several risk factors, LDLs should be under 70 mg/dl. If necessary, the NCEP suggests using cholesterol-busting "statin" drugs such as atorvastatin (Lipitor).

Diet and cholesterol

Most of the cholesterol that you need is made right in your own liver, which churns out about 1 gram (1,000 milligrams) a day from the raw materials in the proteins, fats, and carbohydrates that you consume. But you also get cholesterol from food of animal origin: meat, poultry, fish, eggs, and dairy products. Although some plant foods, such as coconuts and cocoa beans, are high in saturated fats, no plants actually have cholesterol. Table 7-2 lists the amount of cholesterol in normal servings of some representative foods.

Because plants don't contain cholesterol, no plant foods are on this list. No grains. No fruits. No veggies. No nuts and seeds. Of course, you can juice plant food up with cholesterol if you really try: Butter in the bread dough, cheese on the macaroni, cream sauce on the peas and onions, whipped cream on poached peaches, and so on.

Table 7-2	How Much Cholesterol Is on That Plate?	
Food	**Serving Size**	**Cholesterol (mg)**
Meat		
Beef (stewed) lean and fat	3 ounces	87
Beef (stewed) lean	2.2 ounces	66
Beef (ground) lean	3 ounces	74
Beef (ground) regular	3 ounces	76
Beef steak (sirloin)	3 ounces	77
Bacon	3 strips	16
Pork chop, lean	2.5 ounces	71

Food	Serving Size	Cholesterol (mg)
Poultry		
Chicken (roast) breast	3 ounces	73
Chicken (roast) leg	3 ounces	78
Turkey (roast) breast	3 ounces	59
Fish		
Clams	3 ounces	43
Flounder	3 ounces	59
Oysters (raw)	1 cup	120
Salmon (canned)	3 ounces	34
Salmon (baked)	3 ounces	60
Tuna (water canned)	3 ounces	48
Tuna (oil canned)	3 ounces	55
Cheese		
American	1 ounce	27
Cheddar	1 ounce	30
Cream	1 ounce	31
Mozzarella (whole milk)	1 ounce	22
Mozzarella (part skim)	1 ounce	15
Swiss	1 ounce	26
Milk		
Whole	8 ounces	33
2%	8 ounces	18
1%	8 ounces	18
Skim	8 ounces	10
Other dairy products		
Butter	Pat	11

(continued)

Table 7-2 *(continued)*

Food	Serving Size	Cholesterol (mg)
Other		
Eggs, large	1	213
Lard	1 tbsp.	12

Nutritive Value of Foods (Washington, D.C.: U.S. Department of Agriculture)

Chapter 8

Carbohydrates: A Complex Story

*C*arbohydrates — the name means carbon plus water — are sugar compounds that plants make when they're exposed to light. This process of making sugar compounds is called *photosynthesis,* from the Latin words for "light" and "putting together."

In this chapter, I shine a bright light on the different kinds of carbohydrates, illuminating all the nutritional nooks and crannies to explain how each contributes to your vim and vigor — not to mention a yummy daily menu.

Checking Out Carbohydrates

Carbohydrates come in three varieties: simple carbohydrates, complex carbohydrates, and dietary fiber. All are composed of units of sugar. What makes one carbohydrate different from another is the number of sugar units it contains and how the units are linked together.

✔ **Simple carbohydrates:** These carbohydrates have only one or two units of sugar.

- A carbohydrate with one unit of sugar is called a *simple sugar* or a *monosaccharide* (mono = one; saccharide = sugar). Fructose (fruit sugar) is a monosaccharide, and so are glucose (blood sugar), the sugar produced when you digest carbohydrates, and galactose, the sugar derived from digesting lactose (milk sugar).

- A carbohydrate with two units of sugar is called a *double sugar* or a *disaccharide* (di = two). Sucrose (table sugar), which is made of one unit of fructose and one unit of glucose, is a disaccharide.

✔ **Complex carbohydrates:** Also known as *polysaccharides* (poly = many), these carbs have more than two units of sugar linked together. Carbs with three to ten units of sugar are sometimes called *oligosaccharides* (oligo = few).

- Raffinose is a *trisaccharide* (tri = three) that's found in potatoes, beans, and beets. It has one unit each of galactose, glucose, and fructose.

- Stachyose is a *tetrasaccharide* (tetra = four) found in the same vegetables mentioned in the previous item. It has one fructose unit, one glucose unit, and two galactose units.

- Starch, a complex carbohydrate in potatoes, pasta, and rice, is a definite polysaccharide, made of many units of glucose.

Because complex carbohydrates are, well, *complex,* with anywhere from three to a zillion units of sugars, your body takes longer to digest them than it takes to digest simple carbohydrates. As a result, digesting complex carbohydrates releases glucose into your bloodstream more slowly and evenly than digesting simple carbs. (For more about digesting carbs, see the section "Carbohydrates and energy: A biochemical love story," later in this chapter.)

✔ **Dietary fiber:** This term is used to distinguish the fiber in food from the natural and synthetic fibers (silk, cotton, wool, nylon) used in fabrics. Dietary fiber is a third kind of carbohydrate.

- Like the complex carbohydrates, dietary fiber (cellulose, hemicellulose, pectin, beta-glucans, gum) is a polysaccharide. Lignin, a different kind of chemical, is also called a dietary fiber.

- Some kinds of dietary fiber also contain units of soluble or insoluble uronic acids, compounds derived from the sugars fructose, glucose, and galactose. For example, pectin — a soluble fiber in apples — contains soluble galacturonic acid.

Dietary fiber is not like other carbohydrates. The bonds that hold its sugar units together cannot be broken by human digestive enzymes. Although the bacteria living naturally in your intestines convert very small amounts of dietary fiber to fatty acids, dietary fiber is not considered a source of energy. (For more about fatty acids, see Chapter 7.)

In the next section, I talk about how your body gets energy from carbohydrates. Because dietary fiber does not provide energy, I'm going to put it aside for the moment and get back to it in the "Dietary Fiber: The Non-Nutrient in Carbohydrate Foods" section, later in this chapter.

Charting the sweetness of carbs

The information in the following table has absolutely no practical value. It's strictly trivia for your own personal nutrition data bank. Of course, you can call it up for use in social situations. For example, suppose you're standing in line at the hot dog stand at Yankee Stadium, looking for a way to start up a conversation with the trim, attractive person in front of you, who obviously cares about diet and health. "Wow," you may say. "Did you notice the cola over there is sweetened with both fructose and sucrose — a monosaccharide and a disaccharide, both in the same drink? And given how nutrition-savvy they are here, I bet the hot dog rolls are loaded with polysaccharides." Who could resist such a high-minded, intellectual approach?

Naming the Sugar Units in Carbohydrates

Carbohydrate	Composition
Monosaccharides (1 sugar unit)	
Fructose (fruit sugar)	1 unit fructose
Glucose (sugar unit used for fuel)	1 unit glucose
Galactose (made from lactose [milk sugar])	1 unit galactose
Disaccharides (2 sugar units linked together)	
Sucrose (table sugar)	Glucose + fructose
Lactose (milk sugar)	Glucose + galactose
Maltose (malt sugar)	Glucose + glucose
Polysaccharides (many sugar units linked together)	
Raffinose	Galactose + glucose + fructose
Stachyose	Glucose + fructose + galactose + galactose
Starch	Many glucose units
Cellulose	Many glucose units
Hemicellulose	Arabinose* + galactose + mannose* + xylose** plus uronic acids

(continued)

(continued)

(continued)

(continued)	
Carbohydrate	**Composition**
Pectin	Galactose + arabinose + galacturonic acid
Gums	Mainly galacturonic acid

* This sugar is found in many plants.
** This sugar is found in plants and wood.

Carbohydrates and energy: A biochemical love story

Your body runs on glucose, the molecules your cells burn for energy. (For more information on how you get energy from food, check out Chapter 3.)

Proteins, fats, and alcohol (as in beer, wine, and spirits) also provide energy in the form of calories. And protein does give you glucose, but it takes a long time, relatively speaking, for your body to get it.

When you eat carbohydrates, your pancreas secretes insulin, the hormone that enables you to digest starches and sugars. This release of insulin is sometimes called an *insulin spike,* which means the same thing as "insulin secretion" but sounds a whole lot more sinister.

Eating simple carbohydrates such as sucrose (table sugar) provokes higher insulin secretion than eating complex carbohydrates such as starch. If you have a metabolic disorder such as diabetes that keeps you from producing enough insulin, you must be careful not to take in more carbs than you can digest. Unmetabolized sugars circulating through your blood can make you dizzy and maybe even trip you into a diabetic coma.

What makes this interesting is that some perfectly healthful foods, such as carrots, potatoes, and white bread, have more simple carbs than others, such as apples, lentils, peanuts, and whole wheat bread. The Glycemic Index, developed at the University of Toronto in 1981, gives you a handle on this by ranking foods according to how quickly they affect blood sugar levels when compared to glucose (the form of sugar your body uses as energy), the glycemic indicator *par excellence.*

Most people who don't have a metabolic disorder (such as diabetes) that inter-feres with the ability to digest carbs can metabolize even very large amounts of carbohydrate foods easily. Their insulin secretion rises to meet the demand and then quickly settles back to normal. In other words, although some popu-lar weight loss programs, such as the South Beach Diet, rely on the Glycemic Index as a weight loss tool, the fact remains that for most people, a carb is a carb is a carb, regardless of how quickly the sugar enters the bloodstream. Check it out in *Diabetes For Dummies.*

For info on why the difference between simple and complex carbs can matter for athletes, check out the section called "Who needs extra carbohydrates?"

How glucose becomes energy

Inside your cells, the glucose is burned to produce heat and *adenosine triphosphate,* a molecule that stores and releases energy as required by the cell. By the way, nutrition scientists, who have as much trouble pronouncing polysyllabic words as you probably do, usually refer to adenosine triphos-phate by its initials: ATP. Smart cookies!

The transformation of glucose into energy occurs in one of two ways: with oxygen or without it. Glucose is converted to energy with oxygen in the *mito-chondria* — tiny bodies in the jellylike substance inside every cell. This con-version yields energy (ATP, heat) plus water and carbon dioxide — a waste product.

Red blood cells do not have mitochondria, so they change glucose into energy without oxygen. This yields energy (ATP, heat) and lactic acid.

Glucose is also converted to energy in muscle cells. When it comes to produc-ing energy from glucose, muscle cells are, well, double-jointed. They have mito-chondria, so they can process glucose with oxygen. But if the level of oxygen in the muscle cell falls very low, the cells can just go ahead and change glucose into energy without it. This is most likely to happen when you've been exercis-ing so strenuously that you (and your muscles) are, literally, out of breath.

Being able to turn glucose into energy without oxygen is a handy trick, but here's the downside: One byproduct is lactic acid. Why is that a big deal? Too much lactic acid makes your muscles ache.

How pasta ends up on your hips when too many carbs pass your lips

Your cells budget energy very carefully. They do not store more than they need right now. Any glucose the cell does not need for its daily work is converted to glycogen (animal starch) and tucked away as stored energy in your liver and muscles.

Your body can pack about 400 grams (14 ounces) of glycogen into liver and muscle cells. A gram of carbohydrates — including glucose — has four calories. If you add up all the glucose stored in glycogen to the small amount of glucose in your cells and blood, it equals about 1,800 calories of energy.

If your diet provides more carbohydrates than you need to produce this amount of stored calories in the form of glucose and glycogen in your cells, blood, muscles, and liver, the excess will be converted to fat. And that's how your pasta ends up on your hips.

Other ways your body uses carbohydrates

Providing energy is an important job, but it isn't the only thing carbohydrates do for you. Carbohydrates also protect your muscles. When you need energy, your body looks for glucose from carbohydrates first. If none is available, because you're on a carbohydrate-restricted diet or have a medical condition that prevents you from using the carbohydrate foods you consume, your body begins to pull energy out of fatty tissue and then moves on to burning its own protein tissue (muscles). If this use of proteins for energy continues long enough, you run out of fuel and die.

A diet that provides sufficient amounts of carbohydrates keeps your body from eating its own muscles. That's why a carbohydrate-rich diet is sometimes described as *protein sparing*.

What else do carbohydrates do? They

- Regulate the amount of sugar circulating in your blood so that all your cells get the energy they need
- Provide nutrients for the friendly bacteria in your intestinal tract that help digest food
- Assist in your body's absorption of calcium
- May help lower cholesterol levels and regulate blood pressure (these effects are special benefits of dietary fiber, which I discuss in the "Dietary Fiber: The Non-Nutrient in Carbohydrate Foods" section, later in this chapter)

Finding the carbohydrates you need

The most important sources of carbohydrates are plant foods — fruits, vegetables, and grains. Milk and milk products contain the carbohydrate lactose (milk sugar), but meat, fish, and poultry have no carbohydrates at all.

In the fall of 2002, the National Academy of Sciences Institute of Medicine (IOM) released a report recommending that 45 to 65 percent of your daily calories come from carbohydrate foods. The Food Guide Pyramid (see more about that in Chapter 17) makes it easy for you to build a nutritious carb-based diet with portion allowances based on how many calories you consume each day in

- ✔ 6 to 11 servings of grain foods (bread, cereals, pasta, rice), plus

- ✔ 2 to 4 servings of fruit and

- ✔ 3 to 5 servings of vegetables

These foods provide simple carbohydrates, complex carbohydrates, and the natural bonus of dietary fiber. Table sugar, honey, and sweets — which provide simple carbohydrates — are recommended only on a once-in-a-while basis.

One gram of carbohydrates has four calories. To find the number of calories from the carbohydrates in a serving, multiply the number of grams of carbohydrates by four. For example, one whole bagel has about 38 grams of carbohydrates, equal to about 152 calories (38 × 4). (You have to say "about" because the dietary fiber in the bagel provides no calories, because the body can't metabolize it.) *Wait:* That number does not account for all the calories in the serving. Remember, the foods listed here may also contain at least some protein and fat, and these two nutrients add calories.

Some problems with carbohydrates

Some people have a hard time handling carbohydrates. For example, people with Type 1 ("insulin dependent") diabetes do not produce sufficient amounts of insulin, the hormones needed to carry all the glucose produced from carbohydrates into body cells. As a result, the glucose continues to circulate in the blood until it's excreted through the kidneys. That's why one way to tell whether someone has diabetes is to test the level of sugar in that person's urine.

Other people can't digest carbohydrates because their bodies lack the specific enzymes needed to break the bonds that hold a carbohydrate's sugar units together. For example, many (some say most) Asians, Africans, Middle Easterners, South Americans, and Eastern, Central, or Southern Europeans are deficient in lactase, the enzyme that splits lactose (milk sugar) into glucose and galactose. If they drink milk or eat milk products, they end up with a lot of undigested lactose in their intestinal tracts. This undigested lactose makes the bacteria living there happy as clams — but not the person who owns the intestines: As bacteria feast on the undigested sugar, they excrete waste products that give their host gas and cramps.

Time out for the name game!

Here's an interesting bit of nutritional information. The names of all enzymes end in the letters *-ase*. An enzyme that digests a specific substance in food often has a name similar to the substance but with the letters *-ase* at the end.

For example, *proteases* are enzymes that digest protein; *lipases* are enzymes that digest fats (lipids); *galactase* is the enzyme that digests galactose.

To avoid this anomaly, many national cuisines purposely are void of milk as an ingredient. (Quick! Name one native Asian dish that's made with milk. No, coconut milk doesn't count.) Does that mean people living in these countries don't get enough calcium? No. They simply substitute high-calcium foods such as greens or soy products for milk.

TIP

A second solution for people who don't make enough lactase is to use a *predigested milk product* such as yogurt or buttermilk or sour cream, all made by adding friendly bacteria that digest the milk (that is, break the lactose apart) without spoiling it. Other solutions include lactose-free cheeses and enzyme-treated milk.

Who needs extra carbohydrates?

The small amount of glucose in your blood and cells provides the energy you need for your body's daily activities. The 400 grams of glycogen stored in your liver and muscles provides enough energy for ordinary bursts of extra activity.

But what happens when you have to work harder or longer than that? For example, what if you're a long-distance athlete, which means that you use up your available supply of glucose before you finish your competition? (That's why marathoners often run out of gas — a phenomenon called *hitting the wall* — at 20 miles, six miles short of the finish line.)

If you were stuck on an ice floe or lost in the woods for a month or so, after your body exhausts its supply of glucose, including the glucose stored in glycogen, it starts pulling energy first out of fat and then out of muscle. But extracting energy from body fat requires large amounts of oxygen — which is likely to be in short supply when your body has run, swum, or cycled 20 miles. So athletes have to find another way to leap the wall. Here it is: They load up on carbohydrates in advance.

Carbohydrate-loading is a dietary regimen designed to increase temporarily the amount of glycogen stored in your muscles in anticipation of an upcoming event. You start about a week before the event, says the University of Maine's Alfred A. Bushway, Ph.D., exercising to exhaustion so your body pulls as much glycogen as possible out of your muscles. Then, for three days, you eat foods high in fat and protein and low in carbohydrates to keep your glycogen level from rising again.

Three days before the big day, reverse the pattern. Now you want to build and conserve glycogen stores. What you need is a diet that's about 70 percent carbohydrates, providing 6 to 10 grams of carbohydrates for every kilogram (2.2 pounds) of body weight for men and women alike. And not just any carbohydrates, mind you. What you want are the complex carbohydrates in starchy foods like pasta and potatoes, rather than the simple ones more prominent in sugary foods like fruit. And of course, candy.

This carb-loading diet is not for everyday use, nor will it help people competing in events of short duration. It's strictly for events lasting longer than 90 minutes.

What about while you're running, swimming, or cycling? Will consuming simple sugars during the race give you extra short-term bursts of energy? Yes. Sugar is rapidly converted to glycogen and carried to the muscles. But you don't want *straight sugar* (candy, honey) because it's *hydrophilic* (hydro = water; philic = loving), which means that it pulls water from body tissues into your intestinal tract. Using straight sugar can increase dehydration and make you nauseated. Thus, getting the sugar you want from sweetened athletic drinks, which provide fluids along with the energy, is best. The label on the athletic drink also tells you the liquid contains salt (sodium chloride). Why? To replace the salt that you lose when perspiring heavily. Turn to Chapter 13 to find out why this is important.

Dietary Fiber: The Non-Nutrient in Carbohydrate Foods

Dietary fiber is a group of complex carbohydrates that are not a source of energy for human beings. Because human digestive enzymes cannot break the bonds that hold fiber's sugar units together, fiber adds no calories to your diet and cannot be converted to glucose.

Ruminants (animals, such as cows, that chew the cud) have a combination of digestive enzymes and digestive microbes that enable them to extract the nutrients from insoluble dietary fiber (cellulose and some hemicelluloses). But not even these creatures can pull nutrients out of lignin, an insoluble fiber in plant stems and leaves and the predominant fiber in wood. As a result, the U.S. Department of Agriculture specifically prohibits the use of wood or sawdust in animal feed.

But just because you can't digest dietary fiber doesn't mean it isn't a valuable part of your diet. The opposite is true. Dietary fiber is valuable *because* you can't digest it!

The two kinds of dietary fiber

Nutritionists classify dietary fiber as either insoluble fiber or soluble fiber, depending on whether it dissolves in water. (Both kinds of fiber resist human digestive enzymes.)

- ✔ **Insoluble fiber:** This type of fiber includes cellulose, some hemicelluloses, and lignin found in whole grains and other plants. This kind of dietary fiber is a natural laxative. It absorbs water, helps you feel full after eating, and stimulates your intestinal walls to contract and relax. These natural contractions, called *peristalsis,* move solid materials through your digestive tract.

  By moving food quickly through your intestines, insoluble fiber may help relieve or prevent digestive disorders such as constipation or diverticulitis (infection that occurs when food gets stuck in small pouches in the wall of the colon). Insoluble fiber also bulks up stool and makes it softer, reducing your risk of developing hemorrhoids and lessening the discomfort if you already have them.

- ✔ **Soluble fiber:** This fiber, such as pectins in apples and beta-glucans in oats and barley, seems to lower the amount of cholesterol circulating in your blood (your *cholesterol level*). This tendency may be why a diet rich in fiber appears to offer some protection against heart disease.

Here's a benefit for dieters: Soluble fiber forms gels in the presence of water, which is what happens when apples and oat bran reach your digestive tract. Like insoluble fiber, soluble fiber can make you feel full without adding calories.

Ordinary soluble dietary fiber can't be digested, so your body doesn't absorb it. But in 2002, researchers at Detroit's Barbara Ann Karamonos Cancer Institute fed laboratory mice a form of soluble dietary fiber called *modified citrus pectin.* The fiber, which is made from citrus fruit peel, can be digested.

When fed to laboratory rats, it appeared to reduce the size of tumors caused by implanted human breast and colon cancer cells. The researchers believe that the fiber prevents cancer cells from linking together to form tumors. Now, two pharmaceutical companies — one on the East Coast and one on the West Coast — are investigating the effects of modified citrus pectin in human beings. But the product isn't yet ready for prime time. Although it's being sold as a dietary supplement (not as a medicine), experts warn that its effects on human bodies (and human cancers) remain unproven.

Getting fiber from food

You find fiber in all plant foods — fruits, vegetables, and grains. But you find absolutely no fiber in foods from animals: meat, fish, poultry, milk, milk products, and eggs.

A balanced diet with lots of foods from plants gives you both insoluble and soluble fiber. Most foods that contain fiber have both kinds, although the balance usually tilts toward one or the other. For example, the predominant fiber in an apple is pectin (a soluble fiber), but an apple peel also has some cellulose, hemicellulose, and lignin.

Table 8-1 shows you which foods are particularly good sources of specific kinds of fiber. A diet rich in plant foods (fruits, vegetables, grains) gives you adequate amounts of dietary fiber.

Table 8-1	Sources of Different Kinds of Fiber
Fiber	*Where Found*
Soluble fiber	
Pectin	Fruits (apples, strawberries, citrus fruits)
Beta-glucans	Oats, barley
Gums	Beans, cereals (oats, rice, barley), seeds, seaweed
Insoluble fiber	
Cellulose	Leaves (cabbage), roots (carrots, beets), bran, whole wheat, beans
Hemicellulose	Seed coverings (bran, whole grains)
Lignin	Plant stems, leaves, and skin

How much fiber do you need?

According to the U.S. Department of Agriculture, the average American woman gets about 12 grams of fiber a day from food; the average American man, 17 grams. Those figures are well below the new IOM (Institute of Medicine) recommendations that I conveniently list here:

- ✔ 25 grams a day for women younger than 50
- ✔ 38 grams a day for men younger than 50
- ✔ 21 grams a day for women older than 50
- ✔ 30 grams a day for men older than 50

The amounts of dietary fiber recommended by IOM are believed to give you the benefits you want without causing fiber-related — um — unpleasantries.

Unpleasantries? Like what? And how will you know if you've got them?

Trust me: If you eat more than enough fiber, your body will tell you right away. All that roughage may irritate your intestinal tract, which will issue an unmistakable protest in the form of intestinal gas or diarrhea. In extreme cases, if you don't drink enough liquids to moisten and soften the fiber you eat so that it easily slides through your digestive tract, the dietary fiber may form a mass that can end up as an intestinal obstruction (for more about water, see Chapter 13).

If you decide to up the amount of fiber in your diet, follow this advice:

- ✔ Do so *very* gradually, a little bit more every day. That way you're less likely to experience intestinal distress. In other words, if your current diet is heavy on no-fiber foods such as meat, fish, poultry, eggs, milk, and cheese, and low-fiber foods such as white bread and white rice, don't load up on bran cereal (35 grams dietary fiber per 3.5-ounce serving) or dried figs (9.3 grams per serving) all at once. Start by adding a serving of cornflakes (2.0 grams dietary fiber) at breakfast, maybe an apple (2.8 grams) at lunch, a pear (2.6 grams) at mid-afternoon, and a half cup of baked beans (7.7 grams) at dinner. Four simple additions, and already you're up to 15 grams dietary fiber.

- ✔ Always check the nutrition label whenever you shop (for more about the wonderfully informative guides, see Chapter 17). When choosing between similar products, just take the one with the higher fiber content per serving. For example, white pita bread generally has about 1.6 grams dietary fiber per serving. Whole wheat pita bread has 7.4 grams. From a fiber standpoint, you know which works better for your body. Go for it!

- ✔ Get enough liquids. Dietary fiber is like a sponge. It sops up liquid, so increasing your fiber intake may deprive your cells of the water they need to perform their daily work (for more about how your body uses the water you drink, see Chapter 13). That's why the American Academy of Family Physicians (among others) suggests checking to make sure you get plenty fluids when you consume more fiber. How much is enough? Back to Chapter 13.

Table 8-2 shows the amounts of all types of dietary fiber — insoluble plus soluble — in a 100-gram (3.5-ounce) serving of specific foods. By the way, nutritionists like to measure things in terms of 100-gram portions because that makes comparing foods at a glance possible.

To find the amount of dietary fiber in your own serving, divide the gram total for the food shown in Table 8-2 by 3.5 to get the grams per ounce, and then multiply the result by the number of ounces in your portion. For example, if you're having 1 ounce of cereal, the customary serving of ready-to-eat breakfast cereals, divide the gram total of dietary fiber by 3.5; then multiply by one. If your slice of bread weighs ½ ounce, divide the gram total by 3.5; then multiply the result by 0.5 (½).

Or — let's get real! — you can look at the nutrition label on the side of the package that gives the nutrients per portion.

Finally, the amounts on this chart are averages. Different brands of processed products (breads, some cereals, cooked fruits, and vegetables) may have more (or less) fiber per serving.

Fiber factoid

The amount of fiber in a serving of food may depend on whether the food is raw or cooked. For example, as you can see from Table 8-2, a 3.5-ounce serving of plain dried prunes has 7.2 grams of fiber while a 3.5-ounce serving of stewed prunes has 6.6 grams of fiber.

Why? When you stew prunes, they plump up — which means they absorb water. The water adds weight but (obviously) no fiber. So a serving of prunes-plus-water has slightly less fiber per ounce than a same-weight serving of plain dried prunes.

dried prunes

VS.

stewed prunes

Table 8-2	Fiber Content in Common Foods
Food	*Grams of Fiber in a 100-Gram (3.5-Ounce) Serving*
Bread	
Bagel	2.1
Bran bread	8.5
Pita bread (white)	1.6
Pita bread (whole wheat)	7.4
White bread	1.9
Cereals	
Bran cereal	35.3
Bran flakes	18.8
Cornflakes	2.0
Oatmeal	10.6
Wheat flakes	9.0
Grains	
Barley, pearled (minus its outer covering), raw	15.6
Cornmeal, whole grain	11.0
De-germed	5.2
Oat bran, raw	6.6
Rice, raw (brown)	3.5
Rice, raw (white)	1.0–2.8
Rice, raw (wild)	5.2
Wheat bran	15.0
Fruits	
Apple, with skin	2.8
Apricots, dried	7.8
Figs, dried	9.3
Kiwi fruit	3.4

Food	Grams of Fiber in a 100-Gram (3.5-Ounce) Serving
Pear, raw	2.6
Prunes, dried	7.2
Prunes, stewed	6.6
Raisins	5.3
Vegetables	
Baked beans (vegetarian)	7.7
Chickpeas (canned)	5.4
Lima beans, cooked	7.2
Broccoli, raw	2.8
Brussels sprouts, cooked	2.6
Cabbage, white, raw	2.4
Cauliflower, raw	2.4
Corn, sweet, cooked	3.7
Peas with edible pods, raw	2.6
Potatoes, white, baked, w/ skin	5.5
Sweet potato, cooked	3.0
Tomatoes, raw	1.3
Nuts	
Almonds, oil-roasted	11.2
Coconut, raw	9.0
Hazelnuts, oil-roasted	6.4
Peanuts, dry-roasted	8.0
Pistachios	10.8
Other	
Corn chips, toasted	4.4
Tahini (sesame seed paste)	9.3
Tofu	1.2

Provisional Table on the Dietary Fiber Content of Selected Foods (Washington, D.C.: U.S. Department of Agriculture, 1988)

Fiber and your heart:
The continuing saga of oat bran

Oat bran is the second chapter in the fiber fad that started with wheat bran around 1980. Wheat bran, the fiber in wheat, is rich in the insoluble fibers cellulose and lignin. Oat bran's gee-whiz factor is the soluble fiber beta-glucans. For more than 30 years, scientists have known that eating foods high in soluble fiber can lower your cholesterol, although nobody knows exactly why. Fruits and vegetables (especially dried beans) are high in soluble fiber, but ounce for ounce, oats have more. In addition, beta-glucans are a more effective cholesterol-buster than pectin and gum, which are the soluble fibers in most fruits and vegetables.

By 1990, researchers at the University of Kentucky reported that people who add ½ cup dry oat bran (*not* oatmeal) to their regular daily diets can lower their levels of low density lipoproteins (LDLs), the particles that carry cholesterol into your arteries, by as much as 25 percent (see Chapter 7 for more on cholesterol).

Recently, scientists at the Medical School of Northwestern University, funded by Quaker Oats, enlisted 208 healthy volunteers whose normal cholesterol readings averaged about 200 mg/dl for a study involving oat bran. The volunteers' total cholesterol levels decreased an average of 9.3 percent with a low-fat, low-cholesterol diet supplemented by 2 ounces of oats or oat bran every day. About one-third of the cholesterol reduction was credited to the oats.

Oat cereal makers rounded the total loss to 10 percent, and the National Research Council said that a 10 percent drop in cholesterol could produce a 20 percent drop in the risk of a heart attack.

Do I have to tell you what happened next? Books on oat bran hit the bestseller list. Cheerios elbowed Frosted Flakes aside to become the number one cereal in America. And people added oat bran to everything from bagels to orange juice.

Today scientists know that although a little oat bran can't hurt, the link between oats and cholesterol levels is no cure-all.

As a general rule, an adult whose cholesterol level is higher than 250 mg/dl is considered to be at *high risk.* A cholesterol reading between 200 and 250 mg/dl is considered *moderately risky.* A cholesterol level below 200 mg/dl is considered pretty good. No, that's not a technical term, but you get the idea.

If your cholesterol level is above 250 mg/dl, lowering it by 10 percent through a diet that contains oat bran may reduce your risk of heart attack without the use of medication. If your cholesterol level is lower than that to begin with, the effects of oat bran are less dramatic. For example:

✔ If your cholesterol level is below 250 mg/dl, a low-fat, low-cholesterol diet alone may push it down 15 points into the moderately risky range. Adding oats reduces it another 8 points but doesn't take you into okey-dokey territory, under 200 mg/dl.

✔ If your cholesterol is already low, say 199 mg/dl or less, a low-fat, low-cholesterol diet plus oats may drop it to 180 mg/dl, but the oats account for only 6 points of your loss.

Recognizing oat bran's benefits, the Food and Drug Administration now permits health claims on oat product labels. For example, the product label may say: "Soluble fiber from foods such as oat bran, as part of a diet low in saturated fat and cholesterol, may reduce the risk of heart disease."

By the way, the soluble pectin in apples and the soluble beta-glucans (gums) in beans and peas also lower cholesterol levels. The insoluble fiber in wheat bran does not.

Chapter 9

Alcohol: Another Form of Grape and Grain

. . . .

In This Chapter

▶ Finding out how alcohol is made

▶ Categorizing different kinds of alcohol beverages

▶ Digesting alcohol

▶ Revealing alcohol's effect on your health

. . . .

Alcohol beverages are among mankind's oldest home remedies and simple pleasures, so highly regarded that the ancient Greeks and Romans called wine a "gift from the gods," and when the Gaels — early inhabitants of Scotland and Ireland — first produced whiskey, they named it *uisge beatha* (whis-key-ba), a combination of the words for "water" and "life." Today, although you may share their appreciation for the product, you know that alcohol beverages may have risks as well as benefits.

By the way, throughout this chapter I refer to beverages made from alcohol as "alcohol beverages." Yes, I know most people probably think the correct term is "alcoholic beverages," but whenever I write or say those words, I get an immediate image of tipsy beer bottles. Besides, you've heard of "milk beverages" but not "milky" ones, or "cola beverages" but not "cola-y" ones. So do please indulge me.

Revealing the Many Faces of Alcohol

When microorganisms (yeasts) digest (ferment) the sugars in carbohydrate foods, they make two byproducts: a liquid and a gas. The gas is carbon dioxide. The liquid is *ethyl alcohol,* also known as *ethanol,* the intoxicating ingredient in alcohol beverages.

This biochemical process is not an esoteric one. In fact, it happens in your own kitchen every time you make yeast bread. Remember the faint, beer-like odor in the air while the dough is rising? That odor is from the alcohol the yeasts make as they chomp their way through the sugars in the flour. (Don't worry; the alcohol evaporates when you bake the bread.) As the yeasts digest the sugars, they also produce carbon dioxide, which makes the bread rise.

From now on, whenever you see the word *alcohol* alone in this book, unless otherwise noted, it means ethanol, the only alcohol used in alcohol beverages. (Yes, yes, yes. That definition applies backward, too. If you find the word *alcohol* in a previous chapter, it, too, means ethanol. Gee. Some people are sooooooo picky.)

Examining How Alcohol Beverages Are Made

Alcohol beverages are produced either through fermentation or through a combination of fermentation plus distillation.

Fermented alcohol products

Fermentation is a simple process in which yeasts or bacteria are added to carbohydrate foods such as corn, potatoes, rice, or wheat, which are used as starting material. The yeasts digest the sugars in the food, leaving liquid (alcohol); the liquid is filtered to remove the solids, and water is usually added to dilute the alcohol, producing — voilà — an alcohol beverage.

What other alcohols do you have in your home?

Ethanol is the only kind of alcohol used in food and alcohol beverages, but it isn't the only kind of alcohol used in consumer products. Here are the other alcohols that may be sitting on the shelf in your bathroom or workshop (though you definitely don't want to drink them):

Methyl alcohol (methanol): This poisonous alcohol made from wood is used as a *chemical solvent* (a liquid that dissolves other chemicals).

Isopropyl alcohol (rubbing alcohol): This poisonous alcohol is made from *propylene,* a petroleum derivative.

Denatured alcohol: This product is alcohol plus a chemical (denaturant) that makes it taste and smell bad so you won't drink the alcohol. Some denaturants are poisonous.

Beer is made this way. So is wine. *Kumiss,* a fermented milk product, is slightly different because it's made by adding yeasts and friendly bacteria called *lactobacilli* (lacto = milk) to mare's milk. The microorganisms make alcohol, but it isn't separated from the milk, which turns into a fizzy fermented beverage with no water added.

Distilled alcohol products

The second way to make an alcohol beverage is through *distillation.*

As with fermentation, yeasts are added to foods to make alcohol from sugars. But yeasts can't thrive in a place where the concentration of alcohol is higher than 20 percent. To concentrate the alcohol and separate it from the rest of the ingredients in the fermented liquid, distillers pour the fermented liquid into a *still,* a large vat with a wide column-like tube on top. The still is heated so that the alcohol, which boils at a lower temperature than everything else in the vat, turns to vapor, which rises through the column on top of the still, to be collected in containers where it condenses back into a liquid.

This alcohol, called *neutral spirits,* is the base for the alcohol beverages called spirits or distilled spirits: gin, rum, tequila, whiskey, and vodka. Brandy is a special product, a spirit distilled from wine. Fortified wines such as Port and Sherry are wines with spirits added.

The foods used to make beverage alcohol

Beverage alcohol can be made from virtually any carbohydrate food. The foods most commonly used are cereal grains, fruit, honey, molasses, or potatoes. All produce alcohol, but the alcohols have slightly different flavors and colors. Table 9-1 shows you which foods are used to produce the different kinds of alcohol beverages.

Check the spelling

Here's an interesting consumer note: Whiskey is spelled with an *e* if it's made in North America or Ireland, without an *e* — whisky — if it comes from another country (Scotland is the best example).

Why? Nobody knows for sure. But a reasonable assumption is that the Scots may simply have dropped the *e* to differentiate their distilled spirits from the spirits distilled in Ireland. Journeying to the United States, Irish immigrants brought their distillation methods and their *e* with them, so theirs became the name for whiskey made in America.

On its own, alcohol provides energy (7 calories per gram) but no nutrients, so distilled spirits, such as whiskey or plain, unflavored vodka serve up nothing but calories. Beer, wine, cider, and other fermented beverages, such as kumiss (fermented milk), contain some of the food from which they were made, so they contain small amounts of proteins and carbohydrates, vitamins, and minerals.

Table 9-1	Foods Used to Make Alcohol Beverages
Original Food	*Alcohol Beverage Produced*
Fruit and fruit juice	
Agave plant	Tequila
Apples	Hard cider
Grapes and other fruits	Wine
Grain	
Barley	Beer, various distilled spirits, kvass
Corn	Bourbon, corn whiskey, beer
Rice	Sake (a distilled product), rice wine
Rye	Whiskey
Wheat	Distilled spirits, beer
Others	
Honey	Mead
Milk	Kumiss (koumiss), kefir
Potatoes	Vodka
Sugar cane	Rum

How Much Alcohol Is in That Bottle?

No alcohol beverage is 100 percent alcohol. It's alcohol plus water, and — if it's a wine or beer — some residue of the foods from which it was made.

The label on every bottle of wine and spirits shows the alcohol content as *alcohol by volume* (ABV). (For reasons too complicated to discuss in fewer than, say, 50 pages, beer containers may carry this information, but United States law doesn't require it.)

ABV measures the amount of alcohol as a percentage of all the liquid in the container. For example, if your container holds 10 ounces of liquid and 1 ounce of that is alcohol, the product is 10 percent ABV — the alcohol content divided by the total amount of liquid.

Proof — an older term that describes alcohol content —is two times the ABV. For example, an alcohol beverage that is 10 percent alcohol by volume is 20 proof.

By the way, right now, alcohol beverages are the only entries in the food and drink market sold without a Nutrition Facts label. The National Consumers League and the Washington-based Center for Science in the Public Interest are petitioning the Food and Drug Administration to create an ingredients label for alcohol beverages. The label would show the ingredients, the number of standard servings in the container, and the alcohol content and calorie count per serving so you can compare products — and control what you drink. Smart. To see the proposed label, visit `nclnet.org/pressroom/alcoholfactspr.htm`.

Moving Alcohol through Your Body

Other foods must be digested before being absorbed by your cells, but alcohol flows directly through your body's membranes into your bloodstream, which carries alcohol to nearly every organ in your body. Here's a road map to show you the route traveled by the alcohol in every drink you take.

Flowing down the hatch from mouth to stomach

Alcohol is an *astringent;* it coagulates proteins on the surface of the lining of your mouth to make it "pucker." Some alcohol is absorbed through the lining of your mouth and throat, but most of the alcohol you drink spills into your stomach, where an enzyme called *gastric alcohol dehydrogenase* (ADH) begins to metabolize (digest) it.

How much alcohol dehydrogenase your body churns out is influenced by your ethnicity and your gender. For example, Asians, Native Americans, and Inuits appear to secrete less alcohol dehydrogenase than do most Caucasians, and the average woman (regardless of her ethnicity) makes less ADH than the average man does. As a result, more unmetabolized alcohol flows from their tummies into their bloodstreams, and they're likely to become tipsy on smaller amounts of alcohol than an average Caucasian male would need to drink.

While you ponder that, the unmetabolized alcohol is flowing through your stomach walls into your bloodstream and on to your small intestine.

Stopping for a short visit at the energy factory

Most of the alcohol you drink is absorbed through the *duodenum* (small intestine), from which it flows through a large blood vessel (the portal vein) into your liver. There, an enzyme similar to gastric ADH metabolizes the alcohol, which is converted to energy by a coenzyme called *nicotinamide adenine dinucleotide* (NAD). NAD is also used to convert the glucose you get from other carbohydrates to energy; while NAD is being used for alcohol, glucose conversion grinds to a halt.

The normal, healthy liver can process about ½ ounce of pure alcohol (that's 6 to 12 ounces of beer, 5 ounces of wine, or 1 ounce of spirits) in an hour. The rest flows on to your heart.

Taking time out for air

Entering your heart, alcohol reduces the force with which your heart muscle contracts. You pump out slightly less blood for a few minutes, blood vessels all over your body relax, and your blood pressure goes down temporarily. The contractions soon return to normal, but the blood vessels may remain relaxed and your blood pressure lower for as long as half an hour.

At the same time, alcohol flows in blood from your heart through your pulmonary vein to your lungs. Now you breathe out a tiny bit of alcohol every time you exhale, and your breath smells of liquor. Then the newly oxygenated, still alcohol-laden blood flows back through the pulmonary artery to your heart, and up and out through the *aorta* (the major artery that carries blood out to your body).

Rising to the surface

In your blood, alcohol raises your level of high-density lipoproteins (HDLs), although not necessarily the specific *good* ones that carry cholesterol out of your body. (For more about lipoproteins, see Chapter 7.) Alcohol also makes blood less likely to clot, temporarily reducing your risk of heart attack and stroke.

Alcohol makes blood vessels expand, so more warm blood flows up from the center of your body to the surface of the skin. You feel warmer for a while and, if your skin is fair, you may flush and turn pink. (Asians, who — you may remember from a few paragraphs back — tend to make less alcohol dehydrogenase than do Caucasians, often experience a characteristic flushing when they drink even small amounts of alcohol.) At the same time, tiny amounts of alcohol ooze out through your pores, and your perspiration smells of alcohol.

Encountering curves in the road

Alcohol is a sedative. When it reaches your brain, it slows the transmission of impulses between nerve cells that control your ability to think and move. That's why your thinking may be fuzzy, your judgment impaired, your tongue twisted, your vision blurred, and your muscles rubbery.

Do you feel a sudden urge to urinate? Alcohol reduces your brain's production of *antidiuretic hormones,* chemicals that keep you from making too much urine. You may lose lots of liquid, plus vitamins and minerals. You also grow very thirsty, and your urine may smell faintly of alcohol. This cycle continues as long as you have alcohol circulating in your blood, or in other words, until your liver can manage to produce enough ADH to metabolize all the alcohol you've consumed. How long is that? Most people need an hour to metabolize the amount of alcohol (½ ounce) in one drink. But that's an average: Some people have alcohol circulating in their blood for up to three hours after taking a drink.

Alcohol and Health

Beverage alcohol has benefits as well as side effects. The benefits seem to be linked to what is commonly called *moderate drinking* — no more than one drink a day for a woman, two drinks a day for a man — consumed with food. The risks generally appear to flow from alcohol abuse.

Moderate drinking: Some benefits, some risks

Moderate amounts of alcohol reduce stress, so it isn't surprising that recent well-designed scientific studies on large groups of men and women suggest that moderate drinking is heart-healthy, protecting the cardiovascular system (that's science talk for heart and blood vessels). Here are some findings about the cardiovascular benefits and some of the other things moderate drinking can do for you:

> ✔ The American Cancer Society's Cancer Prevention Study 1 followed more than one million Americans in 25 states for 12 years to find that moderate alcohol intake had an "apparent protective effect on coronary heart disease." Translation: Men who drink moderately lower their risk

of heart attack. The risk is 21 percent lower for men who have one drink a day than for men who never drink.

A similar analysis of data for nearly 600,000 women in the long-running (Harvard) Nurses' Health Study showed that women who drink occasionally or have one drink a day are less likely to die of heart attack than those who don't drink at all.

✔ A 2003 study at Tulane University School of Public Health and Tropical Medicine shows that men who drink moderately (two drinks a day) also are less likely to die of clot-related stroke. But because alcohol reduces blood clotting, it increases the risk of *hemorrhagic* stroke (stroke caused by bleeding in the brain). Sorry about that.

✔ According to researchers at USDA's Agricultural Research Service (ARS) laboratory at Beltsville, Maryland, moderate drinking may lower a healthy older woman's risk of developing diabetes.

✔ Contrary to popular opinion, a 15-year, 1,700-person heart disease study at the Institute of Preventive Medicine, Kommunehospitalet in Copenhagen, Denmark, showed that older men and women who regularly consumed up to 21 drinks of wine a week were less likely than teetotalers to develop Alzheimer's disease and other forms of dementia. Similarly, a recent 12-year, 1,488-person survey at Johns Hopkins University in Maryland suggests that regular, moderate drinkers score better over time than teetotalers do on the Mini-Mental State Examination (MMSE), a standard test for memory, reasoning, and decision making.

That's the good news. Here's the bad news: The same studies that applaud the effects of moderate drinking on heart health are less reassuring about the relationship between alcohol and cancer: The American Cancer Society's Cancer Prevention Study 1 shows that people who take more than two drinks a day have a higher incidence of cancer of the mouth and throat (esophagus). In addition;

✔ Researchers at the University of Oklahoma say that men who drink five or more beers a day double their risk of rectal cancer.

✔ American Cancer Society statistics show a higher risk of breast cancer among women who have more than three drinks a week, but newer studies suggest this effect may apply only to older women using hormone replacement therapy.

The physical risks of alcohol abuse

Alcohol abuse is a term generally taken to mean drinking so much that it interferes with your ability to have a normal, productive life. The short-term effects of excessive drinking are well-known to one and all, especially to men who may find that drinking too much decreases sexual desire and makes it impossible to . . . well . . . perform. (No evidence suggests that excessive drinking interferes with female orgasm.)

A lot and a little versus the middle

When scientists talk about the relationship between alcohol and heart disease, the words _J-curve_ often pop up. What's a J-curve? A statistical graph in the shape of the letter J.

In terms of heart disease, the lower peak on the left of the J shows the risk among teetotalers, the high spike on the right shows the risk among those who drink too much, and the curve in the center shows the risk in the moderate middle. In other words, the J-curve says that people who drink moderately have a lower risk of heart disease than people who drink too much or not at all.

That info's nice. This is better: According to a recent report from the Alberta (Canada) Alcohol and Drug Abuse Commission, the J-curve may also describe the relationship between alcohol and stroke, alcohol and diabetes, alcohol and bone loss, and alcohol and longevity. The simple fact is that moderate drinkers appear to live longer, healthier lives than either teetotalers or alcohol abusers. Cheers!

Excessive drinking can also make you feel terrible the next day. _The morning after_ is not fiction. A hangover is a miserable physical fact:

✔ You're thirsty because you lost excess water through copious urination.

✔ Your stomach hurts and you're queasy because even small amounts of alcohol irritate your stomach lining, causing it to secrete extra acid and lots of _histamine,_ the same immune system chemical that makes the skin around a mosquito bite red and itchy.

✔ Your muscles ache and your head pounds because processing alcohol through your liver requires an enzyme — nicotinamide adenine dinucleotide (NAD) — normally used to convert _lactic acid,_ a byproduct of muscle activity, to other chemicals that can be used for energy. The extra, unprocessed lactic acid piles up painfully in your muscles.

Alcoholism: An addiction disease

Alcoholics are people who can't control their drinking. Untreated alcoholism is a life-threatening disease that can lead to death either from an accident or suicide (both are more common among heavy drinkers) or from a toxic reaction (acute alcohol poisoning that paralyzes body organs, including the heart and lungs) or malnutrition or liver damage (cirrhosis).

Alcoholism makes it extremely difficult for the body to get essential nutrients. Here's why:

✔ Alcohol depresses appetite.

✔ An alcoholic may substitute alcohol for food, getting calories but no nutrients.

✔ Even when the alcoholic eats, the alcohol in his or her tissues can prevent the proper absorption of vitamins (notably the B vitamins), minerals, and other nutrients. Alcohol may also reduce the alcoholic's ability to synthesize proteins.

No one knows exactly why some people are able to have a drink once a day or once a month or once a year, enjoy it, and move on, while others become addicted to alcohol. In the past, alcoholism has been blamed on heredity (bad genes), lack of willpower, or even a bad upbringing. But as science continues to unravel the mysteries of body chemistry, it's reasonable to expect that researchers will eventually come up with a rational scientific explanation for the differences between social drinkers and people who can't safely use alcohol. It just hasn't happened yet.

Who should not drink

No one should drink to excess. But some people shouldn't drink at all, not even in moderation. They include

✔ **People who plan to drive or do work that requires both attention and skill.** Alcohol slows reaction time and makes your motor skills — turning the wheel of the car, operating a sewing machine — less precise.

✔ **Women who are pregnant or who plan to become pregnant in the near future.** *Fetal alcohol syndrome* (FAS) is a collection of birth defects including low birth weight, heart defects, retardation, and facial deformities documented only in babies born to female alcoholics. No evidence links FAS to casual drinking — that is, one or two drinks during a pregnancy or even one or two drinks a week. But the fact is that about 7 percent of the babies born in the United States each year are born with birth defects independent of any parental behavior. The parents of these children may feel guilty, even though their behavior had absolutely nothing to do with the birth defect. Your decision about alcohol should take into consideration the possibility of (misplaced) lifelong guilt caused by having had a drink.

✔ **People who take certain prescription drugs or over-the-counter medication.** Alcohol makes some drugs stronger, increases some drugs' side effects, and renders other drugs less effective. At the same time, some drugs make alcohol a more powerful sedative or slow down the elimination of alcohol from your body.

Table 9-2 shows some of the interactions known to occur between alcohol and some common prescription and over-the-counter drugs. This short list gives you an idea of some of the general interactions likely to occur between alcohol and drugs. But the list is far from complete, so if you're taking any kind of medication — over-the-counter or prescription — check with your doctor or pharmacist regarding the possibility of an interaction with alcohol.

Table 9-2	Drug and Alcohol Interactions
Drug	*Possible Interaction with Alcohol*
Analgesics (acetaminophen)	Increased liver toxicity
Analgesics (aspirin and other nonsteroidal inflammatory drugs — NSAIDs)	Increased stomach bleeding; irritation
Antiarthritis drugs	Increased stomach bleeding; irritation
Antidepressants	Increased drowsiness/intoxication; high blood pressure (depends on the type of drug — check with your doctor)
Antidiabetes drugs	Excessively low blood sugar
Antihypertension drugs	Very low blood pressure
Antituberculosis medication (isoniazid)	Decreased drug effectiveness; higher risk of hepatitis
Diet pills	Excessive nervousness
Diuretics	Low blood pressure
Iron supplements	Excessive absorption of iron
Sleeping pills	Increased sedation
Tranquilizers	Increased sedation

James W. Long and James J. Rybacki, The Essential Guide to Prescription Drugs 1995 (New York: Harper Collins, 1995)

Binge drinking: A behavioral no-no

Binge drinkers are "once-in-a-while alcoholics." They don't drink every day, but when they do indulge, they go so far overboard that they sometimes fail to come back up. In simple terms, binge drinking is downing very large amounts of alcohol in a short time, not for a pleasant lift but to get drunk. As a result, binge drinkers may consume so much beer, wine, or spirits that the amount of alcohol in their blood rises to lethal levels, leading to death by alcohol poisoning. Got the picture? Binge drinking is not a sport. It's potentially fatal behavior. Don't do it.

The power of purple (and peanuts)

Grape skin, pulp, and seeds contain *resveratrol,* a naturally occurring plant chemical that seems to reduce the risk of heart disease and some kinds of cancer. The darker the grapes, the higher the concentration of resveratrol.

Dark purple grape juice, for example, has more resveratrol than red grape juice, which has more resveratrol than white grape juice. Because wine is made from grapes, it, too, contains resveratrol (red wine has more resveratrol than white wine).

But you don't need to drink grape juice or wine to get resveratrol. You can simply snack on peanuts. Yes, peanuts. A 1998 analysis from the USDA Agricultural Research Service in Raleigh, North Carolina, showed that peanuts have 1.7 to 3.7 micrograms of resveratrol per gram of nuts. Compare that to the 0.7 micrograms of resveratrol in a glass of red grape juice or 0.6 to 8.0 micrograms of resveratrol per gram of red wine.

This fact may explain data from the long-running Harvard University/Brigham and Women's Hospital Nurses' Health Study, which shows that women who eat an ounce of nuts a day have a lower risk of heart disease. So let's see — wine, grape juice, peanuts . . . decisions, decisions.

Heeding Advice from the Sages: Moderation

Good advice is always current. The folks who wrote Ecclesiastes (a book in the Bible) centuries ago may have been speaking to you when they said, "Wine is as good as life to man if it be drunk moderately." And it's impossible to improve on this slogan from the Romans (actually, one Roman writer named Terence): "Moderation in all things." Hey, you can't get a message more direct — or more sensible — than that.

Chapter 10

Vigorous Vitamins

· ·

In This Chapter

▶ Understanding the value of vitamins

▶ Revealing the best food sources for the vitamins you need

▶ Discovering the consequences of taking too many (or too few) vitamins

▶ Knowing when you may need extra vitamins

· ·

*V*itamins are *organic chemicals,* substances that contain carbon, hydrogen, and oxygen. They occur naturally in all living things, plants and animals alike: flowers, trees, fruits, vegetables, chickens, fish, cows — and you.

Vitamins regulate a variety of bodily functions. They're essential for building body tissues such as bones, skin, glands, nerves, and blood. They assist in metabolizing (digesting) proteins, fats, and carbohydrates so that you can get energy from food. They prevent nutritional deficiency diseases, promote healing, and encourage good health.

This chapter is a guide to where the vitamins are, how you can add them to your diet, how to tell how much is more than enough of any specific vitamin, and ever so much more . . . maybe more than you really want to know.

Taking a Look at the Vitamins Your Body Needs

Your body needs at least 11 specific vitamins: vitamin A, vitamin D, vitamin E, vitamin K, vitamin C, and the members of the B vitamin family: thiamin (vitamin B1), riboflavin (B2), niacin, vitamin B6, folate, and vitamin B12. Two more B vitamins — biotin and pantothenic acid — are now believed valuable to your well-being as well. And one unusual compound called choline has recently received some favorable mention (more about it in the "Choline" section later in this chapter). You need only miniscule quantities of vitamins for good health. In some cases, the recommended dietary allowances (RDAs), determined by the National Research Council, may be as small as several micrograms ($\frac{1}{1,000,000}$ – that's one one-millionth — of a gram).

The father of all vitamins: Casimir Funk

Vitamins are so much a part of modern life you may have a hard time believing they were first discovered less than a century ago. Of course, people have long known that certain foods contain something special. For example, the ancient Greek physician Hippocrates prescribed liver for night-blindness (the inability to see well in dim light). By the end of the 18th century (1795), British Navy ships carried a mandatory supply of limes or lime juice to prevent scurvy among the men, thus earning the Brits once and forever the nickname limeys. Later on, the Japanese Navy gave its sailors whole grain barley to ward off beriberi.

Everyone knew these prescriptions worked, but nobody knew why — until 1912, when

Casimir Funk (1884–1967), a Polish biochemist working first in England and then in the United States, identified "somethings" in food that he called *vitamines* (vita = life; amines = nitrogen compounds).

The following year, Funk and a fellow biochemist, Briton Frederick Hopkins, suggested that some medical conditions such as scurvy and beriberi were simply deficiency diseases caused by the absence of a specific nutrient in the body. Adding a food with the missing nutrient to one's diet would prevent or cure the deficiency disease.

Eureka!

Nutritionists classify vitamins as either *fat soluble* or *water soluble*, meaning that they dissolve either in fat or in water. If you consume larger amounts of fat-soluble vitamins than your body needs, the excess is stored in body fat. Excess water-soluble vitamins are eliminated in urine.

Large amounts of fat-soluble vitamins stored in your body may cause problems (see the section "Fat-soluble vitamins" in this chapter). With water-soluble vitamins, your body simply shrugs its shoulders, so to speak, and urinates away most of the excess.

Medical students often use mnemonic devices — memory joggers — to remember complicated lists of body parts and symptoms of diseases. Here's one I use to remember which vitamins are fat-soluble: "All Dogs Eat Kidneys." This saying helps me remember that vitamins A, D, E, and K are fat-soluble. All the rest dissolve in water.

Fat-soluble vitamins

Vitamin A, vitamin D, vitamin E, and vitamin K are relatives that have two characteristics in common: All dissolve in fat, and all are stored in your fatty tissues. But like members of any family, they also have distinct personalities. One keeps your skin moist. Another protects your bones. A third keeps reproductive organs purring happily. And the fourth enables you to make special proteins.

Which does what? Read on.

Vitamin A

Vitamin A is the moisturizing nutrient that keeps your skin and *mucous membranes* (the slick tissue that lines the eyes, nose, mouth, throat, vagina, and rectum) smooth and supple. Vitamin A is also the vision vitamin, a constituent of *11-cis retinol,* a protein in the *rods* (cells in the back of your eye that enable you to see even when the lights are low) that prevents or slows the development of age-related *macular degeneration,* or progressive damage to the retina of the eye, which can cause the loss of central vision (the ability to see clearly enough to read or do fine work). Finally, vitamin A promotes the growth of healthy bones and teeth, keeps your reproductive system humming, and encourages your immune system to churn out the cells you need to fight off infection.

Two chemicals provide vitamin A: retinoids and carotenoids. *Retinoids* are compounds whose names all start with *ret:* retinol, retinaldehyde, retinoic acid, and so on. These fat-soluble substances are found in several foods of animal origin: liver (again!) and whole milk, eggs, and butter. Retinoids give you *preformed* vitamin A, the kind of nutrient your body can use right away.

The second form of vitamin A is the *vitamin A precursor*, a chemical such as beta-carotene, a deep yellow carotenoid (pigment) found in dark green and bright yellow fruits and vegetables. Your body transforms a vitamin A precursor into a retinol-like substance. So far, scientists have identified at least 500 different carotenoids. Only 1 in 10 — about 50 altogether — are considered, like beta-carotene, to be sources of vitamin A.

Help! I'm turning orange

Because you store retinol in your liver, megadoses of preformed vitamin A can build up to toxic levels. Not so with carotenoids, which serve up another form of that vitamin. They aren't stored in the liver, so these red and yellow pigments in fruits and vegetables are safe even in very large amounts.

But that doesn't mean that excess carotenoids don't have side effects. Carotenoids, like retinoids, are stored in body fat. If you wolf down large quantities of carotenoid-rich foods like carrots and tomatoes every day, day after day, for several weeks, your skin — particularly the palms of your hands and the soles of your feet — will turn a nifty shade of dusty orange, brighter if your skin is naturally light, darker if it's naturally dark. It sounds fantastic, but it has actually happened to people eating two cups of carrots and two whole tomatoes a day for several months. When they cut down on the carrots and tomatoes, the color faded.

Now, let's see . . . it's September 1, and you've been invited to a Halloween party. Maybe this year you'll go as a pumpkin. If you start packing in the carrots and tomatoes right now. . . .

Hand in hand: How vitamins help each other

All vitamins have specific jobs in your body. Some have partners. Here are some examples of nutrient cooperation:

✔ Vitamin E keeps vitamin A from being destroyed in your intestines.

✔ Vitamin D enables your body to absorb calcium and phosphorus.

✔ Vitamin C helps folate build proteins.

✔ Vitamin B1 works in digestive enzyme systems with niacin, pantothenic acid, and magnesium.

Taking vitamins with other vitamins may also improve body levels of nutrients. For example, in 1993, scientists at the National Cancer Institute and the U. S. Department of Agriculture (USDA) Agricultural Research Service gave one group of volunteers a vitamin E capsule plus a multivitamin pill; a second group, vitamin E alone; and a third group, no vitamins at all. The people getting vitamin E plus the multivitamin had the highest amount of vitamin E in their blood — more than twice as high as those who took plain vitamin E capsules.

Sometimes, one vitamin may even alleviate a deficiency caused by the lack of another vitamin. People who do not get enough folate are at risk of a form of anemia in which their red blood cells fail to mature. As soon as they get folate, either by injection or by mouth, they begin making new healthy cells. That's to be expected. What's surprising is the fact that anemia caused by *pellagra,* the niacin deficiency disease, may also respond to folate treatment.

Isn't nature neat?

Traditionally, the recommended dietary allowances of vitamin A are measured in International Units (IU). However, because retinol is the most efficient source of vitamin A, the modern way to measure the RDA for vitamin A is as retinol equivalents, abbreviated as RE. One microgram (mcg) RE = 3.3 IU. However, many vitamin products still list the RDA for vitamin A in IUs.

Vitamin D

If I say "bones" or "teeth," what nutrient springs most quickly to mind? If you answer calcium, you're giving only a partial picture. True, calcium is essential for hardening teeth and bones. But no matter how much calcium you consume, without vitamin D, your body can't absorb and use the mineral. So vitamin D is vital for building — and holding — strong bones and teeth.

Researchers at the Bone Metabolism Laboratory at the Jean Mayer USDA Human Nutrition Research Center on Aging at Tufts University in Boston say vitamin D may also reduce the risk of tooth loss by preventing the inflammatory response that leads to periodontal disease, a condition that destroys the thin tissue (ligaments) that connects the teeth to the surrounding jawbone. Finally, a report in the February 2006 issue of *The American Journal of Public Health* suggests that taking 1,000 international units (IU) of vitamin D a day may cut in half a person's risk of developing some forms of cancer, including cancer of the colon, breast, or ovaries.

Vitamin D comes in three forms: calciferol, cholecalciferol, and ergocalciferol. *Calciferol* occurs naturally in fish oils and egg yolk. In the United States, it's added to margarines and milk. *Cholecalciferol* is created when sunlight hits your skin and ultraviolet rays react with steroid chemicals in body fat just underneath. *Ergocalciferol* is synthesized in plants exposed to sunlight. Cholecalciferol and ergocalciferol justify vitamin D's nickname: the Sunshine Vitamin.

The RDA for vitamin D is measured either in International Units (IUs) or micrograms (mcg) of cholecalciferol: 10 mcg cholecalciferol = 400 IU vitamin D.

Vitamin E

Every animal, including you, needs vitamin E to maintain a healthy reproductive system, nerves, and muscles. You get vitamin E from *tocopherols* and *tocotrienols,* two families of naturally occurring chemicals in vegetable oils, nuts, whole grains, and green leafy vegetables — your best natural sources of vitamin E.

Tocopherols, the more important source, have two sterling characteristics: They're anticoagulants and antioxidants that reduce blood's ability to clot, thus reducing the risk of clot-related stroke and heart attack. *Antioxidants* prevent free radicals (incomplete pieces of molecules) from hooking up with other molecules or fragments of molecules to form toxic substances that can attack tissues in your body. In fact, nutrition scientists at Purdue University released a study showing that vitamin E promotes bone growth by stopping free radicals from reacting with polyunsaturated fatty acids (see Chapter 7 for information on fats) to create molecules that interfere with the formation of new bone cells.

But some claims about E's heart health benefits are now considered iffy. True, a recent clinical trial at Cambridge University in England showed that taking 800 IU (International Units) of vitamin E, two times the RDA, may reduce the risk of nonfatal heart attacks for people who already have heart disease. And, yes, the federal Women's Health Study found that older women taking 600 IU vitamin E per day had a lower risk of heart attack and a lower risk of death from heart disease. But the Heart Outcomes Prevention Evaluation (HOPE) study showed no such benefits. In fact, people taking 400 IU per day vitamin E were more likely to develop heart failure. No one (and no study) has found similar problems among those taking less vitamin E, say 100 IU/day. Whew.

The best sources of vitamin E are vegetables, oils, nuts, and seeds. The RDA is expressed as milligrams *a-tocopherol equivalents* (abbreviated as *a-TE*).

Vitamin K

Vitamin K is a group of chemicals that your body uses to make specialized proteins found in blood *plasma* (the clear fluid in blood), such as prothrombin, the protein chiefly responsible for blood clotting. You also need vitamin K to make bone and kidney tissues. Like vitamin D, vitamin K is essential for healthy bones. Vitamin D increases calcium absorption; vitamin K activates at least three different proteins that take part in forming new bone cells. For example, a report on 888 men and women from the long-running Framingham (Massachusetts) Heart Study shows that those who consumed the least vitamin K each day had the highest incidence of broken bones. The same was true for a 1999 analysis of data from the Nurses' Health Study.

Vitamin K is found in dark green leafy vegetables (broccoli, cabbage, kale, lettuce, spinach, and turnip greens), cheese, liver, cereals, and fruits, but most of what you need comes from resident colonies of friendly bacteria in your intestines, an assembly line of busy bugs churning out the vitamin day and night.

Water-soluble vitamins

Vitamin C and the entire roster of B vitamins (thiamin, riboflavin, niacin, vitamin B6, folate, biotin, and pantothenic acid) are usually grouped together simply because they all dissolve in water.

PQQ, a whole new itty-bitty vitamin

The next time someone tells you to mind your p's and q's, don't take offense. The subject may be nutrition, not manners — pyrroloquinoline quinone (PQQ), the first new vitamin in more than half a century. The water-soluble compound, identified at the University of Texas in 1979 and labeled a vitamin four years later by researchers at Tokyo's Institute of Physical and Chemical Research, is widely available in plant foods such as green tea, green bell peppers, papaya, spinach, carrots, cabbage, and bananas. Animal studies show a connection between PQQ and an enzyme used by mammals to digest lysine, an amino acid found in proteins. The vitamin is essential for some bacteria and maybe even mice. And you? Well, if you need it, you need very, very little. The amounts of other vitamins are measured in milligrams (thousandths of a gram) or micrograms (millionths of a gram). But PQQ is measured in nanograms (billionths of a gram) — 1/1,000,000,000. Which is about as itty-bitty as it gets.

The ability to dissolve in water is an important point, because that means large amounts of these nutrients can't be stored in your body. If you take in more than you need to perform specific bodily tasks, you will simply pee away virtually all the excess. The good news is that these vitamins rarely cause side effects. The bad news is that you have to take enough of these vitamins every day to protect yourself against deficiencies.

Vitamin C

Vitamin C, which also is referred to as ascorbic acid, is essential for the development and maintenance of connective tissue (the fat, muscle, and bone framework of the human body). Vitamin C speeds the production of new cells in wound healing, protects your immune system, helps you fight off infection, reduces the severity of allergic reactions, and plays a role in the syntheses of hormones and other body chemicals. For more on this important nutrient, see the sidebar "A special case: The continuing saga of Vitamin C," further on in this chapter.

Thiamin (vitamin B1)

Call it thiamin. Call it B1. Just don't call it late for lunch (or any other meal). This sulfur *(thia)* and nitrogen *(amin)* compound, the first of the B vitamins to be isolated and identified, helps ensure a healthy appetite. It acts as a *coenzyme* (a substance that works along with other enzymes) essential to at least four different processes by which your body extracts energy from carbohydrates. And thiamin also is a mild diuretic (something that makes you urinate more).

Although thiamin is found in every body tissue, the highest concentrations are in your vital organs — heart, liver, and kidneys.

The richest dietary sources of thiamin are unrefined cereals and grains, lean pork, beans, nuts, and seeds. In the United States, refined flours, stripped of their thiamin, are a nutritional reality, so most Americans get most of their thiamin from breads and cereals enriched with additional B1.

Riboflavin (vitamin B2)

Riboflavin (vitamin B2), the second B vitamin to be identified, was once called "vitamin G." Its present name is derivative of its chemical structure, a carbon-hydrogen-oxygen skeleton that includes *ribitol* (a sugar) attached to a *flavonoid* (a substance from plants containing a pigment called flavone).

Like thiamin, riboflavin is a coenzyme. Without it, your body can't digest and use proteins and carbohydrates. Like vitamin A, it protects the health of mucous membranes — the moist tissues that line the eyes, mouth, nose, throat, vagina, and rectum.

Lemons, limes, oranges — and bacon?

Check the meat label. Right there it is, plain as day — vitamin C in the form of *sodium ascorbate* or *isoascorbate.*

The Food and Drug Administration (FDA) says it has to be there because vitamin C does for meat exactly what it does for your body: It prevents free radicals (incomplete pieces of molecules) from hooking up with each other to form damaging compounds, in this case *carcinogens,* substances that cause cancer.

Processed meats such as bacon and sausages are preserved with sodium nitrite, which protects the meat from *Clostridium botulinum,* microorganisms that cause the potentially fatal food poisoning known as botulism.

On its own, sodium nitrite reacts at high temperatures with compounds in meat to form carcinogens called nitrosamines. But like the Lone Ranger, antioxidant vitamin C rides to the rescue, preventing the chemical reaction and keeping the sausage and bacon safe to eat. How's that for healthy eating, Kemo Sabe?

You get riboflavin from foods of animal origin (meat, fish, poultry, eggs, and milk), whole or enriched grain products, brewer's yeast, and dark green vegetables (like broccoli and spinach).

Niacin

Niacin is one name for a pair of naturally occurring nutrients, nicotinic acid and nicotinamide. Niacin is essential for proper growth, and like other B vitamins, it's intimately involved in enzyme reactions. In fact, it's an integral part of an enzyme that enables oxygen to flow into body tissues. Like thiamin, it gives you a healthy appetite and participates in the metabolism of sugars and fats.

Niacin is available either as a preformed nutrient or via the conversion of the amino acid tryptophan. Preformed niacin comes from meat; tryptophan comes from milk and dairy foods. Some niacin is present in grains, but your body can't absorb it efficiently unless the grain has been treated with lime — the mineral, not the fruit. This is a common practice in Central American and South American countries, where lime is added to cornmeal in making tortillas. In the United States, breads and cereals are routinely fortified with niacin. Your body easily absorbs the added niacin.

The term used to describe the niacin RDA is NE (niacin equivalent): 60 milligrams tryptophan = 1 milligram niacin = 1 niacin equivalent (NE).

Vitamin B6 (Pyridoxine)

Vitamin B6 is another multiple compound, this one comprising three related chemicals: pyridoxine, pyridoxal, and pyridoxamine. Vitamin B6, a component of enzymes that metabolizes proteins and fats, is essential for getting energy and nutrients from food. It also helps lower blood levels of homocysteine (see Chapter 6), an amino acid produced when you digest proteins. The American Heart Association calls a high level of homocysteine an independent (but not major) risk factor for heart disease, and the American Journal of Clinical Nutrition reported in 2005 that a high homocysteine level may be associated with an age-related decline in memory. Alas, follow up studies show no reduction in the risk of heart disease or improvement in memory in those who reduce their blood levels of homocysteine.

The best food sources of vitamin B6 are liver, chicken, fish, pork, lamb, milk, eggs, unmilled rice, whole grains, soybeans, potatoes, beans, nuts, seeds, and dark green vegetables such as turnip greens. In the United States, bread and other products made with refined grains have added vitamin B6.

Folate

Folate, or folic acid, is an essential nutrient for human beings and other *verte-brates* (animals with backbones). Folate takes part in the synthesis of DNA, the metabolism of proteins, and the subsequent synthesis of amino acids used to produce new body cells and tissues. Folate is vital for normal growth and wound healing. An adequate supply of the vitamin is essential for pregnant women to enable them to create new maternal tissue as well as fetal tissue. In addition, an adequate supply of folate dramatically reduces the risk of spinal cord birth defects. Beans, dark green leafy vegetables, liver, yeast, and various fruits are excellent food sources of folate, and all multivitamin supplements must now provide 400 mcg of folate per dose.

Vitamin B12

Vitamin B12 (cyanocobalamin) makes healthy red blood cells. Vitamin B12 protects *myelin,* the fatty material that covers your nerves and enables you to transmit electrical impulses (messages) between nerve cells. These messages make it possible for you to see, hear, think, move, and do all the things a healthy body does each day. In 2005, the Canadian Medical Association Journal reported that low blood levels of B12 in older people are linked to higher levels of homocysteine (a minor risk factor for heart disease; see previous, "Vitamin B6 [Pyridoxine]").

Vitamin B12 is unique. First, it's the only vitamin that contains a mineral, cobalt. (Cyanocobalamin, a cobalt compound, is commonly used as "vitamin B12" in vitamin pills and nutritional supplements.) Second, it's a vitamin that can't be made by higher plants (the ones that give us fruits and vegetables). Like vitamin K, vitamin B12 is made by beneficial bacteria living in your small intestine. Meat, fish, poultry, milk products, and eggs are good sources of vitamin B12. Grains don't naturally contain vitamin B12, but like other B vitamins, it's added to grain products in the United States.

Biotin

Biotin is a B-vitamin, a component of enzymes that ferry carbon and oxygen atoms between cells. Biotin helps you metabolize fats and carbohydrates and is essential for synthesizing fatty acids and amino acids needed for healthy growth. And it seems to prevent a buildup of fat deposits that may interfere with the proper functioning of liver and kidneys. (No, biotin won't keep fat from settling in more visible places, such as your hips.)

The best food sources of biotin are liver, egg yolk, yeast, nuts, and beans. If your diet doesn't give you all the biotin you need, bacteria in your gut will synthesize enough to make up the difference. No RDA exists for biotin, but the Food and Nutrition Board has established an Adequate Intake (AI), which means a safe and effective daily dose.

Pantothenic acid

Pantothenic acid, another B-vitamin, is vital to enzyme reactions that enable you to use carbohydrates and create steroid biochemicals such as hormones. Pantothenic acid also helps stabilize blood sugar levels, defends against infection, and protects *hemoglobin* (the protein in red blood cells that carries oxygen through the body), as well as nerve, brain, and muscle tissue. You get pantothenic acid from meat, fish and poultry, beans, whole grain cereals, and fortified grain products. As with biotin, the Food and Nutrition Board has established an Adequate Intake (AI) for pantothenic acid.

Choline

Choline is not a vitamin, a mineral, a protein, a carbohydrate, or a fat, but it's usually lumped in with the B-vitamins, so heeeeere's choline!

In 1998, 138 years after this nutrient first was identified, the Institute of Medicine (IOM) finally declared it essential for human beings. The IOM had good reasons for doing so. Choline keeps body cells healthy. It's used to make *acetylcholine,* a chemical that enables brain cells to exchange messages. It protects the heart and lowers the risk of liver cancer. And new research at the University of North Carolina (Chapel Hill) shows that choline plays a role in developing and maintaining the ability to think and remember, at least among rat pups and other beasties born to lab animals that were given choline supplements while pregnant. Follow-up studies showed that prenatal choline supplements helped the animals grow bigger brain cells.

True, no one knows whether this would also be true for human pups, er, babies, but some researchers advise pregnant women to eat a varied diet, because getting choline from basic stuff like eggs, meat, and milk is so easy.

IOM's Food and Nutrition Board, the group that sets the RDAs, has established an AI (Adequate Intake) for choline.

Get Your Vitamins Here

One reasonable set of guidelines for good nutrition is the list of Recommended Dietary Allowances (RDAs) established by the National Research Council's Food and Nutrition Board. The RDAs present safe and effective doses for healthy people.

You can find the chart of RDAs for adults (ages 19 and up) in Chapter 4. It's very, very long, with RDAs for 10 different groups of people (men, women, old, young) for 25 specific vitamins and minerals, plus choline. I couldn't possibly ask you to read through it here. Personally, just the thought of retyping the whole thing gives me hives.

Table 10-1 is the easy alternative: It gives you the RDAs for adult men and women (ages 19 to 50) plus a quick, no-brainer guide to food portions that give you at least 25 percent of the recommended dietary allowances of vitamins for healthy adult men and women, ages 25 to 50.

Photocopy this chart. Pin it on your fridge. Tape it to your organizer or appointment book. Stick it in your wallet. Think of it as the truly simple way to see how easy it is to eat healthy.

Table 10-1	Servings That Provide at Least 25% of the RDA
Food	*Serving = 25% of the RDA*
VITAMIN A	**RDA: Women 4,000 IU, Men 5,000 IU***
Breads, cereals, grains	
Oatmeal — instant, fortified	2⅓ cup
Cold cereal	1 ounce
Fruits	
Apricots (dried, cooked)	½ cup
Cantaloupe (raw)	½ cup
Mango (raw)	½ medium
Vegetables	
Carrots, kale, peas and carrots, sweet red pepper (all cooked)	½ cup
Meat, poultry, fish	
Liver — chicken, turkey	½ cup (diced)

(continued)

Table 10-1 *(continued)*

Food	Serving = 25% of the RDA
Dairy products	
Milk — low-fat, skim	2 cups
VITAMIN D	*RDA: Women 5 mcg/200 IU, Men 5 mcg/200 IU*
Meat, poultry, fish	
Salmon (canned)	1½ ounces
Tuna (canned)	2 ounces
Dairy products	
Eggs	3 medium
Milk — enriched	1 cup
VITAMIN E	*RDA: Women 15 mg a-TE, Men 15 mg a-TE*
Breads, cereals, grains	
Cold cereal	1 ounce
Wheat germ — plain	2 tbsp.
Fruits	
Apricots, peaches (canned)	1 cup
Vegetables	
Greens (cooked) — dandelion, mustard, turnip	1 cup
Meat, poultry, fish	
Shrimp	3 ounces
Other	
Almonds, hazelnuts/filberts	2 tbsp.
Peanut butter	2 tbsp.
Sunflower seeds	2 tbsp.
VITAMIN C	*RDA: Women 75 mg, Men 90 mg***
Breads, cereals, grains	
Cold cereal	1 ounce

Food	Serving = 25% of the RDA
Fruits	
Cantaloupe	½ cup, diced
Grapefruit	½ medium
Mango (raw)	½ medium
Orange	1 medium
Strawberries	½ cup
Grape, orange, or tomato juice	¼ cup
Vegetables	
Asparagus, broccoli, Brussels sprouts, kale, kohlrabi, sweet peppers, snow peas (cooked)	½ cup
Sweet potato	1 medium
Meat, poultry, fish	
Liver — beef, pork	3 ounces
THIAMIN (VITAMIN B1)	**RDA: Women 1.1 mg, Men 1.2 mg**
Breads, cereals, grains	
Bagel, English muffin, roll	2 whole
Bread	4 slices
Farina, grits	½ cup
Oatmeal — instant, fortified	⅓ cup
Fruits	
Cantaloupe, honeydew	1 cup
Vegetables	
Corn, peas, peas and carrots (cooked)	1 cup
Meat, poultry, fish	
Ham — roast, smoked, cured, lean	3 ounces
Liver — beef, pork	3 ounces
Pork — all varieties except sausage	3 ounces

(continued)

Table 10-1 *(continued)*

Food	Serving = 25% of the RDA
Other	
Sunflower seeds (hulled, unroasted)	2 tbsp.
RIBOFLAVIN (VITAMIN B2)	**RDA: Women 1.1 mg, Men 1.3 mg**
Breads, cereals, grains	
Bagel, English muffin, pita	2 whole
Cold cereal	1 ounce
Meat, poultry, fish	
Liver — beef, calf, pork	3 ounces
Liver — chicken, turkey	½ cup, diced
Liverwurst	1 ounce
Dairy products	
Milk — all varieties	2 cups
Yogurt — low-fat, nonfat	1 cup
NIACIN	**RDA: Women 14 mg NE, Men 16 mg NE**
Breads, cereals, grains	
Bagel, bran muffin, English muffin, pita, roll	2 whole
Cold cereal — fortified	1 ounce
Lamb, pork, veal — lean	3 ounces
Liver — beef, calf, pork	3 ounces
Chicken (no skin)	3 ounces (½ breast)
Mackerel, mullet, salmon, swordfish	3 ounces
Other	
Peanuts, peanut butter	4 tbsp.
VITAMIN B6	**RDA: Women 1.3 mg, Men 1.3 mg**
Breads, cereals, grains	
Oatmeal — instant, fortified	⅓ cup

Food	Serving = 25% of the RDA
Cold cereal	1 ounce
Fruits	
Banana (raw)	1 medium
Prunes (dried, cooked)	1 cup
Vegetables	
Plantain (boiled)	1 medium
Meat, poultry, fish	
Chicken (roasted, no skin)	½ breast
Lamb — lean only	1 chop
Liver — beef	3 ounces
FOLATE	**RDA: Women 400 mcg, Men 400 mcg**
Breads, cereals, grains	
Whole wheat English muffin, pita	2 whole
Cold cereal	1 ounce
Vegetables	
Asparagus, beets, broccoli, Brussels sprouts, cauliflower, Chinese cabbage, creamed corn, spinach (cooked)	1 cup
Beans (dry, cooked) — black-eyed peas, lentils, red kidney	½ cup
Greens (cooked) — mustard, turnip	1 cup
Meat, poultry, fish	
Liver — beef, calf, pork	3 ounces
VITAMIN B12	**RDA: Women 2.4 mcg, Men 2.4 mcg**
Meat, poultry, fish	
Beef, pork, lamb, veal	3 ounces
Liver — beef, calf, pork	3 ounces
Liver — chicken, turkey	½ cup, diced

(continued)

Table 10-1 *(continued)*

Food	Serving = 25% of the RDA
Catfish, crabmeat, croaker, lobster, mackerel, mussels, oysters, scallops, swordfish, trout, tuna	3 ounces
Dairy products	
Eggs	2 large
Milk — whole, low-fat, skim	2 cups
Yogurt	2 cups
CHOLINE	**Adequate Intake: Women 425 mg, Men 550 mg**
Fruits	
Grape juice (canned)	8 ounces (13 mg)
Vegetables	
Cauliflower (cooked)	1 cup (55 mg)
Potato (baked)	1 medium (18 mg)
Meat, poultry, fish	
Beef (cooked)	3 ounces (59 mg)
Liver (cooked) — beef	3 ounces (453 mg)
Dairy	
Eggs	1 large (200–300 mg)
Milk — whole	8 ounces (10 mg)
Other	
Peanut butter	2 tbsp. (26 mg)

* Although these remain the "official" RDAs, newer recommendations are 900 mcg RE/3,000 IU per day for men and 700 mcg RE/2,300 IU per day for women (the IU amounts are rounded off).
** The Food and Nutrition Board is debating whether to raise the RDA for vitamin C to 200 mg for both men and women.
"Good Sources of Nutrients" (Washington D.C.: U.S. Department of Agriculture/Human Nutrition Service, 1990); "Nutritive Value of Food" (Washington D.C.: U.S. Department of Agriculture, 1991)

Too Much or Too Little: Avoiding Two Ways to Go Wrong with Vitamins

RDAs are broad enough to prevent vitamin deficiencies and avoid the side effects associated with very large doses of some vitamins. If your diet doesn't meet these guidelines, or if you take very large amounts of vitamins as supplements, you may be in for trouble.

Vitamin deficiencies

The good news is that vitamin deficiencies are rare among people who have access to a wide variety of foods and know how to put together a balanced diet. For example, the only people likely to experience a vitamin E deficiency are premature and/or low–birth weight infants and people with a metabolic disorder that keeps them from absorbing fat. A healthy adult may go as long as 10 years on a vitamin E–deficient diet without developing any signs of a problem.

Aha, you say, but what's this subclinical deficiency I hear so much about?

Nutritionists use the term *subclinical deficiency* to describe a nutritional deficit not yet far enough advanced to produce obvious symptoms. In lay terms, however, the phrase has become a handy explanation for common but hard-to-pin-down symptoms such as fatigue, irritability, nervousness, emotional depression, allergies, and insomnia. And it's a dandy way to increase the sale of nutritional supplements.

Simply put, the RDAs protect you against deficiency. If your odd symptoms linger even after you take reasonable amounts of vitamin supplements, probably something other than a lack of any one vitamin is to blame. Don't wait until your patience or your bank account has been exhausted to find out. Get a second opinion as soon as you can. Table 10-2 lists the symptoms of various vitamin deficiencies.

Table 10-2	Vitamin Alert: What Happens When You Don't Get the Vitamins You Need
A Diet Low in This Vitamin	*May Produce These Signs of Deficiency*
Vitamin A	Poor night vision; dry, rough, or cracked skin; dry mucous membranes including the inside of the eye; slow wound healing; nerve damage; reduced ability to taste, hear, and smell; inability to perspire; reduced resistance to respiratory infections

(continued)

Table 10-2 (continued)

A Diet Low in This Vitamin	May Produce These Signs of Deficiency
Vitamin D	In children: rickets (weak muscles, delayed tooth development, and soft bones, all caused by the inability to absorb minerals without vitamin D)In adults: osteomalacia (soft, porous bones that fracture easily)
Vitamin E	Inability to absorb fat
Vitamin K	Blood fails to clot
Vitamin C	Scurvy (bleeding gums; tooth loss; nosebleeds; bruising; painful or swollen joints; shortness of breath; increased susceptibility to infection; slow wound healing; muscle pains; skin rashes)
Thiamin (vitamin B1)	Poor appetite; unintended weight loss; upset stomach; gastric upset (nausea, vomiting); mental depression; an inability to concentrate
Riboflavin (vitamin B2)	Inflamed mucous membranes, including cracked lips, sore tongue and mouth, burning eyes; skin rashes; anemia
Niacin	Pellagra (diarrhea; inflamed skin and mucous membranes; mental confusion and/or dementia)
Vitamin B6	Anemia; convulsions similar to epileptic seizures; skin rashes; upset stomach; nerve damage (in infants)
Folate	Anemia (immature red blood cells)
Vitamin B12	Pernicious anemia (destruction of red blood cells, nerve damage, increased risk of stomach cancer attributed to damaged stomach tissue, neurological/psychiatric symptoms attributed to nerve cell damage)
Biotin	Loss of appetite; upset stomach; pale, dry, scaly skin; hair loss; emotional depression; skin rashes (in infants younger than 6 months)

Big trouble: Vitamin megadoses

Can you get too much of a good thing? Darn right, you can. Some vitamins are toxic when taken in the very large amounts popularly known as *megadoses*. How much is a megadose? Nobody knows for sure. The general consensus, however, is that a megadose is several times the RDA, but the term is so vague that it's in neither my medical dictionary nor the dictionary on my computer.

✔ Megadoses of vitamin A (as retinol) may cause symptoms that make you think you have a brain tumor. Taken by a pregnant woman, megadoses of vitamin A may damage the fetus.

✔ Megadoses of vitamin D may cause kidney stones and hard lumps of calcium in soft tissue (muscles and organs).

✔ Megadoses of niacin (sometimes used to lower cholesterol levels) can damage liver tissue.

✔ Megadoses of vitamin B6 can cause (temporary) damage to nerves in arms and legs, fingers, and toes.

But here's an interesting fact: With one exception, the likeliest way to get a megadose of vitamins is to take supplements (see Chapter 5 for more on supplements). It's pretty much impossible for you to cram down enough food to overdose on vitamins D, E, K, C, and all the Bs. Did you notice the exception? Right: vitamin A. Liver and fish liver oils are concentrated sources of preformed vitamin A (retinol), the potentially toxic form of vitamin A. Liver contains so much retinol that early 20th century explorers to the South Pole made themselves sick on seal and whale liver. Cases of vitamin A toxicity also have been reported among children given daily servings of chicken liver. (See Table 10-3 for more on vitamin A toxicity, this time from supplements.) On the other hand, even very large doses of vitamin E, vitamin K, thiamin (vitamin B1), riboflavin (vitamin B2), folate, vitamin B12, biotin, and pantothenic acid appear safe for human beings. Table 10-3 lists the effects of vitamin overdoses.

Table 10-3	Amounts and Effects of Vitamin Overdoses for Healthy People
Vitamin	*Overdose and Possible Effect*
Vitamin A	15,000 to 25,000 IU retinol a day for adults (2,000 IU or more for children) may lead to liver damage, headache, vomiting, abnormal vision, constipation, hair loss, loss of appetite, low-grade fever, bone pain, sleep disorders, and dry skin and mucous membranes. A pregnant woman who takes more than 10,000 IU a day doubles her risk of giving birth to a child with birth defects.
Vitamin D	2,000 IU a day can cause irreversible damage to kidneys and heart. Smaller doses may cause muscle weakness, headache, nausea, vomiting, high blood pressure, retarded physical growth, and mental retardation in children, and fetal abnormalities.

(continued)

Vitamin	Overdose and Possible Effect
Vitamin E	Large amounts (more than 400 to 800 IU a day) may cause upset stomach or dizziness.
Vitamin C	1,000 mg or higher may cause upset stomach, diarrhea, or constipation.
Niacin	Doses higher than the RDA raise the production of liver enzymes and blood levels of sugar and uric acid, leading to liver damage and an increased risk of diabetes and gout.
Vitamin B6	Continued use of 50 mg or more a day may damage nerves in arms, legs, hands, and feet. Some experts say the damage is likely to be temporary; others say that it may be permanent.
Choline	Very high doses (14 to 37 times the adequate amount) have been linked to vomiting, salivation, sweating, low blood pressure, and — ugh! — fishy body odor.

Table 10-3 *(continued)*

You may not have to go sky-high on vitamin A to run into trouble. In January 2003, new data from a long-running (30-year) study at University Hospital in Uppsala (Sweden) suggested that taking a multivitamin with normal amounts of vitamin A may weaken bones and raise the risk of hip fractures by as much as 700 percent, a conclusion supported by data released in 2004 from the long-running Nurses' Health Study. A high blood level of retinol — from large amounts of vitamin A from food or supplements — apparently inhibits special cells that usually make new bone, revs up cells that destroy bone, and interferes with vitamin D's ability to help you absorb calcium. Of course, confirming studies are needed, but you can bet the debate about lowering the amount of A in your favorite supplement will be vigorous. The new recommendations for vitamin A are 700 RE/2,300 IU of vitamin A for women and 900 RE/3,000 IU for men, but many popular multivitamins still contain 750–1500 RE/2,500–5,000 IU. Oooops?

Exceeding the RDAs: Taking Extra Vitamins as Needed

Who needs extra vitamins? Maybe you. The RDAs are designed to protect healthy people from deficiencies, but sometimes the circumstances of your life (or your lifestyle) mean that you need something extra. Are you taking medication? Do you smoke? Are you on a restricted diet? Are you pregnant? Are you a nursing mother? Are you approaching menopause? Answer "yes" to any of these questions, and you may be a person who needs larger amounts of vitamins than the RDAs provide.

A special case: The continuing saga of vitamin C

In 1970, chemist Linus Pauling published *Vitamin C and the Common Cold,* a small book (just about 100 pages) made weightier by the fact that Pauling had not one, but two Nobel prizes on his shelf — one for chemistry and one for peace. Ever since, people have been fighting over Pauling's message that very large doses of vitamin C — called *gram doses* because they provide more than 1,000 milligrams (1 gram) — prevent or cure the common cold or his later (unfounded) claim that these doses may also cure advanced cancer.

Over the past decade, the argument has switched to vitamin C's reputed ability to protect heart health. For example, an April 2004 report in the *Journal of the American College of Nutrition* said vitamin C could lower blood levels of CRP, an inflammation-related protein that increases the risk of heart disease. University of California, Berkeley, researchers gave 160 healthy adult volunteers either 500 milligrams vitamin C or a mixture of antioxidant nutrients or a look-alike pill with no nutrients once a day for two months. In the end, the folks who got the vitamin C experienced a 24 percent drop in CRP blood levels versus a statistically insignificant 4.7 percent for the cocktail and no change at all for those on the placebo. Not surprisingly, UC epidemiologists thought vitamin C may become an important aid to heart health.

Unless, that is, you're taking medicines to knock down your "bad" cholesterol and boost the "good" kind. As the American Heart Association (AHA) Council on Nutrition Physical Activity and Metabolism points out, when 20 volunteers in an HDL-Atherosclerosis Treatment Study were given vitamin C supplements along with their anti-cholesterol meds, they ended up with lower-than-expected levels of heart healthy high density lipoproteins (HDLs). In another small study, women taking antioxidant vitamins along with post-menopausal estrogens were more likely than those taking look-alike pills to die from their heart disease.

Oh, well. Nothing's perfect.

I'm taking medication

Many valuable medicines interact with vitamins. Some drugs increase or decrease the effectiveness of vitamins; some vitamins increase or decrease the effectiveness of drugs. For example, a woman who's using birth control pills may absorb less than the customary amount of the B vitamins. For more about vitamin and drug interactions, see Chapter 25.

I'm a smoker

It's a fact — you probably have abnormally low blood levels of vitamin C. More trouble: Chemicals from tobacco smoke create more free radicals in your body. Even the National Research Council, which is tough on vitamin overdosing, says that regular smokers need to take about 66 percent more vitamin C — up to 100 mg a day — than nonsmokers.

I never eat animals

On the other hand, if you're nuts for veggies but follow a vegan diet — one that shuns all foods from animals (including milk, cheese, eggs, and fish oils) — you simply cannot get enough vitamin D without taking supplements. Vegans also benefit from extra vitamin C because it increases their ability to absorb iron from plant food. And vitamin B12–enriched grains or supplements are a must to supply the nutrient found only in fish, poultry, milk, cheese, and eggs.

I'm a couch potato who plans to start working out

When you do head for the gym, take it slow, and take an extra dose of vitamin E. A study at the USDA Center for Human Nutrition at Tufts University (Boston) suggests that an 800 milligram vitamin E supplement every day for the first month after you begin exercising minimizes muscle damage by preventing reactions with free radicals (parts of molecules) that cause inflammation. After that, you're on your own: The vitamin doesn't help conditioned athletes whose muscles have adapted to workout stress.

I'm pregnant

Keep in mind that "eating for two" means that you're the sole source of nutrients for the growing fetus, not that you need to double the amount of food you eat. If you don't get the vitamins you need, neither will your baby.

The RDAs for many nutrients are the same as those for women who aren't pregnant. But when you're pregnant, you need extra

- ✔ **Vitamin D:** Every smidgen of vitamin D in a newborn's body came from his or her mom. If the mother doesn't have enough D, neither will the baby. Are vitamin pills the answer? Yes. And no. The qualifier is how many pills, because although too little vitamin D can weaken a developing fetus, too much can cause birth defects. That's why until new recommendations for vitamin D are issued, the second important *d*-word is "doctor." As in, check with yours to see what's right for you.

- ✔ **Vitamin E:** To create all that new tissue (the woman's as well as the baby's), a pregnant woman needs an extra 2 a-TE each day, the approximate amount in one egg.

✔ **Vitamin C:** The level of vitamin C in your blood falls as your vitamin C flows across the placenta to your baby, who may — at some point in the pregnancy — have vitamin C levels as much as 50 percent higher than yours. So you need an extra 10 milligrams vitamin C each day (½ cup cooked zucchini or 2 stalks of asparagus).

✔ **Riboflavin (vitamin B2):** To protect the baby against structural defects such as cleft palate or a deformed heart, a pregnant woman needs an extra 0.3 milligrams riboflavin each day (slightly less than 1 ounce of ready-to-eat cereal).

✔ **Folate:** Folate protects the child against cleft palate and neural tube (spinal cord) defects. As many as two of every 1,000 babies born each year in the United States have a neural tube defect such as spina bifida because their mothers didn't get enough folate to meet the RDA standard. The accepted increase in folate for pregnant women has been 200 micrograms (slightly more than the amount in 8 ounces of orange juice). But new studies show that taking 400 micrograms folate before becoming pregnant and through the first two months of pregnancy significantly lowers the risk of giving birth to a child with cleft palate. Taking 400 micrograms folate each day through an entire pregnancy reduces the risk of neural tube defect.

✔ **Vitamin B12:** To meet the demands of the growing fetus, a pregnant woman needs an extra 0.2 micrograms vitamin B12 each day (just 3 ounces of roast chicken).

I'm breast-feeding

You need extra vitamin A, vitamin E, thiamin, riboflavin, and folate to produce sufficient quantities of nutritious breast milk, about 750 milliters (¾ liter) each day. You need extra vitamin D, vitamin C, and niacin as insurance to replace the vitamins you lose — that is, the ones you transfer to your child in your milk.

I'm approaching menopause

Information about the specific vitamin requirements of older women is as hard to find as, well, information about the specific vitamin requirements about older men. It's enough to make you wonder what's going on with the people who set the RDAs. Don't they know that everyone gets older? Right now, just about all anybody can say for sure about the nutritional needs of older women is that they require extra calcium to stem the natural loss of bone that occurs when women reach menopause and their production of the female hormone estrogen declines. They may also need extra vitamin D to enable their bodies to absorb and use the calcium. Gender Bias Alert! No similar studies are available for older men. But adding vitamin D supplements to calcium supplements increases bone density in older people. The current RDA for vitamin D is set at 5 micrograms/200 IU for all adults, but the new AI (Adequate Intake) for vitamin D is 10 micrograms/400 IU for people ages 51 to 70 and 15 micrograms/600 IU or more for people 71 and older. Some researchers suggest that even these amounts may be too low to guarantee maximum calcium absorption.

Check with your doctor before adding vitamin D supplements. In very large amounts, this vitamin can be toxic.

I have very light skin or very dark skin

Sunlight — yes, plain old sunlight — transforms fats just under the surface of your skin to vitamin D. So getting what you need should be a cinch, right? Not necessarily. Getting enough vitamin D from sunlight is hard to do when you have very light skin and avoid the sun for fear of skin cancer. Even more difficult is getting enough vitamin D when you have very dark skin, which acts as a kind of natural sunblock. When Centers for Disease Control and Prevention researchers surveyed the vitamin D status of more than 2,000 African American and Caucasian women ages 15 to 49, they found low body levels of vitamin D in 42 percent of the African American women and 4.2 percent of the Caucasian women. Based on these numbers, Boston University researchers suggest that the Recommended Dietary Amount for adults who don't get enough sunlight may be as much as four times the current recommended amount. Check this out with your doctor; it's very important news for women who are or hope to be pregnant and need extra vitamin D (check back a few paragraphs for this information).

Chapter 11

Mighty Minerals

• •

In This Chapter

▶ Explaining how your body uses minerals

▶ Getting the minerals you need from foods

▶ Finding out what happens when you don't get enough (or you get too much) minerals

▶ Knowing when you need a little extra

• •

Minerals are *elements,* substances composed of only one kind of atom. They're inorganic (translation: They don't contain the carbon, hydrogen, and oxygen atoms found in all organic compounds, including vitamins). Minerals occur naturally in nonliving things such as rocks and metal ores. Although minerals also are present in plants and animals, they're imported: Plants get minerals from soil; animals get minerals by eating plants.

Most minerals have names reflecting the places where they're found or characteristics such as their color. For example, the name calcium comes from *calx,* the Greek word for "lime" (chalk), where calcium is found; chlorine comes from *chloros,* the Greek word for "greenish-yellow," which just happens to be the color of the mineral. Other minerals, such as americium, curium, berkelium, californium, fermium, and nobelium, are named for where they were found or to honor an important scientist.

This chapter tells you which minerals your body requires to stay in tiptop shape, where to find these minerals in food, and precisely how much of each mineral a healthy person needs.

Taking Inventory of the Minerals You Need

Think of your body as a house. Vitamins (all about them in Chapter 10) are like tiny little maids and butlers, scurrying about to turn on the lights and make sure that the windows are closed to keep the heat from escaping. Minerals are more sturdy stuff, the mortar and bricks that strengthen the frame of the house and the current that keeps the lights running.

Nutritionists classify the minerals essential for human life as either major minerals (including the principal electrolytes — see Chapter 13) or trace elements. *Major minerals* and *trace elements* are both minerals. The difference between them, nutritionally speaking, is how much you have in your body and how much you need to take in to maintain a steady supply.

Your body stores varying amounts of minerals but keeps more than 5 grams (about ⅙ of an ounce) of each of the major minerals and principal electrolytes on hand; you need to consume more than 100 milligrams a day of each major mineral to maintain a steady supply and to make up for losses. You store less than 5 grams of each trace element and need to take in less than 100 milligrams a day to stay even.

Some minerals interact with other minerals or with medical drugs. For example, calcium binds tetracycline antibiotics into compounds your body can't break apart so that the antibiotic moves out of your digestive tract, unabsorbed and unused. That's why your doctor warns you off milk and dairy products when you're taking this medicine. For more about interactions between minerals and medicines, turn to Chapter 25.

Introducing the major minerals

The following major minerals are essential for human beings:

- Calcium
- Phosphorus
- Magnesium
- Sulfur
- Sodium
- Potassium
- Chloride

Note: Sodium, potassium, and chloride, also known as the principal electrolytes, are covered in Chapter 13.

Although sulfur, a major mineral, is an essential nutrient for human beings, it's almost never included in nutritional books and/or charts. Why? Because it's an integral part of all proteins. Any diet that provides adequate protein also provides adequate sulfur. (For more on proteins, bookmark this page and turn back to Chapter 6.)

After you've checked out proteins, come on back to look at the major minerals in minute detail.

An elementary guide to minerals

The early Greeks thought that all material on Earth was constructed of a combination of four basic elements: earth, water, air, and fire. Wrong. Centuries later, alchemists looking for the formula for precious metals, such as gold, decided that the essential elements were sulfur, salt, and mercury. Wrong again.

In 1669, a group of German chemists isolated phosphorus, the first mineral element to be accurately identified. After that, things moved a bit more swiftly. By the end of the 19th century, scientists knew the names and chemical properties of 82 elements. Today, 112 elements have been identified.

The classic guide to chemical elements is the periodic table, a chart devised in 1869 by Russian chemist Dmitri Mendeleev (1834–1907), for whom mendelevium was named. The table was revised by British physicist Henry Moseley (1887–1915), who came up with the concept of *atomic numbers,* numbers based on the number of *protons* (positively charged particles) in an elemental atom.

The periodic table is a clean, crisp way of characterizing the elements, and if you are now or ever were a chemistry, physics, or premed student, you can testify firsthand to the joy (maybe that's not the best word?) of memorizing the information it provides. Personally, I'd rather be forced to watch reruns of *The Dating Game.*

Calcium

When you step on the scale in the morning, you can assume that about three pounds of your body weight is calcium, most of it packed into your bones and teeth.

Calcium is also present in extracellular fluid (the liquid around body cells), where it performs the following duties:

- ✔ Regulating fluid balance by controlling the flow of water in and out of cells
- ✔ Enabling cells to send messages back and forth from one to another
- ✔ Keeping muscles moving smoothly and preventing cramping

An adequate amount of calcium is important for controlling high blood pressure — and not only for the person who takes the calcium directly. At least one study shows that when a pregnant woman gets a sufficient amount of calcium, her baby's blood pressure stays lower than average for at least the first seven years of life, meaning a lower risk of developing high blood pressure later on.

Your best food sources of calcium are milk and dairy products, plus fish such as canned sardines and salmon. Calcium also is found in dark green leafy vegetables, but the calcium in plant foods is bound into compounds that are less easily absorbed by your body.

Calcium: The bone team player

The toe bone's connected to the foot bone. The foot bone's connected to the anklebone. The anklebone's connected to the knee bone. And what holds them together all the way up to the head bone is connected to your diet.

Like all body tissues, bones are constantly being replenished. Old bone cells break down, and new ones are born. Specialized cells called osteoclasts start the process by boring tiny holes into solid bone so that other specialized cells, called osteoblasts, can refill the open spaces with fresh bone. At that point, crystals of calcium, the best-known dietary bone builder, glom onto the network of new bone cells to harden and strengthen the bone.

Calcium begins its work on your bones while you're still in your mother's womb. But it's not the only mineral at play. You should also think zinc. Based on a survey of 242 pregnant women in Peru, where zinc deficiency is common, Johns Hopkins researchers found the babies born to women who got prenatal supplements with iron, folic acid, and zinc had longer, stronger legs bones than did babies born to women who got the same supplement minus the zinc.

After you're born, calcium continues to build your bones, but only with the help of vitamin D, which produces a calcium-binding protein that enables you to absorb the calcium in the milk Mummy feeds you. To make sure you get your D, virtually all milk sold in the United States is fortified with the vitamin. And because you may outgrow your taste for milk but never outgrow your need for calcium, calcium supplements for adults frequently include vitamin D.

But vitamin D isn't milk's only contribution. Remember the iron in the Peruvian (and American) prenatal supplements? It isn't there by accident. Iron increases the production of collagen, the most important protein in bone. Milk contains lactoferrin (lacto = milk; ferri = iron), an iron-binding compound that stimulates the production of the cells that promote bone growth.

When researchers at the University of Auckland in New Zealand added lactoferrin from cow's milk to a dish of osteoblasts, the bone cells grew more quickly. When they injected lactoferrin into the skulls of five lab mice, the bone at the site of the injection also grew faster, leading the team to suggest in the journal *Endocrinology* that lactoferrin may play a role in treating osteoporosis.

No surprise to the Department of Nutrition Sciences at the University of Arizona, where a study done with scientists from the University of Arkansas and Columbia University shows that women in their 40s, 50s, and 60s who get about 18 milligrams of iron a day have stronger, denser bones than women who get less iron. What makes this intriguing is that 18 milligrams a day is more than double the current RDA (8 milligrams) for older women.

But the iron/calcium dance is a balancing act. In your body, iron and calcium appear to compete to see which one gets absorbed. So the extra iron works only for women who get about 800 to 1,200 milligrams calcium a day — women who get less and women who get more don't seem to benefit from extra iron.

Finally, please note that the word *bones* begins with *b* — as in vitamin B12. The female sex hormone estrogen preserves bone; the male sex hormone testosterone builds new bone. As people age and their supply of sex hormones diminishes, they lose bone faster than they can replace it. One complicating factor may be low levels of vitamin B12. A report in the *Journal of Clinical Endocrinology and Metabolism* says that researchers at the University of California, San Francisco, found that women with lower levels of this vitamin also have less dense hip bones.

So to protect your bones, you need calcium, zinc, iron, and vitamins D and B12, all found most abundantly in milk, cheese, eggs, and red meat. Which sounds like a cardiologist's nutritional high-fat, high-cholesterol nightmare — unless you edit the menu to read: skim milk, low-fat cheese, egg whites, and lean beef. Way to go.

Phosphorus

Like calcium, phosphorus is essential for strong bones and teeth. For tiptop performance, you need about half as much phosphorus as calcium. Phosphorus also enables a cell to transmit the *genetic code* (genes and chromosomes that carry information about your special characteristics) to the new cells created when a cell divides and reproduces. In addition, phosphorus

✔ Helps maintain the pH balance of blood (that is, keeps it from being too acidic or too alkaline)

✔ Is vital for metabolizing carbohydrates, synthesizing proteins, and ferrying fats and fatty acids among tissues and organs

✔ Is part of *myelin,* the fatty sheath that surrounds and protects each nerve cell

Phosphorus is in almost everything you eat, but the best sources are high-protein foods such as meat, fish, poultry, eggs, and milk. These foods provide more than half the phosphorus in a nonvegetarian diet; grains, nuts, seeds, and dry beans also provide respectable amounts.

Magnesium

Your body uses magnesium to make body tissues, especially bone. The adult human body has about an ounce of magnesium, and three-quarters of it is in the bones. Magnesium also is part of more than 300 different enzymes that trigger chemical reactions throughout your body. You use magnesium to

✔ Move nutrients in and out of cells

✔ Send messages between cells

✔ Transmit the genetic code (genes and chromosomes) when cells divide and reproduce

An adequate supply of magnesium also is heart-healthy because it enables you to convert food to energy using less oxygen.

Bananas are a good source of magnesium and so are many other plant foods, including dark green fruits and vegetables (magnesium is part of chlorophyll, the green pigment in plants), whole seeds, nuts, beans, and grains.

Introducing the trace elements

Trace elements also are minerals, but they're present in much, much smaller amounts. That's why they are called *trace minerals.* You need just a trace. Get it? Good! Trace elements include:

- ✔ Iron
- ✔ Zinc
- ✔ Iodine
- ✔ Selenium
- ✔ Copper
- ✔ Manganese
- ✔ Fluoride
- ✔ Chromium
- ✔ Molybdenum

Step up to meet and greet the trace elements.

Iron

Iron is an essential constituent of hemoglobin and myoglobin, two proteins that store and transport oxygen. You find hemoglobin in red blood cells (it's what makes them red). Myoglobin (myo = muscle) is in muscle tissue. Iron also is part of various enzymes.

Your best food sources of iron are organ meats (liver, heart, kidneys), red meat, egg yolks, wheat germ, and oysters. These foods contain heme (heme = blood) iron, a form of iron that your body can easily absorb.

Whole grains, wheat germ, raisins, nuts, seed, prunes and prune juice, and potato skins contain nonheme iron. Because plants contain substances called *phytates,* which bind this iron into compounds, your body has a hard time getting at the iron. Eating plant foods with meat or with foods that are rich in vitamin C (like tomatoes) increases your ability to split away the phytates and get iron out of plant foods.

Zinc

Zinc protects nerve and brain tissue, bolsters the immune system, and is essential for healthy growth. Zinc is part of the enzymes (and hormones such as insulin) that metabolize food, and you can fairly call it the macho male mineral.

The largest quantities of zinc in the male human body are in the testes, where it's used in making a continuous supply of *testosterone,* the hormone a man needs to produce plentiful amounts of healthy, viable sperm. Without enough zinc, male fertility falters. So, yes, the old wives' tale is true: Oysters — a rich source of zinc — are useful for men. By the way, women also need zinc . . . just not as much as men do. How much is that? Aha! Check Table 11-1 or leaf back to Chapter 4.

Other good sources of zinc are meat, liver, and eggs. Plenty of zinc is in nuts, beans, miso, pumpkin and sunflower seeds, whole-grain products, and wheat germ. But the zinc in plants, like the iron in plants, occurs in compounds that your body absorbs less efficiently than the zinc in foods from animals.

Iodine

Iodine is a component of the thyroid hormones thyroxine and triiodothyronine, which help regulate cell activities. These hormones are also essential for protein synthesis, tissue growth (including the formation of healthy nerves and bones), and reproduction.

The best natural sources of iodine are seafood and plants grown near the ocean, but modern Americans are most likely to get the iodine they need from iodized salt (plain table salt with iodine added). And here's an odd nutritional note: You may get substantial amounts of iodine from milk. Are the cows consuming iodized salt? No. The milk is processed and stored in machines and vessels kept clean and sanitary with iodates and *iodophors,* iodine-based disinfectants. Tiny trace amounts get into the products sent to the stores. Iodates are also used as dough conditioners (additives that make dough more pliable), so you're also likely to find some iodine in most bread sold in supermarkets.

Selenium

Selenium was identified as an essential human nutrient in 1979 when Chinese nutrition researchers discovered that people with low body stores of selenium were at increased risk of *Keshan disease,* a disorder of the heart muscle with symptoms that include rapid heartbeat, enlarged heart, and (in severe cases) heart failure, a consequence most common among young children and women of childbearing age.

How does selenium protect your heart? One possibility is that it works as an antioxidant in tandem with vitamin E. A second possibility, raised by U.S. Department of Agriculture studies with laboratory rats, is that it prevents viruses from attacking heart muscle.

Here's some exciting news: The results of a four-year study involving 1,312 patients previously treated for skin cancer strongly suggests that daily doses of selenium in amounts 3.8 times the current recommended daily allowance (RDA) (55 micrograms) may reduce the incidence of cancers of the lung, prostate, colon, and rectum. The University of Arizona study was designed to see whether taking selenium lowered the risk of skin cancer. It didn't. But among the patients who got selenium rather than a placebo, 45 percent fewer lung cancers, 58 percent fewer colon and rectal cancers, 63 percent fewer prostate cancers, and a 50 percent lower death rate from cancer overall were recorded. Now a follow-up study will determine whether these results hold up.

Although fruits and vegetables grown in selenium-rich soils are themselves rich in this mineral, the best sources of selenium are seafood, meat and organ meats (liver, kidney), eggs, and dairy products.

Copper

Copper is an antioxidant found in enzymes that deactivate free radicals (pieces of molecules that can link up to form compounds that damage body tissues) and make it possible for your body to use iron. Copper also may play a role in slowing the aging process by decreasing the incidence of *protein glycation,* a reaction in which sugar molecules (gly = sugar) hook up with protein molecules in your bloodstream, twist the protein molecules out of shape, and make them unusable. Protein glycation may result in bone loss, high cholesterol, cardiac abnormalities, and a slew of other unpleasantries. In people with diabetes, excess protein glycation may also be one factor involved in complications such as loss of vision.

In addition, copper

✔ Promotes the growth of strong bones

✔ Protects the health of nerve tissue

✔ Prevents your hair from turning gray prematurely

But, no no, a thousand times, no: Large amounts of copper absolutely, and I repeat, *absolutely* will not turn gray hair back to its original color. Besides, megadoses of copper are potentially toxic.

You can get the copper you need from organ meats (such as liver and heart), seafood, nuts, and dried beans, including cacao beans (the beans used to make chocolate).

Manganese

Most of the manganese in your body is in glands (pituitary, mammary, pancreas), organs (liver, kidneys, intestines), and bones. Manganese is an essential constituent of the enzymes that metabolize carbohydrates and synthesize fats (including cholesterol). Manganese is important for a healthy reproductive system. During pregnancy, manganese speeds the proper growth of fetal tissue, particularly bones and cartilage.

You get manganese from whole grains, cereal products, fruits, and vegetables. Tea is also a good source of manganese.

Fluoride

Fluoride is the form of fluorine (an element) in drinking water. Your body stores fluoride in bones and teeth. Although researchers still have some questions about whether fluoride is an essential nutrient, it's clear that it hardens dental enamel, reducing your risk of getting cavities. In addition, some nutrition researchers suspect (but cannot prove) that some forms of fluoride strengthen bones.

Small amounts of fluoride are in all soil, water, plants, and animal tissues. You also get a steady supply of fluoride from fluoridated drinking water.

Chromium

Very small amounts of *trivalent chromium,* a digestible form of the very same metallic element that decorates your car and household appliances, are essential for several enzymes that you need to metabolize fat.

Chromium is also a necessary partner for glucose tolerance factor (GTF), a group of chemicals that enables insulin (an enzyme from the pancreas) to regulate your use of glucose, the end product of metabolism and the basic fuel for every body cell (see Chapter 8). In a recent joint study by USDA and the Beijing Medical University, adults with noninsulin-dependent diabetes who took chromium supplements had lower blood levels of sugar, protein, and cholesterol, which are all good signs for people with diabetes. In a related study, chromium reduced blood pressure in laboratory rats bred to develop hypertension (high blood pressure), a common complication in diabetes.

Right now, little information exists about the precise amounts of chromium in specific foods. Nonetheless, yeast, calves' liver, American cheese, wheat germ, and broccoli are regarded as valuable sources of this trace element.

Molybdenum

Molybdenum (pronounced mo-*lib*-de-num) is part of several enzymes that metabolize proteins. You get molybdenum from beans and grains. Cows eat grains, so milk and cheese have some molybdenum. Molybdenum also leeches into drinking water from surrounding soil. The molybdenum content of plants and drinking water depends entirely on how much molybdenum is in the soil.

Getting the Minerals You Need

Table 11-1 is a handy guide to foods that provide the minerals and trace elements your body needs. This chart is the easy way to figure out which foods (and how much) provide at least 25 percent of the recommended dietary allowance (RDA) for healthy adults ages 25 to 50.

No muss, no fuss, no calculators. Just photocopy these pages and stick them on the fridge. What an easy way to eat right! Wait! One more important note: When you see "men" or "women" in the following chart, it means "men and women ages 25 to 50" — unless otherwise noted.

Table 11-1 Get Your Minerals Here! — Foods and Serving Sizes	
Food	*Serving*
CALCIUM and PHOSPHORUS	**RDA: Calcium — men and women 1,000 mg** **RDA: Phosphorus — men and women 700 mg**
Breads, cereals, grains	
Bran muffin, English muffin	2 whole
Vegetables	
Broccoli, spinach, turnip greens (cooked)	1 cup
Dairy products	
Natural Gruyère, Romano, Swiss, Parmesan cheeses	1 ounce
Processed cheddar or Swiss cheeses	1½ ounces
Natural blue, brick, Camembert, feta, Gouda, Monterey, mozzarella, Muenster, provolone, Roquefort cheeses	2 ounces
Ricotta cheese	½ cup
Ice cream/ice milk	1 cup
Milk — all varieties, including chocolate	1 cup
Yogurt — all varieties	1 cup (8 ounces)
Other	
Tofu	½ cup, cubed

Food	Serving
MAGNESIUM	**RDA: Men 400-420 mg,* women 310-320 mg***
Breads, cereals, grains	
Bread — whole wheat	4 slices
Bran muffin, English muffin, pita — whole wheat	2 whole
Cold cereal	2 ounces
Vegetables	
Artichoke	2 medium
Black-eyed peas, chickpeas, soybeans, white beans (dry, cooked)	1 cup
Dairy products	
Milk — chocolate, made with skim milk	2 cups
Yogurt — plain nonfat	2 cups
Other	
Nuts and seeds	2 tbsp.
Tofu	½ cup cubed
IRON	**RDA: Men 8 mg, women 18 mg, 8 mg***
Breads, cereals, grains	
Bagel, bran muffin, pita	2 whole
Farina, oatmeal — instant, fortified	⅓ cup
Cold cereal	1 ounce
Fruits	
Apricots (dried, cooked)	1 cup
Vegetables	
Black-eyed peas, chickpeas, lentils, red and white beans (dried, cooked)	1 cup
Soybeans (cooked)	½ cup
Meat, poultry, fish	
Liver — beef, pork	3 ounces
Liver — chicken, turkey	1 cup, diced

(continued)

Table 11-1 *(continued)*

Food	Serving
Clams (raw) — meat only	3–4 ounces
Oysters (raw) — meat only	1–2 ounces
Other	
Pine nuts, seeds — pumpkin or squash	4 tbsp.
ZINC	**RDA: Men 11 mg, women 8 mg**
Breads, cereals, grains	
Cold cereals — fortified	2 ounces
Meat, poultry, fish	
Beef — all varieties, lean	3 ounces
Lamb — all varieties, lean	3 ounces
Tongue (braised)	3 ounces
Veal — roast, lean only	3 ounces
Chicken (no skin)	2 legs
Oysters	3 ounces
Dairy products	
Yogurt — all varieties	2 cups
Other	
Seeds — pumpkin or squash	4 tbsp.
COPPER	**AI: Men and women 900 mg.**
Breads, cereals, grains	
Barley (cooked)	⅓ cup
Bran muffin, English muffin, pita	2 whole
Fruits	
Prunes (dried, cooked)	1 cup
Vegetables	
Black-eyed peas, lentils, soybeans (cooked)	1 cup

Food	Serving
Meat, poultry, fish	
Liver — beef, calf	3 ounces
Liver — chicken, turkey	½ cup, diced
Crabmeat, lobster, oysters, shrimp	3 ounces
Other	
Almonds, Brazil nuts, cashews, hazelnuts/filberts, peanuts, pistachios, walnuts, mixed nuts	4 tbsp.
Seeds — pumpkin, sesame, squash, sunflower	4 tbsp.

*The lower numbers are for people age 19-30; the higher numbers, for people age 31+.
Good Sources of Nutrients (Washington, D.C.: U.S. Department of Agriculture/Human Nutrition
Service, 1990); Nutritive Value of Food (Washington, D.C.: USDA, 1991); DRI reports 1998-2004

Did you notice something missing from this list? Right you are. There are no entries for the essential trace elements chromium, fluoride, iodine, molybdenum, and selenium, because a healthful, varied diet provides sufficient quantities of these nutrients. Iodized salt and fluoridated water are extra insurance.

Overdoses and Underdoses: Too Much and Too Little

The Recommended Dietary Allowances (RDAs) and Adequate Intakes (AIs) for minerals and trace elements are generous allowances, large enough to prevent deficiency but not so large that they trigger toxic side effects. (Read more about RDAs and AIs in Chapter 4.)

Avoiding mineral deficiency

What happens if you don't get enough minerals and trace elements? Some minerals, such as phosphorus and magnesium, are so widely available in food that deficiencies are rare to nonexistent. No nutrition scientist has yet been able to identify a naturally occurring deficiency of sulfur, manganese, chromium, or molybdenum in human beings who follow a sensible diet. Most drinking water contains adequate fluoride, and Americans get so much copper (can it be from chocolate bars?) that deficiency is practically unheard of in the United States.

But other minerals are more problematic:

- **Calcium:** Without enough calcium, a child's bones and teeth don't grow strong and straight, and an adult's bones lose minerals and weaken. Calcium is a team player. To protect against deficiency, you also need adequate amounts of vitamin D, the nutrient that allows you to absorb the calcium you get from food or supplements. Milk fortified with vitamin D has done much to eliminate rickets (see Chapter 10 on vitamins).

- **Iron:** *Iron deficiency anemia* is not just an old advertising slogan. Lacking sufficient iron, your body can't make the hemoglobin it requires to carry energy-sustaining oxygen to every tissue. As a result, you're often tired and feel weak. Mild iron deficiency may also inhibit intellectual performance. In one Johns Hopkins study, high school girls scored higher verbal, memory, and learning test scores when they took supplements providing Recommended Dietary Amounts of iron.

  Check with your doctor before downing iron supplements or cereals fortified with 100 percent of your daily iron requirement, the *Environmental Nutrition* newsletter warns. Hemochromatosis, a common but often-undiagnosed genetic defect affecting one in every 250 Americans, can lead to *iron overload,* an increased absorption of the mineral linked to arthritis, heart disease, and diabetes, as well as an increased risk of infectious diseases and cancer (viruses and cancer cells thrive in iron-rich blood).

- **Zinc:** An adequate supply of zinc is vital for making testosterone and healthy sperm. Men who don't get enough zinc may be temporarily infertile. Zinc deprivation can make you lose your appetite and your ability to taste food. It may also weaken your immune system, increasing your risk of infections. Wounds heal more slowly when you don't get enough zinc. That includes the tissue damage caused by working out. In plain language: If you don't get the zinc you need, your charley horse may linger longer. And, yes, zinc may fight the symptoms of the common cold. To date, several studies have confirmed that sucking on lozenges containing one form of zinc (zinc gluconate) shortens a cold — by a day or two. Others show no differences. Your choice.

  These results are for adults, not children, and the zinc tablets are meant just for the several days of your cold. To find out more about zinc excess, see the section "Knowing how much is too much" later in this chapter.

- **Iodine:** A moderate iodine deficiency leads to *goiter* (a swollen thyroid gland) and reduced production of thyroid hormones. A more severe deficiency early in life may cause a form of mental and physical retardation called *cretinism.*

✔ **Selenium:** Not enough selenium in your diet? Watch out for muscle pain or weakness. To protect against selenium problems, make sure that you get plenty of vitamin E. Some animal studies show that a selenium deficiency responds to vitamin E supplements. And vice versa.

Knowing how much is too much

Like some vitamins, some minerals are potentially toxic in large doses:

✔ **Calcium:** Though clearly beneficial in amounts higher than the current RDAs, calcium is not problem-free:

- Constipation, bloating, nausea, and intestinal gas are common side effects among healthy people taking supplements equal to 1,500 to 4,000 milligrams of calcium a day.

- Doses higher than 4,000 milligrams a day may be linked to kidney damage.

- Megadoses of calcium can bind with iron and zinc, making it harder for your body to absorb these two essential trace elements.

✔ **Phosphorus:** Too much phosphorus can lower your body stores of calcium.

✔ **Magnesium:** Megadoses of magnesium appear safe for healthy people, but if you have kidney disease, the magnesium overload can cause weak muscles, breathing difficulty, irregular heartbeat and/or cardiac arrest (your heart stops beating).

✔ **Iron:** Overdosing on iron supplements can be deadly, especially for young children. The lethal dose for a young child may be as low as 3 grams (3,000 milligrams) elemental iron at one time. This is the amount in 60 tablets with 50 milligrams elemental iron each. For adults, the lethal dose is estimated to be 200 to 250 milligrams elemental iron per kilogram (2.2 pounds) of body weight. That's about 13,600 milligrams for a 150-pound person — the amount you'd get in 292 tablets with 50 milligrams elemental iron each. New FDA rules require individual blister packaging for supplements containing more than 30 milligrams iron to foil tiny fingers and prevent accidental overdoses.

✔ **Zinc:** Moderately high doses of zinc (up to 25 milligrams a day) may slow your body's absorption of copper. Doses 27 to 37 times the RDA (11 mg/males; 8 mg/females) may interfere with your immune function and make you more susceptible to infection, the very thing that normal doses of zinc protect against. Gram doses (2,000 milligrams/2 grams) of zinc cause symptoms of zinc poisoning: vomiting, gastric upset, and irritation of the stomach lining.

✔ **Iodine:** Overdoses of iodine cause exactly the same problems as iodine deficiency: goiter. How can that be? When you consume very large amounts of iodine, the mineral stimulates your thyroid gland, which swells in a furious attempt to step up its production of thyroid hormones. This reaction may occur among people who eat lots of dried seaweed for long periods of time.

✔ **Selenium:** In China, nutrition researchers have linked doses as high as 5 milligrams of selenium a day (90 times the RDA) to thickened but fragile nails, hair loss, and perspiration with a garlicky odor. In the United States, a small group of people who had accidentally gotten a supplement that mistakenly contained 27.3 milligrams selenium (436 times the RDA) fell victim to *selenium intoxication* — fatigue, abdominal pain, nausea and diarrhea, and nerve damage. The longer they used the supplements, the worse their symptoms were.

✔ **Fluoride:** Despite decades of argument, no scientific proof exists that the fluorides in drinking water increase the risk of cancer in human beings. But there's no question that large doses of fluoride — which you're unlikely to consume unless you drink well or groundwater in the western United States — causes fluorosis (brown patches on your teeth), brittle bones, fatigue, and muscle weakness. Over long periods of time, high doses of fluoride may also cause *outcroppings* (little bumps) of bone on the spine.

Fluoride levels higher than 6 milligrams a day are considered hazardous.

✔ **Molybdenum:** Doses of molybdenum two to seven times the Adequate Intake (AI) (45 micrograms) may increase the amount of copper you excrete in urine.

Exceeding the RDAs: People who need extra minerals

If your diet provides enough minerals to meet the RDAs, you're in pretty good shape most of the time. But a restrictive diet, the circumstances of your reproductive life, and just plain getting older can increase your need for minerals. Here are some scenarios.

You're a strict vegetarian

Vegetarians who pass up fish, meat, and poultry must get their iron either from fortified grain products such as breakfast cereals or commercial breads or naturally from foods such as seeds, nuts, blackstrap molasses, raisins, prune juice, potato skins, green leafy vegetables, tofu, miso, or brewer's yeast. Because iron in plant foods is bound into compounds that are difficult for the human body to absorb, iron supplements are pretty much standard fare.

NUTRITION SPEAK

I'm looking for an iron supplement. What's this "ferrous" stuff?

The iron in iron supplements comes in several different forms, each one composed of elemental iron (the kind of iron your body actually uses) coupled with an organic acid that makes the iron easy to absorb.

The iron compounds commonly found in iron supplements are:

- Ferrous citrate (iron plus citric acid)

- Ferrous fumarate (iron plus fumaric acid)

- Ferrous gluconate (iron plus a sugar derivative)

- Ferrous lactate (iron plus lactic acid, an acid formed in the fermentation of milk)

- Ferrous succinate (iron plus succinic acid)

- Ferrous sulfate (iron plus a sulfuric acid derivative)

In your stomach, these compounds dissolve at different rates, yielding different amounts of elemental iron. So supplement labels list the compound and the amount of elemental iron it provides, like this:

Ferrous gluconate 300 milligrams

Elemental iron 34 milligrams

This tells you that the supplement has 300 milligrams of the iron compound ferrous gluconate, which gives you 34 milligrams of usable elemental iron. If the label just says "iron," that's shorthand for elemental iron. The elemental iron number is what you look for in judging the iron content of a vitamin/mineral supplement.

Vegans — vegetarians who avoid all foods from animals, including dairy products — have a similar problem getting the calcium they need. Calcium is in vegetables, but it, like iron, is bound into hard-to-absorb compounds. So vegans need calcium-rich substitutes. Good food choices are soybean milk fortified with calcium, orange juice with added calcium, and tofu processed with calcium sulfate.

You live inland, away from the ocean

Now here's a story of 20th century nutritional success. Seafood and plants grown near the ocean are exposed to iodine-rich seawater. Freshwater fish, plants grown far from the sea, and the animals that feed on these fish and plants are not exposed to iodine. So people who live inland and get all their food from local gardens and farms cannot get the iodine they need from food.

American savvy and technology rode to the rescue in 1924 with the introduction of iodized salt. Then came refrigerated railroad cars and trucks to carry food from both coasts to every inland city and state. Together, modern salt and efficient shipment virtually eliminated goiter, the iodine deficiency disease, in this country. Nonetheless, millions of people worldwide still suffer from chronic iodine deficiency.

You're a man

Just as women lose iron during menstrual bleeding, men lose zinc at ejaculation. Men who are extremely active sexually may need extra zinc. The trouble is, no one has ever written down standards for what constitutes "extremely active." Check this one out with your doctor.

Men who take a daily supplement of 200 micrograms selenium seem to cut their risk of prostate cancer by two-thirds. The selenium supplement also produces an overall drop in cancer mortality, plus a significantly lower risk of prostate cancer, colon cancer, and lung cancer in both men and women.

You're a woman

The average woman loses about 2 to 3 teaspoons of blood during each menstrual period, a loss of 1.4 milligrams of iron. Women whose periods are very heavy lose more blood and more iron. Because getting the iron you need from a diet providing fewer than 2,000 calories a day may be virtually impossible, you may develop a mild iron deficiency. To remedy this, some doctors prescribe a daily iron supplement.

Women who use an intrauterine device (IUD) may also be given a prescription for iron supplements because IUDs irritate the lining of the uterus and cause a small but significant loss of blood and iron.

You're pregnant

The news about pregnancy is that women may not need extra calcium. This finding, released late in 1998, is so surprising that it probably pays to stay tuned for more — and definitely check with your own doctor. Meanwhile, pregnant women still need supplements to build not only fetal tissues but also new tissues and blood vessels in their own bodies. Animal studies suggest (but don't prove) that you may also need extra copper to protect nerve cells in the fetal brain. Nutritional supplements for pregnant women are specifically formulated to provide the extra nutrients they need.

NUTRITION SPEAK

Calcium supplements: What kind of calcium is in that pill?

Calcium-rich foods give you calcium paired with natural organic acids, a combination that your body easily digests and absorbs.

The form of calcium most commonly found in supplements, however, is calcium carbonate, the kind of calcium that occurs naturally in limestone and oyster shells.

Calcium carbonate is a versatile compound. Not only does it build strong bones and teeth, but it also neutralizes stomach acid and relieves heartburn. Calcium carbonate antacids can be used as calcium supplements. They're nutritionally sound and generally cost less than products designed solely as nutritional supplements.

Some calcium supplements contain compounds that mix calcium with an organic acid. Calcium lactate is calcium plus lactic acid, the combination that occurs naturally in milk. Calcium citrate is calcium plus citric acid, an acid found in fruits.

These compounds are easier to digest, but they're sometimes more expensive than calcium carbonate products. Calcium carbonate is nearly half calcium, a very high percentage. But unless your stomach is very acidic, it's hard for your digestive system to break the compound open and get at the elemental calcium (the kind of calcium your body can use). You can increase your absorption of calcium from calcium carbonate by taking the tablets with meals.

Because different calcium compounds yield different amounts of elemental calcium, the label lists both the calcium compound and the amount of elemental calcium provided, like this:

Calcium carbonate, 500 milligrams, providing 200 milligrams elemental calcium.

Whenever you see the word calcium alone, it stands for elemental calcium.

The human body absorbs calcium most efficiently in amounts of 500 milligrams or less. You get more calcium from one 500-milligram calcium tablet twice a day than one 1,000-milligram tablet. If the 1,000-milligram tablets are a better buy, break them in half.

Warning: Not all antacids double as dietary supplements. Antacids containing magnesium or aluminum compounds are safe for neutralizing stomach acid, but they won't work as supplements. In fact, just the opposite is true. Taking magnesium antacids reduces your absorption of calcium, and taking aluminum antacids reduces your absorption of phosphorus. Because manufacturers sometimes change the ingredients in their products without notice, you always need to read the product label before assuming that an antacid can double as a calcium supplement.

You're breast-feeding

Nursing mothers need extra calcium, phosphorus, magnesium, iron, zinc, and selenium to protect their own bodies while producing nutritious breast milk. The same supplements that provide extra nutrients for pregnant women will meet a nursing mother's needs.

Wow — You think that was a hot flash?

Then you need extra calcium. Both men and women produce the sex hormones testosterone and estrogen, although men make proportionately more testosterone and women, more estrogen. Testosterone builds bone; estrogen preserves it.

At menopause, a woman's production of estrogen drops precipitously, and her bones rapidly become less dense. As men age and their testosterone levels drop, they're also at risk of losing bone tissue, but the loss is less rapid and dramatic than a woman's.

For both men and woman, severe loss of bone density can lead to osteoporosis and an increased risk of bone fractures, a condition more common among women of Caucasian and Asian ancestry. Estrogen supplements can help a woman maintain bone tissue, but taking the hormone may have serious side effects, including an increased risk of breast cancer.

Twenty years ago, nutritionists thought it impossible to stop age-related loss of bone density — that your body ceased to absorb calcium when you passed your mid-20s. Today, medications such as alendronate (Fosamax) protect an aging woman's bones without estrogen's potentially harmful effects. Increasing your consumption of calcium plus vitamin D may also be helpful, regardless of your gender. But the most recent studies — by which I mean the study released in February 2006 as I am typing these words — says the value of extra calcium may not be as high as once believed. What can I say? Stay tuned for more on this one.

Chapter 12

Phabulous Phytochemicals

. . . .

In This Chapter

▶ Explaining what phytochemicals are and why they're important

▶ Eying accelerating research on phytochemicals

▶ Using phytochemicals every day

. . . .

*J*ust when you think you have a handle on a big issue like nutrition, the Folks in Charge of Everything toss something new on the table.

I thought I included something about every aspect of food and health in the first edition of *Nutrition For Dummies.* Then a new word started showing up in nutrition articles and reports. The word is *phytochemicals,* a five-syllable mouthful meaning chemicals from plants. In addition, I thought it was so interesting that I wrote an entirely new chapter on the subject for *NFD*/2E (which is what my editor calls the second edition) and *NFD*/3E. Now here we are in *NFD*/4E, and by golly, finding a nutrition junkie who hasn't heard of phytochemicals is difficult. But what people are hearing has turned around a bit.

Phytochemicals (chemicals manufactured only in plants) are the substances that produce many of the beneficial effects associated with a diet that includes lots of fruits, vegetables, beans, and grains. This chapter gives you a brief summary of the nature of phytochemicals, tells where to find them, and explains how they work.

Phytochemicals Are Everywhere

Did you take French literature in high school or college? If your answer is no, you may as well skip to the third sentence in the paragraph that follows. But if your answer's yes, then you're probably familiar with Molière's *The Bourgeois Gentleman.* The bourgeois gentleman is a lovable but pompous character who's surprised to discover he's been speaking prose all his life without knowing it.

Your relationship with phytochemicals is probably something like that. You've been eating them all your life without knowing it. The following are all phytochemicals:

- ✔ *Carotenoids,* the pigments that make fruits and vegetables orange, red, and yellow (dark green vegetables and fruits like kiwi contain these pigments, too, but green chlorophyll masks the carotenoids' colors)

- ✔ *Thiocyanates,* the smelly sulfur compounds that make you turn up your nose at the aroma of boiling cabbage

- ✔ *Daidzein* and *genistein,* hormonelike compounds in many fruits and vegetables

- ✔ Dietary fiber

These and other phytochemicals, such as vitamins (yes, vitamins), perform beneficial housekeeping chores in your body. They

- ✔ Keep your cells healthy

- ✔ Help prevent the formation of *carcinogens* (cancer-producing substances)

- ✔ Reduce cholesterol levels

- ✔ Help move food through your intestinal tract

The undeniable value of phytochemicals is one reason the U.S. Department of Agriculture/Health and Human Services *Dietary Guidelines for Americans* urges you to have at least five servings of fruits and vegetables and several servings of grains every day.

Did you notice that no minerals appear in the list of phytochemicals? The omission is deliberate. Plants don't manufacture minerals; they absorb them from the soil. Therefore, minerals aren't phytochemicals.

Perusing the Different Kinds of Phytochemicals

The most interesting phytochemicals in plant foods appear to be antioxidants, hormonelike compounds, and enzyme-activating sulfur compounds. Each group plays a specific role in maintaining health and reducing your risk of certain illnesses.

Antioxidants

Antioxidants are named for their ability to prevent a chemical reaction called *oxidation,* which enables molecular fragments called *free radicals* to join together, forming potentially carcinogenic (cancer-causing) compounds in your body.

Antioxidants also slow the normal wear-and-tear on body cells, so some researchers noted that a diet rich in plant foods (fruits, vegetables, grains, and beans) seems likely to reduce the risk of heart disease and maybe reduce the risk of some kinds of cancer. For example, consuming lots of lycopene (the red carotenoid in tomatoes) has been linked to a lower risk of prostate cancer — as long as the tomatoes are mixed with a dab of oil, which makes the lycopene easy to absorb.

However (you knew this was coming, right?), recent studies show that although a diet rich in fruits and veggies is healthful as all get-out, stuffing yourself with the antioxidant vitamins A and C has ab-so-lute-ly no effect on the risk of heart disease.

Hormonelike compounds

Many plants contain compounds that behave like *estrogens,* the female sex hormones. Because only animal bodies can produce true hormones, these plant chemicals are called *hormonelike compounds* or *phytoestrogens* (plant estrogen). Seems fair.

The three kinds of phytoestrogens are

- ✔ Isoflavones, in fruits, vegetables, and beans
- ✔ Lignans, in grains
- ✔ Coumestans, in sprouts and alfalfa

The most-studied phytoestrogens are the isoflavones known as *daidzein* and *genistein* (found in soy), two compounds with a chemical structure similar to *estradiol,* which is the estrogen produced by mammalian ovaries.

Like natural or synthetic estrogens, daidzein and genistein hook onto sensitive spots in reproductive tissue (breast, ovary, uterus, prostate) called estrogen receptors. But phytoestrogens have weaker estrogenic effects than natural or synthetic estrogens. It takes about 100,000 molecules of daidzein or genistein to produce the same estrogenic effect as one molecule of estradiol. Every phytoestrogen molecule that hooks onto an estrogen receptor displaces a stronger estrogen molecule. As a result, researchers suggested that consuming isoflavone-rich foods such as soy products may provide post-menopausal women with the benefits of estrogen (stronger bones and relief from hot flashes) without the higher risk of reproductive cancers (of the breast, ovary, or uterus) associated with hormone replacement therapy (HRT). The theory was supported by the fact that the incidence of breast and uterine cancer, heart disease, osteoporosis, and menopausal discomfort is lower in countries where soy — a primary source of phytoestrogens — is a significant part of the diet.

However, recent animal and human studies offer conflicting evidence. On the one hand, these studies

✔ Raise questions about the safety of phytoestrogen-rich foods for women with hormone-sensitive tumors

✔ Show that phytoestrogen may stimulate tumor growth in animals whose ovaries have been removed

✔ Demonstrate that isoflavone-rich foods have only modest effects on preserving bone and relieving "hot flashes" at menopause

One the other hand, including isoflavone-rich soy foods such as tofu, miso, tempeh, soy milk, soy flour, and soy protein in a healthful diet

✔ May reduce total cholesterol, lower LDL ("bad cholesterol"), and maintain or even increase blood levels of HDL ("good cholesterol"). In 2005, researchers at the Johns Hopkins University School of Nursing announced the results of a 216-woman study funded by the National Heart, Lung, and Blood Institute in which women consuming 20 grams of soy proteins per day had significant decreases in LDLs, while women who were given the same amount of milk protein did not.

✔ Helps people feel full longer so they can stick to a lower-calorie diet for managing weight loss.

Bottom Line? According to the International Food Information Council, "Further clinical studies will continue to increase understanding of the role of soy in maintaining and improving health." Couldn't have said it better myself.

Sulfur compounds

Slide an apple pie in the oven, and soon the kitchen fills with a yummy aroma that makes your mouth water and your digestive juices flow. But boil some cabbage and — yuck! What is that awful smell? It's sulfur, the same chemical that identifies rotten eggs.

Cruciferous vegetables (named for the Latin word for "cross," in reference to their *x*-shaped blossoms) — such as broccoli, Brussels sprouts, cauliflower, kale, kohlrabi, mustard seed, radishes, rutabaga, turnips, and watercress — all contain stinky sulfur compounds, such as *sulforaphane glucosinolate (SGSD), glucobrassicin, gluconapin, gluconasturtin, neoglucobrassicin,* and *sinigrin,* that seem to tell your body to rev up its production of enzymes that inactivate and help eliminate carcinogens.

These smelly sulfurs may be one reason why people who eat lots of cruciferous veggies generally have a lower risk of cancer. In animal studies at Johns Hopkins University School of Medicine, rats given chemicals known to cause breast tumors were less likely to develop tumors when they were given broccoli sprouts, a food that's unusually high in sulforaphane. In 2005, a human trial conducted in China by researchers from Johns Hopkins, Qidong Liver Cancer Institute, Jiao Tong University (Shanghai), and the University of Minnesota Cancer Center showed that the sulforaphane-rich sprouts appear to help the body defang aflatoxins produced by molds that grow on grains such as rice. *Aflatoxins,* which damage cells and raise the risk of cancer, may be linked to the high incidence of stomach and liver cancer in China. Further studies are in the planning phases. (But of course.)

Dietary fiber

Dietary fiber is a special bonus found only in plant foods. You can't get it from meat or fish or poultry or eggs or dairy foods.

Soluble dietary fiber, such as the pectins in apples and the gums in beans, mops up cholesterol and lowers your risk of heart disease. Insoluble dietary fiber, such as the cellulose in fruit skins, bulks up stool and prevents constipation, moving food more quickly through your gut so there's less time for food to create substances thought to trigger the growth of cancerous cells. (Turn to Chapter 4 to find out how much dietary fiber you need to get each day and to Chapter 8 to read everything you ever wanted to know about dietary fiber — maybe even more.)

Phorecasting the Phuture of Phytochemicals

Yes, I know that misspelling *forecasting* as "phorecasting" and *future* as "phuture" is gross. Yes, I know I already named this chapter "Phabulous Phytochemicals" and that should have been enough, but I just couldn't resist the tempting play on words.

Please don't let my lack of semantic restraint turn you away from the fact that phytochemical research is serious stuff that eventually should enable people to identify biochemical reactions that trigger — or prevent — specific medical conditions.

While you're waiting for final analyses, the best nutrition advice is to dig into those veggies, fruits, and grains — and turn to Chapter 13 to find out why you need to wash them down with plenty of cold, clear water.

Chapter 13

Water Works

*Y*our body is mostly (50 to 70 percent) water. Exactly how much water depends on how old you are and how much muscle and fat you have. Muscle tissue has more water than fat tissue. Because the average male body has proportionately more muscle than the average female body, it also has more water. For the same reason — more muscle — a young body has more water than an older one.

You definitely won't enjoy the experience, but if you have to, you can live without food for weeks at a time, getting subsistence levels of nutrients by digesting your own muscle and fat. But water's different. Without it, you'll die in a matter of days — more quickly in a place warm enough to make you perspire and lose water more quickly.

This chapter clues you in on why water is so important, not to mention how you can manage to keep your body's water level, well, *level*.

Investigating the Many Ways Your Body Uses Water

Water is a solvent. It dissolves other substances and carries nutrients and other material (such as blood cells) around the body, making it possible for every organ to do its job. You need water to

✔ Digest food, dissolving nutrients so that they can pass through the intestinal cell walls into your bloodstream, and move food along through your intestinal tract

✔ Carry waste products out of your body

✔ Provide a medium in which biochemical reactions such as metabolism (digesting food, producing energy, and building tissue) occur

✔ Send electrical messages between cells so that your muscles can move, your eyes can see, your brain can think, and so on

✔ Regulate body temperature — cooling your body with moisture (perspiration) that evaporates on your skin

✔ Lubricate your moving parts

Maintaining the Right Amount of Water in Your Body

As much as three-quarters of the water in your body is in *intracellular fluid,* the liquid inside body cells. The rest is in *extracellular fluid,* which is all the other body liquids, such as

✔ Interstitial fluid (the fluid between cells)

✔ Blood plasma (the clear liquid in blood)

✔ Lymph (a clear, slightly yellow fluid collected from body tissues that flows through your lymph nodes and eventually into your blood vessels)

✔ Bodily secretions such as sweat, seminal fluid, and vaginal fluids

✔ Urine

A healthy body has just the right amount of fluid inside and outside each cell, a situation medical folk call *fluid balance.* Maintaining your fluid balance is essential to life. If too little water is inside a cell, it shrivels and dies. If there's too much water, the cell bursts.

A balancing act: The role of electrolytes

Your body maintains its fluid balance through the action of substances called *electrolytes,* which are mineral compounds that, when dissolved in water, become electrically charged particles called *ions.*

Many minerals, including calcium, phosphorus, and magnesium, form compounds that dissolve into charged particles. But nutritionists generally use the term electrolyte to describe sodium, potassium, and chlorine. The most familiar electrolyte is the one found on every dinner table: sodium chloride — plain old table salt. (In water, its molecules dissolve into two ions: one sodium ion and one chloride ion.)

Fluoridated water: The real Tooth Fairy

Except for the common cold, dental cavities are the most common human medical problem.

You get cavities from *mutans streptococci,* bacteria that live in dental plaque. The bacteria digest and ferment carbohydrate residue on your teeth (plain table sugar is the worst offender) leaving acid that eats away at the mineral surface of the tooth. This eating away is called *decay.* When the decay gets past the enamel to the softer pulp inside of the tooth, your tooth hurts. And you head for the dentist even though you hate it so much you'd almost rather put up with the pain. But almost doesn't count, so off you go.

Brushing and flossing help prevent cavities by cleaning your teeth so that bacteria have less to feast on. Another way to reduce your susceptibility to cavities is to drink *fluoridated water* — water containing the mineral fluorine.

Fluoride — the form of fluorine found in food and water — combines with other minerals in teeth and makes the minerals less soluble (harder to dissolve). You get the most benefit by drinking water containing 1 part fluoride to every 1 million parts water (1 ppm) from the day you're born until the day you get your last permanent tooth, usually around age 11 to 13.

Some drinking water, notably in the American Southwest, is fluoridated naturally when it flows through rocks containing fluorine. Sometimes so much fluoride is in this water that it causes a brownish spotting (or mottling) that occurs while teeth are developing and accumulating minerals. This effect doesn't occur with drinking water artificially supplemented with fluoride at the approved standard of one part fluoride to every million parts of water.

Because fluorides concentrate in bones, some people believe that drinking fluoridated water raises the risk of bone cancers, but no evidence to support this claim has ever been found in human beings. However, in 1990, a U.S. Public Health Service's National Toxicology Program (NTP) study of the long-term effects of high fluoride consumption on laboratory rats and mice added fuel to the fire: Four of the 1,044 laboratory rats and mice fed high doses of fluoride for two years developed *osteosarcoma,* a form of bone cancer.

The study sent an immediate *frisson* (shiver of fear) through the health community, but within a year, federal officials reviewing the study issued an opinion endorsing the safety and effectiveness of fluoridated water.

Here's why: First, the number of cancers among the laboratory animals was low enough to have occurred simply by chance. Second, the cancers occurred only in male rats; no cases were reported in female rats or mice of either sex. Finally, the amount of fluorides the animals ingested was 50 to 100 times higher than what you get in drinking water. To get as much fluoride as those rats did, human beings would have to drink more than 380 8-ounce glasses of fluoridated water a day.

Today, more than half the people living in the United States have access to adequately fluoridated public water supplies. The result is a lifelong 50 percent to 70 percent reduction in cavities among the residents of these communities.

Under normal circumstances, the fluid inside your cells has more potassium than sodium and chloride. The fluid outside is just the opposite: more sodium and chloride than potassium. The cell wall is a *semipermeable membrane;* some things pass through, but others don't. Water molecules and small mineral molecules flow through freely, unlike larger molecules such as proteins.

The process by which sodium flows out and potassium flows in to keep things on an even keel is called the *sodium pump.* If this process were to cease, sodium ions would build up inside your cells. Sodium attracts water; the more sodium there is inside the cell, the more water flows in. Eventually, the cell would burst and die. The sodium pump, regular as a clock, prevents this imbalance from happening so you can move along, blissfully unaware of those efficient, electric ions.

Dehydrating without enough water and electrolytes

Drink more water than you need, and your healthy body simply shrugs its shoulders, so to speak, urinates more copiously, and readjusts the water level. It's hard for a healthy person on a normal diet to drink himself or herself to death on water.

But if you don't get enough water, your body lets you know pretty quickly.

The first sign is thirst, that unpleasant dryness in your mouth caused by the loss of water from cells in your gums, tongue, and cheeks. The second sign is reduced urination.

What else do those electrolytes do?

In addition to keeping fluid levels balanced, sodium, potassium, and chloride (the form of chlorine found in food) ions create electrical impulses that enable cells to send messages back and forth between themselves so you can think, see, move, and perform all the bioelectrical functions that you take for granted.

Sodium, potassium, and chloride are also major minerals (see Chapter 11) and essential nutrients. Like other nutrients, they're useful in these bodily processes:

✔ Sodium helps digest proteins and carbohydrates and keeps your blood from becoming too acidic or too alkaline.

✔ Potassium is used in digestion to synthesize proteins and starch and is a major constituent of muscle tissue.

✔ Chloride is a constituent of hydrochloric acid, which breaks down food in your stomach. It's also used by white blood cells to make *hypochlorite,* a natural antiseptic.

Reduced urination is a protective mechanism triggered by *ADH,* a hormone secreted by the hypothalamus, a gland at the base of your brain. The initials are short for *antidiuretic hormone.* Remember, a diuretic is a substance, such as caffeine, that increases urine production. ADH does just the opposite, helping your body conserve water rather than eliminate it.

If you don't heed these signals, your tissues will begin to dry out. In other words, you're dehydrating, and if you don't — or can't — get water, you won't survive.

Getting the Water You Need

Because you don't store water, you need to take in a new supply every day, enough to replace what you lose when you breathe, perspire, urinate, and defecate. On average, this needed amount adds up to 1,500 to 3,000 milliliters (50 to 100 ounces; 6 to 12.5 cups) a day. Here's where the water goes:

- ✔ 850 to 1,200 milliliters (28 to 40 ounces) is lost in breath and perspiration.

- ✔ 600 to 1,600 milliliters (20 to 53 ounces) is lost in urine.

- ✔ 50 to 200 milliliters (1.6 to 6.6 ounces) is lost in feces.

Toss in some extra ounces for a safe margin, and you get the current recommendations that women age 19 and up consume about 11 cups of water a day and men age 19 and up, about 15. But not all that water must come in a cup from the tap. About 15 percent of the water that you need is created when you digest and metabolize food. The end products of digestion and metabolism are carbon dioxide (a waste product that you breathe out of your body) and water composed of hydrogen from food and oxygen from the air that you breathe. The rest of your daily water comes directly from what you eat and drink. You can get water from, well, plain water. Eight 10-ounce glasses give you 2,400 milliliters, approximately enough to replace what your body loses every day, so everyone from athletes to couch potatoes knows that a healthy body needs eight full glasses of water a day. Or at least they thought they knew, but then Dartmouth Medical School kidney specialist Heinz Valtin turned off the tap.

Yes, the National Research Council's Food and Nutrition Board says each of us needs about 1 milliliter (ml) of water for each calorie of food we consume. On a 2,000-calorie-a-day diet, that's about 74 fluid ounces, or slightly more than nine 8-ounce glasses a day. Fair enough, Valtin said, but who says that it all has to come from, well, water? His report in the *American Journal of Physiology* (2003) points out that some of the water you require is right there in your food. Fruits and vegetables are full of water. Lettuce, for example, is 90 percent water. Furthermore, you get water from foods that you'd never think of as water sources: hamburger (more than 50 percent), cheese (the softer the cheese, the higher the water content — Swiss cheese is 38 percent water; skim milk ricotta, 74 percent), a plain, hard bagel (29 percent water), milk powder (2 percent), and even butter and margarine (10 percent). Only oils have no water.

How does water know where to go?

Osmosis is the principle that governs how water flows through a semipermeable membrane (one that lets only certain substances pass through) such as the one surrounding a body cell.

Here's the principle: Water flows through a semipermeable membrane from the side where the liquid solution is least dense to the side where it's denser. In other words, the water, acting as if it has a mind of its own, tries to equalize the densities of the liquids on both sides of the membrane.

How does the water know which side is more dense? Now that one's easy: Wherever the sodium content is higher. When more sodium is inside the cell, more water flows in to dilute it. When more sodium is in the fluid outside the

cell, water flows out of the cell to dilute the liquid on the outside.

Osmosis explains why drinking seawater doesn't hydrate your body. When you drink seawater, liquid flows out of your cells to dilute the salty solution in your intestinal tract. The more you drink, the more water you lose. When you drink seawater, you're literally drinking yourself into dehydration.

Of course, the same thing happens — though certainly to a lesser degree — when you eat salted pretzels or nuts. The salt in your mouth makes your saliva saltier. This draws liquid out of the cells in your cheeks and tongue, which feel uncomfortably dry. You need . . . a drink of water!

In other words (actually in Valtin's words), a healthy adult in a temperate climate who isn't perspiring heavily can get enough water simply by drinking only when he or she is thirsty. Gulp. Or by drinking water when he or she is also drinking lots of coffee, tea, soft drinks, or alcohol.

Not all liquids are equally liquefying. The caffeine in coffee and tea and the alcohol in beer, wine, and spirits are *diuretics,* chemicals that make you urinate more copiously. Although caffeinated and alcohol beverages provide water, they also increase its elimination from your body — which is why you feel thirsty the morning after you've had a glass or two of wine. And when you feel thirsty, what do you do? Drink some water.

Taking in Extra Water and Electrolytes As Needed

In the United States, most people regularly consume much more sodium than they need. In fact, some people who are sodium-sensitive may end up with high blood pressure that can be lowered if they reduce their sodium intake. For more about high blood pressure, check out *High Blood Pressure For Dummies* (published by Wiley) by Alan L. Rubin, M.D.

Potassium and chloride are found in so many foods that here, too, a dietary deficiency is a rarity. In fact, the only recorded case of chloride deficiency was among infants given a formula liquid from which the chloride was inadvertently omitted.

In 2004, the Adequate Intake (AI) for sodium, potassium, and chloride were set at one-size-fits-all averages for a healthy adult age 19–50 weighing 70 kilograms (154 pounds; see Chapter 4 for more on AI):

- ✔ **Sodium:** 1,500 milligrams
- ✔ **Potassium:** 4,700 milligrams
- ✔ **Chloride:** 2,300 milligrams

Most Americans get much more as a matter of course, and sometimes you actually need extra water and electrolytes. The next sections tell you when.

Death by dehydration: Not a pretty sight

Every day, you lose an amount of water equal to about 4 percent of your total weight. If you don't take in enough water to replace what you lose naturally by breathing, perspiring, urinating, and defecating, warning signals go off loud and clear.

Early on, when you've lost just a little water, equal to about 1 percent of your body weight, you feel thirsty. If you ignore thirst, it grows more intense.

When water loss rises to about 2 percent of your weight, your appetite fades. Your circulation slows as water seeps out of blood cells and blood plasma. And you experience a sense of emotional discomfort, a perception that things are, well, not right.

By the time your water loss equals 4 percent of your body weight (5 pounds for a 130-pound woman; 7 pounds for a 170-pound man), you're slightly nauseated, your skin is flushed, and you're very, very tired. With less water circulating through your tissues, your hands and feet tingle, your head aches, your temperature rises, you breathe more quickly, and your pulse quickens.

After this, things begin spiraling downhill. When your water loss reaches 10 percent of your body weight, your tongue swells, your kidneys start to fail, and you're so dizzy that you can't stand on one foot with your eyes closed. In fact, you probably can't even try: Your muscles are in spasm.

When you lose enough water to equal 15 percent of your body weight, you're deaf and pretty much unable to see out of eyes that are sunken and covered with stiffened lids. Your skin has shrunk, and your tongue has shriveled.

When you've lost water equal to 20 percent of your body weight, you've had it. You're at the limit of your endurance. Deprived of life-giving liquid, your skin cracks, and your organs grind to a halt. And — sorry about this — so do you. *Ave atque vale,* as the Romans say. Or as the Romans say when in the U.S.A, Canada, Great Britain, Australia, or any place where English is the mother tongue: "Hail and Farewell."

When ginger ale won't cut it

Serious dehydration calls for serious medicine, such as the World Health Organization's handy-dandy, two-tumbler electrolyte replacement formula.

Wait! Stop! If you're reading this while lying in bed exhausted by some variety of *turista,* the traveler's diarrhea acquired from impure drinking water, do not make the formula without absolutely clean glasses, washed in bottled water. Better yet, get paper cups.

Now here's what you need:

Glass No. 1

8 ounces orange juice

A pinch of salt

½ teaspoon sweetener (honey, corn syrup)

Glass No. 2

8 ounces boiled or bottled or distilled water

¼ teaspoon baking soda

Take a sip from one glass, then the other, and continue until finished. If diarrhea continues, contact your doctor.

You're sick to your stomach

Repeated vomiting or diarrhea drains your body of water and electrolytes. Similarly, you also need extra water to replace the liquid lost in perspiration when you have a high fever.

When you lose enough water to be dangerously dehydrated, you also lose the electrolytes you need to maintain fluid balance, regulate body temperature, and trigger dozens of biochemical reactions. Plain water doesn't replace those electrolytes. Check with your doctor for a drink that will hydrate your body without upsetting your tummy.

You're exercising or working hard in a hot environment

When you're warm, your body perspires. The moisture evaporates and cools your skin so that blood circulating up from the center of your body to the surface is cooled. The cooled blood returns to the center of your body, lowering the temperature (your *core temperature*) there, too.

If you don't cool your body down, you continue losing water. If you don't replace the lost water, things can get dicey because not only are you losing water, you're also losing electrolytes. The most common cause of temporary sodium, potassium, and chloride depletion is heavy, uncontrolled perspiration.

Deprived of water and electrolytes, your muscles cramp, you're dizzy and weak, and perspiration, now uncontrolled, no longer cools you. Your core body temperature begins rising, and without relief — air conditioning or a cool shower, plus water, ginger ale, or fruit juice — you may progress from heat cramps to heat exhaustion to heat stroke. The latter is potentially fatal.

But — and it's a big one — drinking *too much* water while exercising can also be hazardous to your health. Flooding your body with liquid dilutes the sodium in your bloodstream and may make your brain and other body tissues swell, a condition known as *hyponaturemia* or "water intoxication." The New Rule from the American College of Sports Medicine is to drink just enough water to maintain your body weight while working out. How much is that? Step on a scale before exercising. Exercise for an hour. Step back on the scale. You need 16 ounces of water to replace every pound lost in your one hour's exercise. Lose one pound, drink 16 ounces. Lose ½ pound, drink 8 ounces. That was easy!

You're on a high-protein diet

You need extra water to eliminate the nitrogen compounds in protein. This is true of infants on high-protein formulas and adults on high-protein weight-reducing diets. See Chapter 6 to find out why too much protein may be so harmful.

You're taking certain medications

Because some medications interact with water and electrolytes, always ask whether you need extra water and electrolytes whenever your doctor prescribes

- **Diuretics:** They increase the loss of sodium, potassium, and chloride.
- **Neomycin (an antibiotic):** It binds sodium into insoluble compounds, making it less available to your body.
- **Colchicine (an antigout drug):** It lowers your absorption of sodium.

You have high blood pressure

In 1997, when researchers at Johns Hopkins analyzed the results of more than 30 studies dealing with high blood pressure, they found that people taking daily supplements of 2,500 mg (2.5 grams) of potassium were likely to have blood pressure several points lower than people not taking the supplements. Ask your doctor about this one, and remember: Food is also a good source of potassium. One whole banana has up to 470 milligrams of potassium, one cup of dates — 1,160 milligrams, and one cup of raisins — 1,239 milligrams.

Water is water. Or is it?

Chemically speaking, water's an odd duck. It's the only substance on Earth than can exist as a liquid (water) and a solid (ice) — but not a bendable plastic. No, snow is not plastic water. It's a grouping of solids (ice crystals).

Water may be hard or soft, but these terms have nothing to do with how the water feels on your hand. They describe the liquid's mineral content:

✔ *Hard water* has lots of minerals, particularly calcium and magnesium. This water rises to the Earth's surface from underground springs, usually picking up calcium carbonate as it moves up through the ground.

✔ *Soft water* has fewer minerals. In nature, soft water is surface water, the runoff from rain-swollen streams or rainwater that falls directly into reservoirs. "Water softeners" are products that attract and remove the minerals in water.

What you get at the supermarket is another thing altogether:

✔ *Distilled water* is tap water that has been *distilled,* or boiled until it turns to steam, which is then collected and condensed back into a liquid free of impurities, chemicals, and minerals. The name may also be used to describe a liquid produced by *ultrafiltration,* a process that removes everything from the water except water molecules. Distilled water is very important in chemical and pharmaceutical processing. You'll appreciate the fact that it doesn't clog your iron; makes clean, clear ice cubes; and serves as a flavor-free mixer or base for tea and coffee.

✔ *Mineral water* is spring water. It's naturally alkaline, which makes it a natural antacid and a mild diuretic (a substance that increases urination). The term *spring water* is used to describe water from springs nearer to the Earth's surface, so it has fewer mineral particles and what some people describe as a "cleaner taste" than mineral water.

✔ *Still water* is spring water that flows up to the surface on its own. *Sparkling water* is pushed to the top by naturally occurring gases in the underground spring. So, you ask, what's the big difference? Sparkling water has bubbles; still water doesn't.

✔ *Springlike* or *spring fresh* are terms designed to make something sound more highfalutin than it really is. These products aren't spring water; they're probably filtered tap water.

Part III
Healthy Eating

In this part . . .

You find out how to put foods together to build a healthy diet right here. The chapters in this part are chock-full of guidelines from the Dietary Guidelines for Americans 2005 and strategies based on MyPyramid, the Official Word on making selections that enhance your body while pleasing your palate. And, oh yes, there's an explanation of why you get hungry and why you find some foods more appetizing than others — an important factor in creating a nutritious diet. (Hey, if it doesn't taste good, why would you want to eat it?)

Chapter 14

Why You Eat When You Eat

*B*ecause you need food to live, your body is no slouch at letting you know that it's ready for breakfast, lunch, dinner, and maybe a few snacks in between. This chapter explains the signals your body uses to get you to the table, to the drive-through of your favorite restaurant, or to the vending machine down the hall.

Understanding the Difference between Hunger and Appetite

People eat for two main reasons. The first reason is hunger; the second is appetite. Hunger and appetite are *not* synonyms. In fact, hunger and appetite are entirely different processes.

Hunger is the need for food. It is

✔ A physical reaction that includes chemical changes in your body related to a naturally low level of glucose in your blood several hours after eating

✔ An instinctive, protective mechanism that makes sure that your body gets the fuel it requires to function reasonably well

Appetite is the desire for food. It is

✔ A sensory or psychological reaction (looks good! smells good!) that stimulates an involuntary physiological response (salivation, stomach contractions)

✔ A conditioned response to food (see the sidebar on Pavlov's dogs)

Pavlov's performing puppies

Ivan Petrovich Pavlov (1849–1936) was a Russian physiologist who won the Nobel Prize in physiology/medicine in 1904 for his research on the digestive glands. Pavlov's Big Bang, though, was his identification of respondent conditioning — a fancy way of saying that you can train people to respond physically (or emotionally) to an object or stimulus that simply reminds them of something that they love or hate.

Pavlov tested respondent conditioning on dogs. He began by ringing a bell each time he offered food to his laboratory dogs so that the dogs learned to associate the sound of the bell with the sight and smell of food.

Then he rang the bell without offering the food, and the dogs responded as though food were on tap — salivating madly, even though the dish was empty.

Respondent conditioning applies to many things other than food. For example, it can make a winning Olympic athlete teary at the sight of the flag that represents his country. Food companies are great at using respondent conditioning to encourage you to buy their products: When you see a picture of a deep, dark, rich chocolate bar, doesn't your mouth start to water, and. . . . Hey, come back! Where are you going?

The practical difference between hunger and appetite is this: When you're hungry, you eat one hot dog. After that, your appetite may lead you to eat two more hot dogs just because they look appealing or taste good.

In other words, appetite is the basis for the familiar saying: "Your eyes are bigger than your stomach." Not to mention the well-known advertising slogan: "Bet you can't eat just one." Hey, these guys know their customers.

Refueling: The Cycle of Hunger and Satiety

Your body does its best to create cycles of activity that parallel a 24-hour day. Like sleep, hunger occurs at pretty regular intervals, although your lifestyle may make it difficult to follow this natural pattern — even when your stomach loudly announces it's empty!

Recognizing hunger

The clearest signals that your body wants food, right now, are the physical reactions from your stomach and your blood that let you know it's definitely time to put more food in your mouth and — eat!

Growling and rumbling: Your stomach speaks

An empty belly has no manners. If you do not fill it right away, your stomach will issue an audible — sometimes embarrassing — call for food. This rumbling signal is called a *hunger pang*.

Hunger pangs actually are plain old muscle contractions. When your stomach's full, these contractions and their continual waves down the entire length of the intestine — known as *peristalsis* — move food through your digestive tract (see Chapter 2 for more about digestion). When your stomach's empty, the contractions just squeeze air, and that makes noise.

This phenomenon first was observed in 1912 by an American physiologist named Walter B. Cannon. (Cannon? Rumble? Could I make this up?) Cannon convinced a fellow researcher to swallow a small balloon attached to a thin tube connected to a pressure-sensitive machine. Then Cannon inflated and deflated the balloon to simulate the sensation of a full or empty stomach. Measuring the pressure and frequency of his volunteer's stomach contractions, Cannon discovered that the contractions were strongest and occurred most frequently when the balloon was deflated and the stomach empty. Cannon drew the obvious conclusion: When your stomach is empty, you feel hungry.

Getting that empty feeling

Every time you eat, your pancreas secretes *insulin,* a hormone that enables you to move blood sugar (glucose) out of the blood and into cells where it's needed for various chores. *Glucose* is the basic fuel your body uses for energy. (See Chapter 8.) As a result, the level of glucose circulating in your blood rises and then declines naturally, producing a vague feeling of emptiness, and perhaps weakness, that prompts you to eat. Most people experience the natural rise and fall of glucose as a relatively smooth pattern that lasts about four hours.

What meal is this, anyway?

Breakfast and lunch leave no doubt. The first comes right after you wake up in the morning; the second, in the middle of the day, sometime around noon.

But when do you eat dinner? And what about supper?

According to *Webster's New International Dictionary of the English Language* (2nd edition, 1941 — 15 pounds, including the new binding I put on when the old one crumbled after I dropped the darned thing on its spine once too often), dinner is the main meal of the day, usually eaten around midday, although (get this) some people, "especially in cities," have their dinner between 6 p.m. and 8 p.m. — which probably makes it their supper, because Webster's calls that a meal you eat at the end of the day.

In other words, dinner is lunch except when it's supper. Help!

Knowing when you're full

The satisfying feeling of fullness after eating is called *satiety,* the signal that says, okay, hold the hot dogs, I've had plenty, and I need to push back from the table.

As nutrition research and the understanding of brain functions have become more sophisticated, scientists have discovered that your *hypothalamus,* a small gland on top of the *brain stem* (the part of the brain that connects to the top of the spinal cord), seems to house your appetite controls in an area of the brain where hormones and other chemicals that control hunger and appetite are made (see Figure 14-1). For example, the hypothalamus releases neuropeptide Y (NPY), a chemical that latches onto brain cells and then send out a signal: More food!

Figure 14-1:
Your hypothalamus is in charge of your appetite!

Other body cells also play a role in making your body say, "I'm full." In 1995, researchers at Rockefeller University discovered a gene in *fat cells* (the body cells where fat is stored) that directs the production of a hormone called *leptin* (from the Greek word for *thin*). Leptin appears to tell your body how much fat you have stored, thus regulating your hunger (need for food to provide fuel). Leptin also reduces the hypothalamus's secretion of NPY, the hormone that signals hunger. When the Rockefeller folks injected leptin into specially bred fat mice, the mice ate less, burned food faster, and lost significant amounts of weight.

Eventually, researchers hope that this kind of information can lead to the creation of safe and effective drugs to combat obesity.

Beating the four-hour hungries

Throughout the world, the cycle of hunger (namely, of glucose rising and falling) prompts a feeding schedule that generally provides four meals during the day: breakfast, lunch, *tea* (a mid-afternoon meal), and supper.

In the United States, a three-meal-a-day culture forces people to fight their natural rhythm by going without food from lunch at noon to supper at 6 p.m. or later. The unpleasant result is that when glucose levels decline around 4 p.m., and people in many countries are enjoying afternoon tea, many Americans get really testy and try to satisfy their natural hunger by grabbing the nearest food, usually a high-fat, high-calorie snack.

In 1989, David Jenkins, M.D., Ph.D., and Tom Wolever, M.D., Ph.D., of the University of Toronto, set up a "nibbling study" designed to test the idea that if you even out digestion — by eating several small meals rather than three big ones — you can spread out insulin secretion and keep the amount of glucose in your blood on an even keel all day long.

The theory turned out to be right. People who ate five or six small meals rather than three big ones felt better and experienced an extra bonus: lower cholesterol levels. After two weeks of nibbling, the people in the Jenkins-Wolever study showed a 13.5 percent lower level of low-density lipoproteins (LDL) than people who ate exactly the same amount of food divided into three big meals. As a result, many diets designed to help you lose weight or control your cholesterol (what? you haven't got a copy of *Controlling Cholesterol For Dummies?* Impossible!) now emphasize a daily regimen of several small meals rather than the basic big three. Smart cookies. Low-fat, low-cholesterol, low-cal, of course.

Maintaining a healthy appetite

The best way to deal with hunger and appetite is to find out how to recognize and follow your body's natural cues.

If you're hungry, eat — in reasonable amounts that support a realistic weight. (Confused about how much you should weigh? Check out the weight table in Chapter 3.) And remember: Nobody's perfect. Make one day's indulgence guilt-free by reducing your calorie intake proportionately over the next few days. A little give here, a little take there, and you'll stay on target overall.

Responding to Your Environment on a Gut Level

Your physical and psychological environments definitely affect appetite and hunger, sometimes leading you to eat more than normal, sometimes less.

Baby, it's cold outside

You're more likely to feel hungry when you're in a cool place than you are when you're in a warm one. And you're more likely to want high-calorie dishes in cold weather than in hot weather. Just think about the foods that tempt you in winter — stews, roasts, thick soups — versus those you find pleasing on a simmering summer day — salads, chilled fruit, simple sandwiches.

This difference is no accident. Food gives you calories. Calories keep you warm. Making sure that you get what you need, your body even processes food faster when it's cold out. Your stomach empties more quickly as food speeds along through the digestive tract, which means those old hunger pangs show up sooner than expected, which, in turn, means that you eat more and stay warmer and . . . well, you get the picture.

Exercising more than your mouth

Everybody knows that working out gives you a big appetite, right? Well, everybody's wrong (it happens all the time). Yes, people who exercise regularly are likely to have a healthy (read: normal) appetite, but they're rarely hungry immediately after exercising because

- ✔ Exercise pulls stored energy — glucose and fat — out of body tissues, so your glucose levels stay steady and you don't feel hungry.

- ✔ Exercise slows the passage of food through the digestive tract. Your stomach empties more slowly and you feel fuller longer.

> *Caution:* If you eat a heavy meal right before heading for the gym or the stationary bike in your bedroom, the food sitting in your stomach may make you feel stuffed. Sometimes, you may develop cramps. Or — as *Heartburn & Reflux For Dummies* (Wiley) explains — heartburn. Ouch.

✔ Exercise (including mental exertion) reduces anxiety. For some people, that means less desire to reach for a snack.

Nursing your appetite back to health

Severe physical stress or trauma — a broken bone, surgery, a burn, a high fever — reduces appetite and slows the natural contractions of the intestinal tract. If you eat at times like this, the food may back up in your gut or even stretch your bowel enough to tear it. In situations like this, intravenous feeding — fluids with nutrients sent through a needle directly into a vein — give you nutrition without irritation.

Taking medicine, changing your appetite

Taking some medicines may make you more (or less) likely to eat. Some drugs used to treat common conditions affect your appetite. When you use these medicines, you may find yourself eating more (or less) than usual. This side effect is rarely mentioned when doctors hand out prescriptions, perhaps because it isn't life-threatening and usually disappears when you stop taking the drug.

Some examples of appetite uppers are certain antidepressants (mood elevators), antihistamines (allergy pills), diuretics (drugs that make you urinate more frequently), steroids (drugs that fight inflammation), and tranquilizers (calming drugs). Appetite reducers include some antibiotics, anti-cancer drugs, anti-seizure drugs, blood pressure medications, and cholesterol-lowering drugs.

Of course, not every drug in a particular class of drugs (that is, antibiotics or antidepressants) has the same effect on appetite. For example, the antidepressant drug amitriptyline (Elavil) increases your appetite and may cause weight gain; another antidepressant drug, fluoxetine (Prozac) usually does not.

The fact that a drug affects appetite is almost never a reason to avoid using it. But knowing that a relationship exists between the drug and your desire for food can be helpful. Plain common sense dictates that you ask your doctor about possible drug/appetite interactions whenever a drug is prescribed for you. If the drug package the pharmacist gives you doesn't come with an insert, ask for one. Read the fine print about side effects and other interesting details — such as the direction to avoid alcohol or driving or using heavy machinery.

When Your Appetite Goes Haywire: Eating Disorders

An eating disorder is a psychological illness that leads you to eat either too much or too little. Indulging in a hot fudge sundae once in a while is not an eating disorder. Neither is dieting for three weeks so that you can fit into last year's dress this New Year's Eve.

The difference between normal indulgence and normal dieting to lose weight versus an eating disorder is that the first two are acceptable, healthy behavior while an eating disorder is a potentially life-threatening illness that requires immediate medical attention.

Eating too much

Although many recent studies document an alarming worldwide increase in obesity, particularly among young children, not everyone who is larger or heavier than the current American ideal has an eating disorder. Human bodies come in many different sizes, and some healthy people are just naturally larger or heavier than others. An eating disorder may be present, though, when

- A person continually confuses the desire for food (appetite) with the need for food (hunger)

- A person who has access to a normal diet experiences psychological distress when denied food

- A person uses food to relieve anxiety provoked by what he or she considers a scary situation — a new job, a party, ordinary criticism, or a deadline

Traditionally, doctors have found that treating obesity successfully is difficult (see Chapter 3). However, recent research suggests that some people overeat in response to irregularities in the production of chemicals that regulate satiety (your feeling of fullness). This research may open the path to new kinds of drugs that can control extreme appetite, thus reducing the incidence of obesity-related disorders such as arthritis, diabetes, high blood pressure, and heart disease.

Bingeing, purging, and starving: Unhealthy relationships to food

Some people relieve their anxiety not by eating but by refusing to eat or by regurgitating food after they've eaten it. The first kind of behavior is called anorexia nervosa; the second, bulimia.

Anorexia nervosa (voluntary starvation), the eating disorder that sidelined Mary-Kate Olsen in 2004, is virtually unknown in places where food is hard to come by. It seems to be an affliction of affluence, most likely to strike the young and well-to-do. It's nine times more common among women than among men.

Many doctors who specialize in treating people with eating disorders suggest that anorexia nervosa may be an attempt to control one's life by rejecting a developing body. In other words, by starving themselves, anorexic girls avoid developing breasts and hips, and anorexic boys avoid developing the broad wedge-shape adult male body. By not growing wide, both hope to avoid growing up.

Left untreated, anorexia nervosa can end in death by starvation.

A second form of eating disorder is *bulimia.* Unlike people with anorexia, individuals with bulimia don't refuse to eat. In fact, they may often binge (consume enormous amounts of food in one sitting: a whole chicken, several pints of ice cream, a whole loaf of bread).

But bulimic people don't want to keep the food they eat in their bodies. They may use laxatives to increase defecation, but the more common method they use for getting rid of food is regurgitation. Bulimic people may simply retire to the bathroom after eating and stick their fingers into their throats to make themselves throw up. Or they may use *emetics* (drugs that induce vomiting). Either way, danger looms.

The human body is not designed for repeated stuffing followed by regurgitation. Bingeing may dilate the stomach to the point of rupture; constant vomiting may severely irritate or even tear through the lining of the esophagus (throat). In addition, the continued use of large quantities of emetics may result in a life-threatening loss of potassium that triggers irregular heartbeat or heart failure, factors that contributed to the 1983 death of singer Karen Carpenter, an anorexic/bulimic who — at one point in her disease — weighed only 80 pounds but still saw herself as overweight. One symptom of anorexia and/or bulimia is the inability to look in a mirror and see yourself as you really are. Even at their most skeletal, people with these eating disorders perceive themselves as grossly fat.

As you can see, eating disorders are life-threatening conditions. But they can be treated. If you (or someone you know) experience any of the signs and symptoms just described, the safest course is to seek immediate medical advice and treatment. For more info about eating conditions, contact the National Eating Disorders Association, 603 Stewart St., Suite 803, Seattle, WA 98101; phone 800-931-2237; e-mail `info@NationalEatingDisorders.org`; Web site `www.nationaleatingdisorders.org`.

Chapter 15

Why You Like the Foods You Like

*N*utritionally speaking, *taste* is the ability to perceive flavors in food and beverages. *Preference* is the appreciation of one food and distaste of another. Decisions about taste are physical reactions that are dependent on specialized body organs called taste buds. Although your culture has a decided influence on what you think is good to eat, decisions about food preferences may also depend on your genes, your medical history, and your personal reactions to specific foods.

Tackling Taste: How Your Brain and Tongue Work Together

Your *taste buds* are sensory organs that enable you to perceive different flavors in food — in other words, to taste the food you eat.

Taste buds (also referred to as *taste papillae*) are not flowers. They're tiny bumps on the surface of your tongue (see Figure 15-1). Each one contains groups of receptor cells that anchor an antennalike structure called a *microvillus,* which projects up through a gap (or pore) in the center of the taste bud, sort of like a thread sticking through the hole in Life Savers candy. (For more about the microvilli and how they behave in your digestive tract, see Chapter 2.)

The microvilli in your taste buds transmit messages from flavor chemicals in the food along nerve fibers to your brain, which translates the messages into perceptions: "Oh, wow, that's good," or "Man, that's awful."

The four (maybe five) basic flavors

Your taste buds definitely recognize four basic flavors: *sweet, sour, bitter,* and *salty.* Some people add a fifth basic flavor to this list. It's called *umami,* a Japanese word describing richness or a savory flavor associated with certain amino acids such as glutamates — I talk more about monosodium glutamate (MSG) later in this section — and soy products such as tofu.

Early on, scientists thought that everyone had specific taste buds for specific flavors: sweet taste buds for sweets, sour taste buds for sour, and so on. However, the prevailing theory today is that groups of taste buds work together so that flavor chemicals in food link up with chemical bonds in taste buds to create patterns that you recognize as sweet, sour, bitter, and salt. The technical term for this process is *across-fiber pattern theory of gustatory coding.* Receptor patterns for the fave four (sweet, sour, bitter, salt) have been tentatively identified, but the pattern for umami remains elusive.

Flavors are not frivolous. They're one of the factors that enable you to enjoy food. In fact, flavors are so important that MSG is used to make food taste better. MSG, most often found in food prepared in Chinese restaurants, stimulates brain cells. People who are sensitive to MSG may actually develop *Chinese restaurant syndrome,* which is characterized by tight facial muscles, headache, nausea, and sweating caused by overbouncy brain cells. Very large doses of MSG given to lab rats have been lethal, and the compound is banned from baby food. However, no real evidence indicates that a little MSG is a problem for people who aren't sensitive to it. Which leaves only one question: How does MSG work? Does it enhance existing flavors or simply add that umami flavor on its own? Believe it or not, right now nobody knows. Sorry about that.

Your health and your taste buds

Some illnesses and medicines alter your ability to taste foods. The result may be partial or total *ageusia* (the medical term for loss of taste). Or you may experience *flavor confusion* — meaning that you mix up flavors, translating sour as bitter, or sweet as salt, or vice versa.

Table 15-1 lists some medical conditions that affect your sense of taste.

Table 15-1	These Things Make Tasting Food Difficult
This Condition	*May Lead to This Problem*
A bacterial or viral infection of the tongue	Secretions that block your taste buds
Injury to your mouth, nose, or throat	Damage to the nerves that transmit flavor signals
Radiation therapy to mouth and throat	Damage to the nerves that transmit flavor

The nose knows — and the eyes have it

Your nose is important to your sense of taste. Just like the taste of food, the aroma of food also stimulates sensory messages. Think about how you sniff your brandy before drinking and how the wonderful aroma of baking bread warms the heart and stirs the soul — not to mention the salivary glands. When you can't smell, you can't really taste. As anyone who's ever had a cold knows, when your nose is stuffed and your sense of smell is deadened, almost everything tastes like plain old cotton. Don't have a cold? You can test this theory by closing your eyes, pinching your nostrils shut, and having someone put a tiny piece of either a raw onion or a fresh apple into your mouth. Bet you can't tell which is which without looking — or sniffing!

Food color is also an important clue to what you'll enjoy eating. Repeated studies show that when testers change the expected color of foods, people find them (the foods, not the testers) less appealing. For example, blue mashed potatoes or green beef lose to plain old white mashed potatoes and red meat every time.

Tricking your taste buds

Combining foods can short-circuit your taste buds' ability to identify flavors correctly. For example, when you sip wine (even an apparently smooth and silky one), your taste buds say, "Hey, that alcohol's sharp." Take a bite of cheese first, and the wine tastes smoother (less acidic) because the cheese's fat and protein molecules coat your receptor cells so that acidic wine molecules cannot connect.

A similar phenomenon occurs during serial wine tastings (tasting many wines, one after another). Try two equally dry, acidic wines, and the second seems mellower because acid molecules from the first one fill up space on the chemical bonds that perceive acidity. Drink a sweet wine after a dry one, and the sweetness often is more pronounced.

Here's another way to fool your taste buds: Eat an artichoke. The meaty part at the base of the artichoke leaves contains *cynarin,* a sweet-tasting chemical that makes any food you taste after the artichoke taste sweeter.

Determining Deliciousness

When it comes to deciding what tastes good, all human beings and most animals have four things in common: They like sweets, crave salt, go for the fat, and avoid the bitter (at least at first).

These choices are rooted deep in biology and evolution. In fact, you can say that whenever you reach for something that you consider good to eat, the entire human race — especially your own individual ancestors — reaches with you.

Listening to your body

Here's something to chew on: The foods that taste good — sweet foods, salty foods, fatty foods — are essential for a healthy body.

✔ Sweet foods are a source of quick energy because their sugars can be converted quickly to glucose, the molecule that your body burns for energy. (Check out Chapter 8 for an explanation of how your body uses sugars.)

Better yet, sweet foods make you feel good. Eating them tells your brain to release natural painkillers called *endorphins.* Sweet foods may also stimulate an increase in blood levels of *adrenaline,* a hormone secreted by the adrenal glands. Adrenaline sometimes is labeled the *fight-or-flight hormone* because it's secreted more heavily when you feel threatened and must decide whether to stand your ground — *fight* — or hurry away — *flight.*

✔ Salt is vital to life. As Chapter 13 explains, salt enables your body to maintain its fluid balance and to regulate chemicals called electrolytes that give your nerve cells the power needed to fire electrical charges that energize your muscles, power up your organs, and transmit messages from your brain.

✔ Fatty foods are even richer in calories (energy) than sugars. So the fact that you want them most when you're very hungry comes as no surprise. (Chapter 2 and Chapter 7 explain how you use fats for energy.)

✔ Which fatty food you want may depend on your sex. Several studies suggest that women like their fats with sugar — Hey, where's the chocolate? Men, on the other hand, seem to prefer their fat with salt — Bring on the fries!

Loving the food you're with: Geography and taste

Marvin Harris was an anthropologist with a special interest in the history of food. In a perfectly delightful book called *Good to Eat: Riddles of Food and Culture* (Simon & Schuster, 1986), Harris posed this interesting situation:

Creepy crawly nutrients

Who's to say grilled grasshopper is less appetizing than a lobster? After all, both have long skinny bodies and plenty of legs. But the difference is in the nutrients: The bug beats the lobster hands (legs?) down.

Food 3.5 oz	Protein (g)	Fat (g)	Carbohydrates (g)	Iron (mg)
Water Beetle	19.8	8.3	2.1	13.6
Red Ant	13.9	3.5	2.9	5.7
Cricket	12.9	5.5	5.1	9.5
Small Grasshopper	20.6	6.1	3.9	5.0
Large Grasshopper	14.3	3.3	2.2	3.0
Lobster	22	<1	<1	0.4
Blue crab	20	<1	0	0.8

USDA and Iowa State University (www.ent.iastate.edu/misc/insectnutrition.html)

Suppose you live in a forest where someone has pinned $20 and $1 bills to the upper branches of the trees. Which will you reach for? The $20 bills, of course. But wait. Suppose that only a couple of $20 bills are pinned to branches among millions and millions of $1 bills. Does that change the picture? You betcha.

Searching for food is hard work. You don't want to spend so much time and energy searching for food that you end up using more calories than the food that you find can provide. Substitute "chickens" for $20 bills and "large insects" for $1 bills, and you can see why people who live in places where insects far outnumber the chickens spend their time and energy on picking off the plentiful high-protein bugs rather than chasing after the occasional chicken — although they wouldn't turn it down if it fell into the pot.

So, you may say that Harris's first rule of food choice is that people tend to eat and enjoy what is easily available, which explains the differences in cuisines in different parts of the world.

Here's a second rule: For a food to be appealing (good to eat), it must be both nutritious and relatively easy or economical to produce.

A food that meets one test but not the other is likely to be off the list. For example:

- The human stomach cannot extract nutrients from grass. So even though grass grows here, there, and everywhere, under ordinary circumstances, grass never ends up in your salad.

- Cows are harder to raise than plants, especially under the hot South Asian sun; pigs eat what people do, so they compete for your food supply. In other words, although they're highly nutritious, sometimes neither the cow nor the pig is economical to produce. This anthropological explanation is a reasonable argument for why some cultures have prohibited the use of pigs and cows as food.

Taking offense to tastes

Virtually everyone instinctively dislikes bitter foods, at least at first tasting. This dislike is a protective mechanism. Bitter foods are often poisonous, so disliking stuff that tastes bitter is a primitive but effective way to eliminate potentially toxic food.

According to Linda Bartoshuk, Ph.D., professor of surgery (otolaryngology) at the Yale University School of Medicine, about two-thirds of all human beings carry a gene that makes them especially sensitive to bitter flavors. This gene may have given their ancestors a leg up in surviving their evolutionary food trials.

People with this gene can taste very small concentrations of a chemical called phenylthiocarbamide (PTC). Because PTC is potentially toxic, Dr. Bartoshuk tests for the trait by having people taste a piece of paper impregnated with 6-n-propylthiouracil, a thyroid medication whose flavor and chemical structure are similar to PTC. People who say the paper tastes bitter are called *PTC tasters*. People who taste only paper are called *PTC nontasters*.

If you're a PTC taster, you're likely to find the taste of saccharin, caffeine, the salt substitute potassium chloride, and the food preservatives sodium benzoate and potassium benzoate really nasty. The same is true for the flavor chemicals common to cruciferous vegetables — members of the mustard family, including broccoli, Brussels sprouts, cabbage, cauliflower, and radishes.

No such ambivalence exists among people who've gotten truly sick — I'm talking nausea and vomiting here — after eating a specific food. When that happens, you'll probably come to like its flavor less. Sometimes, says psychologist Alexandra W. Logue, author of *The Psychology of Eating and Drinking,* your revulsion may be so strong that you'll never try the food again — even when you know that what actually made you sick was something else entirely, like riding a roller coaster just before eating, or having the flu, or taking a drug whose side effects upset your stomach.

If you're allergic to a food or have a metabolic problem that makes digesting it hard for you, you may eat the food less frequently, but you'll enjoy it as much as everyone else does. For example, people who cannot digest lactose, the sugar in milk, may end up gassy every time they eat ice cream, but they still like the way the ice cream tastes.

Does it matter whether you like your food? Yes, of course, it does. The simple act of putting food into your mouth needs to stimulate the flow of saliva and the secretion of enzymes that you need to digest the food. Some studies suggest that if you really like your food, your pancreas may release as much as 30 times its normal amount of digestive enzymes.

However, if you truly loathe what you're eating, your body may refuse to take it in. No saliva flows; your mouth becomes so dry that you may not even be able to swallow the food. If you do manage to choke it down, your stomach muscles and your digestive tract may convulse in an effort to be rid of the awful stuff.

Changing the Menu: Adapting to Exotic Foods

New foods are an adventure. As a rule, people may not like them the first time around, but in time — and with patience — what once seemed strange can become just another dish at dinner.

Learning to like unusual foods

Exposure to different people and cultures often expands your taste horizons. Some taboos — horsemeat, snake, dog — may simply be too emotion-laden to be overcome. Others with no emotional baggage fall to experience. Most people hate very salty, very bitter, very acidic, or very slippery foods such as caviar, coffee, Scotch whisky, and oysters on first taste, but many later learn to enjoy them.

Coming to terms with these foods can be both physically and psychologically rewarding:

- Many bitter foods, such as coffee and unsweetened chocolate, are relatively mild stimulants that temporarily improve mood and physical performance.

- Strongly flavored foods, such as salty caviar, offer a challenge to the taste buds.

- Foods such as oysters, which may seem totally disgusting the first time you see or taste them, are symbols of wealth or worldliness. Trying them implies a certain sophistication in the way you face life.

Happily, an educated, adventurous sense of taste can be a pleasure that lasts as long as you live. Professional tea tasters, wine tasters, and others (maybe you?) who have developed the ability to recognize even the smallest differences among flavors continue to enjoy their gift well into old age. Although your sense of taste declines as you grow older, you can keep it perking as long as you supply the stimuli in the form of tasty, well-seasoned food.

In other words, as they say about adult life's other major sensory delight, "Use it or lose it."

Stirring the stew: The culinary benefits of immigration

If you're lucky enough to live in a place that attracts many immigrants, your dining experience is flavored by the favorite foods of other people (meaning the foods of other cultures). In the United States, for example, the *melting pot* is not an idle phrase. American cooking literally bubbles with contributions from every group that's ever stepped ashore in what President Lyndon Baines Johnson used to call the "good ole U. S. of A."

Table 15-2 lists some of the foods and food combinations characteristic of specific ethnic/regional cuisines. Imagine how few you might sample living in a place where everybody shares exactly the same ethnic, racial, or religious backgrounds. Just thinking about it is enough to make me want to stand up and shout, "Hooray for diversity at the dinner table!" (Check out Figure 15-2 for the visuals!)

Table 15-2	Geography and Food Preference
If Your Ancestors Came From	*You're Likely to Be Familiar with This Flavor Combination*
Central and Eastern Europe	Sour cream and dill or paprika
China	Soy sauce plus wine and ginger
Germany	Meat roasted in vinegar and sugar
Greece	Olive oil and lemon
India	Cumin and curry
Italy	Tomatoes, cheese, and olive oil
Japan	Soy sauce plus rice wine and sugar
Korea	Soy sauce plus brown sugar, sesame, and chile
Mexico	Tomatoes and chile peppers
Middle Europe	Milk and vegetables
Puerto Rico	Rice and fish
West Africa	Peanuts and chile peppers

A. W. Logue, The Psychology of Eating and Drinking, 2nd edition (New York: W. H. Freeman and Company, 1991)

Figure 15-2:
Ethnic and
regional
cuisines
abound.

Of course, enjoying other peoples' foods doesn't mean you don't have your own special treats. Table 15-3 is a flag-waver: A list of made-in-America taste sensations, many created here by immigrant chefs whose talents flowered in American kitchens.

Table 15-3	Foods Born in the USA
This Food Item	*Was Born Here*
Baked beans	Boston (Pilgrim adaptation of Native American dish)
Clam chowder	Boston (named for *la chaudière,* a large copper soup pot, used by fishermen to make a communal soup)
Hamburger	Everywhere (originally called a Hamburg steak, except in Hamburg, Germany)
Jambalaya	Louisiana (combination of French Canadian with native coastal cookery)
Potato chips	Saratoga Springs, New York (credited to a chef at Moon's Lake House hotel)
Spoon bread	Southern United States (adapted from Native American corn pudding)
Vichyssoise	New York (Ritz Carlton Hotel; created by a chef born near Vichy, France)

James Trager, *The Foodbook (New York: Grossman Publishers, 1970)*

Chapter 16

What Is a Healthful Diet?

The American Heart Association says to limit your consumption of fats and cholesterol. The American Cancer Society says to eat more fiber. The National Research Council says to watch out for fats, sugar, and salt. The American Diabetes Association says to eat regular meals so your blood sugar stays even. The Food Police say if it tastes good, forget it!

The U.S. Departments of Agriculture and Health and Human Services have incorporated virtually all but the "tastes good, forget it" rule into the *Dietary Guidelines for Americans 2005* and even added some advisories of their own. Before you begin reading this chapter, make sure you have a couple bookmarks or something else to hold your place — the material here often refers to information in other chapters, so you may have to skip back and forth.

What Are Dietary Guidelines for Americans?

The *Dietary Guidelines for Americans* is a collection of sensible suggestions first published by the Departments of Agriculture and Health and Human Services (USDA/HHS) in 1980, with five revised editions since then (1985, 1990, 1995, 2000, 2005).

Comparing Guidelines

My personal favorite among the many editions of the *Dietary Guidelines* is the 2000 edition. Its greatest virtue is that it seemed to have been written by real people who actually liked food. You could see this right up front in the very first paragraph, which began: "Eating is one of life's greatest pleasures." Hallelujah!

Contrast that with the first sentence of the *Dietary Guidelines for Americans 2005:* "The *Dietary Guidelines for Americans* [*Dietary Guidelines*], first published in 1980, provides science-based advice to promote health and reduce risk for chronic disease through diet and physical activity."

Alas, what you see is what you get: A frankly cranky, bare bones, chilly presentation of the facts. Where the section and chapter section titles in 2000 were nicely encouraging ("Aim for a healthy weight," "Build a Healthy Base," and so on) 2005's are plain clunky ("Weight Management," "Adequate Nutrients within Calorie Need," and the like).

Perhaps sensing a small disconnect between *them* (the people who wrote the *Guidelines*) and *you* (the person who's supposed to read them), the USDA/HHA team put its shoulders back to the wheel and its fingers back on the keyboard to create *Finding Your Way to a Healthier You,* a neat little brochure that summarizes the *Guidelines* for civilians. Well, one out of two ain't bad.

To read and/or download the *Dietary Guidelines for Americans 2005* and *Finding Your Way to a Healthier You,* click on www.health.gov/dietaryguidelines, scroll to *2005 Edition* and choose the appropriate listing.

To compare 2000 with 2005, scroll down to *2000 Edition* on the same page and choose "Nutrition and Your Health: Dietary Guidelines for Americans." To track the evolution of the guidelines, choose "Summary chart of guidelines, 1980-2000."

Prefer print? You can order a hard copy of the 2005 *Guidelines* (Stock Number 001-000-04719-1) from the U.S. Government Printing Office either by phone (866-512-1800) or online at bookstore.gpo.gov. And, no, there's no "www" in that Net address.

As the first chapter of the 2005 edition explains, the *Guidelines* lay out food and lifestyle choices that promote good health, provide the energy for an active life, and may reduce the risk or severity of chronic illnesses, such as diabetes and heart disease. These suggestions are organized as nine stand-alone chapters, but for convenience's sake — and because it seems logical — I've grouped them into three categories: "Controlling Your Weight," "Making Smart Food Choices," and "Keeping Food Safe to Eat."

From now on, when I refer you to a chapter — such as "check back in Chapter 8" — I'm talking about a chapter in *Nutrition For Dummies,* not in *Dietary Guidelines for Americans 2005.* Onward!

Controlling Your Weight

During the past two decades, as the number of overweight Americans has bounced upward like a rubber ball, the incidence of obesity-related conditions such as Type 2 diabetes, high blood pressure, and heart disease also has risen.

The challenge (as always) is to set, reach, and hold a healthful weight. Three chapters in the new *Dietary Guidelines* ("Adequate Nutrients within Calorie Needs," "Weight Management," and "Physical Activities") lay out some clear, um, guidelines.

Getting the most nutritious calories

Some foods provide lots of nutrients per calorie. Some don't. The former are called "nutrient-dense foods." The latter aren't.

As you may expect, the *Guidelines* recommend choosing foods from the first group to meet your calorie needs each day, while limiting the amount of

- ✔ Foods high in saturated fat
- ✔ Foods high in trans fats
- ✔ Foods high in cholesterol
- ✔ Foods with added sugar
- ✔ Foods with added salt
- ✔ Alcohol beverages

In other words, stick to a balanced diet. No surprise there. And for a list of superstar foods, check out Chapter 28, which is — this *is* a surprise! — titled "Twelve Superstar Foods."

Managing your weight

To reach and keep a healthful weight, follow a few realistic rules:

- ✔ **Evaluate your weight.** The best test of who's actually overweight is the *Body Mass Index (BMI),* a measure of body fat versus body lean mass (in other words, muscle) that can be used to predict health outcomes. You can read all about BMI in Chapter 3. So if you haven't already done so, turn back to Chapter 3 and read, read, read, but come right back here when you're done.

- **If you need to lose weight, do so gradually.** Forget the "lose 30 pounds in 30 days" jazz. Depending on how much weight you have to lose, your long-term goal needs to be losing about 10 percent of your total weight over a 6-month period. Losing ½ to 2 pounds a week is a safe and practical way of doing so.

- **Encourage healthy weight in children.** One unhappy fact is that overweight kids become overweight adults. Helping children stick to a healthy weight pays large dividends down the road of life.

- **Check with your doctor before starting a weight loss diet.** This advice is most important for women who are pregnant or nursing, for children, and for anyone — young or old — who has a chronic disease and/or is on medication.

Being physically active

When you take in more calories from food than you use up running your body systems (heart, lungs, brain, and so forth) and doing a day's physical work, you end up storing the extra calories as body fat. In other words, you gain weight. The reverse also is true. When you spend more energy in a day than you take in as food, you pull the extra energy you need out of stored fat and you lose weight.

I'm no mathematician, but I can reduce this principle to two simple equations in which *E* stands for *energy* (in calories), > stands for *greater than*, < stands for *less than,* and *W* stands for the change in *weight:*

If $E_{in} > E_{out}$: $E_{total} = +W$

If $E_{in} < E_{out}$: $E_{total} = -W$

It ain't Einstein's theory of relativity, but you get the picture!

For real-life examples of how the *energy-in, energy-out theory* works, stick your bookmark in this page and go to Table 3-1 in Chapter 3 to find out how to calculate the number of calories a person can consume each day without pushing up the poundage. Even being mildly active increases the number of calories you can wolf down without gaining weight. The more strenuous the activity, the more plentiful the calorie allowance. Suppose that you're a 25-year-old man who weighs 140 pounds. The formula in Table 3-1 shows that you require 1,652 calories a day to run your body systems. Clearly, you need more calories for doing your daily physical work, simply moving around, or exercising.

Other reasons to exercise

Weight control is a good reason to step up your exercise level, but it isn't the only one. Here are four more:

✔ **Exercise increases muscles.** When you exercise regularly, you end up with more muscle tissue than the average bear. Because muscle tissue weighs more than fat tissue, athletes (even weekend warrior types) may end up weighing more than they did before they started exercising to lose weight. But a higher muscle-to-fat ratio is healthier and more important in the long run than actual weight in pounds. Exercise that changes your body's ratio of muscle to fat gives you a leg up in the longevity race.

✔ **Exercise reduces the amount of fat stored in your body.** People who are fat around the middle as opposed to the hips (in other words an apple shape versus a pear shape) are at higher risk of weight-related illness. Exercise helps reduce abdominal fat and thus lowers your risk of weight-related diseases. Use a tape measure to identify your own body type by comparing your waistline to your hips (around the buttocks). If your waist (abdomen) is bigger, you're an apple. If your hips are bigger, you're a pear.

✔ **Exercise strengthens your bones.** *Osteoporosis* (thinning of the bones that leads to repeated fractures) doesn't happen only to little old ladies. True, on average, a woman's bones thin faster and more dramatically than a man's, but after the mid-30s, everybody — male and female — begins losing bone density. Exercise can slow, halt, or in some cases even reverse the process. In addition, being physically active develops muscles that help support bones. Stronger bones equal less risk of fracture, which, in turn, equals less risk of potentially fatal complications.

✔ **Exercise increases brainpower.** You know that aerobic exercise increases the flow of oxygen to the heart, but did you also know that it increases the flow of oxygen to the brain?

When a rush job (or a rush of anxiety) keeps you up all night, a judicious exercise break can keep you bright until dawn. According to Massachusetts Institute of Technology nutrition research scientist Judith J. Wurtman, Ph.D., when you're awake and working during hours that you'd normally be asleep, your internal body rhythms tell your body to cool down, even though your brain is racing along. Simply standing up and stretching, walking around the room, or doing a couple of sit-ups every hour or so speeds up your metabolism, warms up your muscles, increases your ability to stay awake, and, in Dr. Wurtman's words, "prolongs your ability to work smart into the night." Eureka!

After you decide to start moving, the *Guidelines* say, do it every day. How much should you do? Per the *Guidelines*:

✔ Most people will benefit from 30 minutes of moderate physical activity — such as a brisk walk — per day.

 ✔ To manage body weight and/or prevent gradual weight gain, make it 60
    minutes of moderate-to-vigorous-intensity activity several days a week.

 ✔ To keep weight off, try 60 to 90 minutes of daily moderate physical activity.

 ✔ To reach true physical fitness, your regimen should include cardiovascu-
    lar conditioning, stretching exercises for flexibility, and resistance exer-
    cises or calisthenics for muscle strength and endurance.

Not everybody can — or should — run right out and start chopping down
trees or throwing touchdown passes to control his or her weight. In fact, if
you have gained a lot of weight recently, have been overweight for a long
time, haven't exercised in a while, or have a chronic medical condition, you
need to check with your doctor before starting any new regimen. (***Caution:***
Check out of any health club that puts you right on the floor without first
checking your vital signs — heartbeat, respiration, and so forth.)

Making Smart Food Choices

Okay. So you have your weight goals firmly in mind and three, or four, or even
seven times a week, you manage to *Hup! Two, three, four* at home, or in the
gym, or on a walk around the block. The next task set forth by the *Guidelines*
is to put together a diet that supports your new healthy lifestyle.

The *Guidelines* has five chapters designed to simplify your task: "Food Groups
to Encourage," "Fats," "Carbohydrates," "Sodium and Potassium," and
"Alcoholic Beverages."

Picking the perfect plants

From the beginning, way back in 1980, the various editions of the *Guidelines*
have recommended that you build your diet on a base of plant foods. Why?
Because plant foods

 ✔ Add plenty of bulk but few calories to your diet, so you feel full without
    adding weight

 ✔ Are usually low in fat and have no cholesterol, which means they reduce
    your risk of heart disease

 ✔ Are high in fiber, which reduces the risk of heart disease; prevents con-
    stipation; reduces the risk of developing hemorrhoids (or at least makes
    existing ones less painful); moves food quickly through your digestive
    tract, thus reducing the risk of diverticular disease (inflammation
    caused by food getting caught in the folds of your intestines and causing

tiny out-pouchings of the weakened gut wall); and may lower your risk of some gastrointestinal cancers.

✔ Are rich in beneficial substances called phytochemicals, which may reduce your risk of heart disease and some forms of cancer (for more, see Chapter 12)

For all these reasons, the *Guidelines* recommend that a basic 2,000 calorie daily diet include

✔ 2 cups of fruit

✔ 2.5 cups of vegetables (include dark green, orange, and starchy veggies, plus beans)

✔ 3 or more 1-ounce servings of whole grain products

To protect your bones, the *Guidelines* advise washing down your plants with 3 daily cups of low-fat milk (349 milligrams calcium) or fat-free milk (306 milligrams calcium) or the equivalent amount of milk products such as cheddar cheese, which has 204 milligrams calcium per ounce. For more on calcium, mark this page and flip to Chapter 11.

Figuring out fats

As you can plainly see in Chapter 7, dietary fat (the fat in foods) is an essential nutrient. Infants need these fats to thrive, and the same cholesterol that may increase an adult's risk of heart disease is vital to an embryo's healthy development, triggering the action of genes that tells cells to become specialized body structures — arms, legs, backbone, and so forth.

Grown-ups, however, need to control fat intake so they can control calories and reduce the risk of obesity-related illnesses, such as heart disease, diabetes, and some forms of cancer.

Overall, the *Guidelines* suggest that your adult diet derive no more than 35 percent of its calories from fat and no more than 10 percent of calories from saturated fat and that it deliver 300 milligrams or less of cholesterol a day. To reach these goals

✔ Most of your fat calories should come from foods such as fish, nuts, and vegetable oils that are rich in polyunsaturated and monounsaturated fats.

✔ Dairy products, such as milk, should be low- or no-fat (skim).

✔ Poultry and meat should be lean (yes, trim off that visible fat).

✔ With trans fats, less is always better.

Counting on carbs

Carbs are your fastest source of energy, but the trick here is to get your carbs complex (I explain complex versus simple carbs in Chapter 8), which means from plant foods: fruits and vegetables and whole grains. The companion stratagem is to buy and prepare foods with little added sugar.

Together, these two simple steps help control weight, provide vital nutrients, and — as the *Guidelines* slyly note — "reduce the incidence of dental caries" (cavities). Next!

Limiting salt, balancing potassium

Sodium is a mineral that helps regulate your body's fluid balance, the flow of water into and out of every cell described in Chapter 13. This balance keeps just enough water inside the cell so that it can perform its daily jobs but not so much that the cell — packed to bursting — explodes.

Most people have no problems with sodium. They eat a lot one day, a little less the next, and their bodies adjust. Others, however, don't react so evenly. For them, a high-sodium diet appears to increase the risk of high blood pressure. When you already have high blood pressure, you can tell fairly quickly whether lowering the amount of salt in your diet lowers your blood pressure. But no test is available at this point for telling whether someone who doesn't have high blood pressure will develop it by consuming a diet that's high in sodium.

Because limiting sodium intake to a moderate level won't harm anyone, the guidelines advocate avoiding excessive amounts of salt. Doing so helps reduce blood pressure levels for people who are salt-sensitive.

What's moderate use? According to the *Guidelines,* you should consume less than 2,300 milligrams (approximately 1 teaspoon of salt) of sodium per day. The easiest way to reach that goal is to choose and prepare foods with very little added salt. At the same time, it pays to consume potassium-rich foods, such as (what else?) fruits and vegetables, because an adequate supply of potassium helps control blood pressure.

By the way, moderating your salt intake has another, unadvertised benefit. It may lower your weight a bit. Why? Because sodium is *hydrophilic* (hydro = water; philic = loving). Sodium attracts and holds water. When you eat less salt, you retain less water, you're less bloated, and you feel thinner.

Don't reduce salt intake drastically without first checking with your doctor. Remember, sodium is an essential nutrient, and the *Guidelines* advocate moderate use, and not no use at all.

Where's the sodium?

The foods with the highest amounts of naturally occurring sodium are natural cheeses, sea fish, and shellfish. Some foods are low in sodium but pick up plenty of salt when they're processed. For example, one cup of cooked fresh green peas has about 2 milligrams (mg) sodium, but one cup of canned peas may have 493 mg sodium. To be fair, most canned and processed vegetables are now available in low-sodium versions, too. The difference is notable: One cup of low-sodium canned peas has 8 mg of sodium, 485 mg less than regular canned peas.

You also get added sodium in the salt on snack foods, such as potato chips and peanuts, not to mention the salt you add yourself from the shaker that's on virtually every American table. Not all the sodium you swallow is sodium chloride. Sodium compounds also are used as preservatives, thickeners, and buffers (chemicals that smooth down acidity).

Table 16-1 lists several different kinds of sodium compounds in food. Table 16-2 lists sodium compounds in over-the-counter (OTC) drug products.

Table 16-1	Sodium Compounds in Food
Sodium Compound	*Function*
Monosodium glutamate (MSG)	Flavor enhancer
Sodium benzoate	Keeps food from spoiling
Sodium caseinate	Thickens foods and provides protein
Sodium chloride (table salt)	Flavoring agent
Sodium citrate	Holds carbonation in soft drinks
Sodium hydroxide	Makes peeling the skin off tomatoes and fruits before canning easier
Sodium nitrate/nitrite	Keeps food (cured meats) from spoiling — and gives these foods their distinctive red color
Sodium phosphates	Mineral supplement
Sodium saccharin	No-calorie sweetener

"The Sodium Content of Your Food," Home and Garden Bulletin, No. 233 (Washington, D.C.: U.S. Department of Agriculture, August 1980); Ruth Winter, A Consumer's Dictionary of Food Additives (New York: Crown, 1978)

Table 16-2	Sodium Compounds in OTC Drug Products
Sodium Compound	*Function*
Sodium ascorbate	A form of vitamin C used in nutritional supplements
Sodium bicarbonate	Antacid
Sodium biphosphate	Laxative
Sodium citrate	Antacid
Sodium fluoride	Mineral used in nutritional supplements and as a decay preventative in tooth powders
Sodium phosphates	Laxative
Sodium saccharin	Sweetener
Sodium salicylate	Analgesic (similar to aspirin)

Handbook of Nonprescription Drugs, 9th ed. (Washington, D.C.: American Pharmaceutical Association, 1990); Physicians' Desk Reference, 48th ed. (Montvale, N.J.: Medical Economics Data Production, 1994)

Moderating alcohol consumption

Telling someone to drink alcohol beverages in moderation sounds like Mom-and-apple-pie advice, right? Right. But — and you've heard this song before — what's *moderation,* anyway? Laypersons (you and me, babe) may define moderate in terms of the effects that alcohol has on the ability to perform simple tasks, such as speaking and thinking clearly or moving in a straight line. Obviously, if the amount of alcohol you drink makes you slur your words or bump into the furniture, that isn't moderation.

The *Dietary Guidelines* define moderate drinking as one drink a day for a woman and two drinks a day for a man. Aha, you say, but what's one drink? Good question. Here's the answer:

- 12 ounces of regular beer (150 calories)
- 5 ounces of wine (100 calories)
- 1½ ounces of 80-proof (40 percent alcohol) distilled spirits (100 calories)

Dietary Guidelines for Americans 2005 (Washington, D.C.: U.S. Department of Agriculture, 2005)

Some people shouldn't drink at all, not even in moderation, including people who suffer from alcoholism, people who plan to drive a car or take part in other activities that require attention to detail or real physical skill, and people using medication (prescription drugs or over-the-counter products). For information about who should and should not drink, as well as a list of drugs that interact with alcohol, take a look at Chapter 9.

Keeping Food Safe to Eat

In 2000, the Centers for Disease Control and Prevention (CDC) estimated that spoiled or contaminated food causes about 76 million illnesses — 325,000 of them serious enough to require hospitalization — and 5,000 deaths every year in the United States. Three years later, the USDA blamed *Salmonella* organisms alone for more than 3.5 million American stomachaches — or worse.

Clearly, keeping food safe to eat is an important goal. To do that, here's an equation any careful cook can rely on:

> Clean stores + clean hands + clean kitchen + proper storage + proper temperature = safe food

That's the short version of the *Guidelines'* guidelines. For more details about exactly how to keep food safe from store to dinner plate, stick a bookmark in this page and flip forward to Chapters 19, 20, and 21. Imagine! Four chapters with info about one subject. Sort of tells you how important it is, doesn't it?

 Right now, raw is in but not — as the *Guidelines* explain — necessarily healthful. To reduce your risk of picking up an icky bacterial disease along with dinner, the *Guidelines* advise avoiding raw (unpasteurized) milk or any products made from unpasteurized milk; raw or partially cooked eggs or any dish containing raw eggs; raw or undercooked meat and poultry; unpasteurized juices; and raw sprouts.

Okay, Now Relax

Life is not a test. You don't lose points for failing to follow the *Dietary Guidelines for Americans 2005* every single day of your life. Nobody's perfect, and the *Guidelines* are meant to be broken — once in a while.

For example, ideally you should hold your daily intake of dietary fat to 20 to 35 percent of your total calories. But you can bet that you'll exceed that amount this Saturday when you stroll by the buffet at your best friend's wedding and see Camembert cheese (70 percent of the calories from fat), sirloin steak (56 percent of the calories from fat), salad with Thousand Island dressing (90 percent of the calories from fat), and whipped cream cake (I can't count that high).

Is this a crisis? Should you stay home? Must you keep your mouth shut tight all night? Are you kidding? Here's the Real Rule: Let the good times roll every once in a while. After the party's over, compensate.

For the rest of the week, go back to your exercise regimen and back to your healthful menu emphasizing lots of the nutritious, delicious, low- or no-fat foods that should make up most of your regular diet.

In the end, you're likely to have averaged out to a desirable amount with no fuss and no muss and be right in line with that headline from the first page of the 2000 *Guidelines* that I mention at the beginning of this chapter: "Eating is one of life's greatest pleasures." Amen to that.

Chapter 17

Making Wise Food Choices

*T*his chapter features the new Food Guide Pyramid and the Nutrition Facts labels — and it tells you how to use them to create a healthful diet.

But consider yourself warned: The following pages are packed with numbers and details, maybe more than you ever wanted to know about your daily bread — and everything else on your plate. Don't let the many, many facts and stats turn you off. The information you find here really is useful for making good food choices. Take a deep breath, keep your highlighter handy, and jump right in.

Playing with Blocks: Basics of the Food Pyramids

Food pyramids are comprised of building blocks for grown-ups. Instead of letters in the alphabet, these blocks represent food groups that you can put together to create a picture of a healthful diet.

The essential message of all good guides to healthful food choices is that no one food is either good or bad — how much and how often you eat a food is what counts. With that in mind, a food pyramid delivers three important messages:

✔ **Variety:** The fact that the pyramid contains several blocks tells you that no single food gives you all the nutrients you need.

✔ **Moderation:** Having blocks smaller than others tells you that although every food is valuable, some — such as fats and sweets — are best consumed in small amounts.

✔ **Balance:** You can't build a pyramid with a set of identical blocks. Blocks of different sizes show that a healthful diet is balanced: the right amount from each food group.

Clearly, the virtue of a food pyramid is that using it enables you to eat practically everything you like — as long as you follow the recommendations on how much and how frequently (or infrequently) to eat it.

The original USDA Food Guide Pyramid

The first food pyramid was created by the U.S. Department of Agriculture (USDA) in 1992 in response to criticism that the previous government guide to food choices — the Four Food Group Plan (vegetables and fruits, breads and cereals, milk and milk products, meat and meat alternatives) — was too heavily weighted toward high-fat, high-cholesterol foods from animals.

Figure 17-1 depicts the original USDA Food Guide Pyramid. As you can see, this pyramid is based on daily food choices, showing you which foods are in what groups. Unlike the Four Food Group Plan, the pyramid separates fruits and vegetables into two distinct groups and lists the number of servings from each food group that you should have each day. (The number of servings is provided in ranges. The lower end is for people who consume about 1,600 calories a day, and the upper end is for people whose daily dietary intake nears 3,000 calories.)

How much is a serving? Not to worry. That's spelled out in Table 17-1.

Table 17-1	**Standard Serving Sizes**
Food Group	*Serving Size*
Bread	1 slice bread
Cereal	1 ounce ready-to-eat cereal ½ cup cooked cereal
Rice, pasta, crackers	½ cup cooked rice or pasta 5–6 small crackers
Vegetables	1 cup raw leafy vegetables ½ cup chopped raw vegetables ½ cup cooked chopped vegetables ¾ cup vegetable juice
Fruits	1 medium piece of fresh fruit (apple, banana, orange, peach) ½ cup cooked or canned chopped fruit ¾ cup fruit juice

Food Group	Serving Size
Milk products	1 cup milk 1 cup yogurt 1½ ounces natural cheese 2 ounces processed cheese
Meat	2–3 ounces cooked lean meat
Fish	2–3 ounces cooked fish
Poultry	2–3 ounces cooked lean poultry
Dry beans	½ cup cooked dry beans
Eggs	1 egg (1 ounce)
Nuts, seeds	2 tablespoons peanut butter ⅓ cup nuts or seeds
Fats, oils, sweets	No specific amount; very little

The Food Guide Pyramid (Washington, D.C.: International Food Information Council Foundation, U.S. Department of Agriculture, Food Marketing Institute, 1995)

Figure 17-1:
The original
USDA Food
Guide
Pyramid.

U.S. Department of Agriculture/U.S. Department of Health and Human Services

One useful aspect of the original USDA Food Guide Pyramid is its recommendation of different numbers of daily servings for people consuming different amounts of calories each day. For example, consider how the recommended number of servings from the bread group varies at different levels of calorie consumption.

Table 17-2 lists the original USDA serving recommendations for three levels of calorie consumption:

- 1,600 calories per day (sufficient for women who don't exercise and for many older adults)

- 2,200 calories per day (meets the needs of most children, active women, and many sedentary men)

- 2,800 calories per day (provides the energy required by most teenage boys, many active men, and some very active women)

Table 17-2	How Many Servings: Daily Choices Based on the Original USDA Food Guide Pyramid		
Food	*1,600 Calories/Day*	*2,200 Calories/Day*	*2,800 Calories/Day*
Bread group	6 servings	9 servings	11 servings
Fruit group	2 servings	3 servings	4 servings
Vegetable group	3 servings	4 servings	5 servings
Milk group*	2–3 servings	2–3 servings	2–3 servings
Meat group	5 ounces	6 ounces	7 ounces

* Requirements higher for women who are pregnant or nursing
The Food Guide Pyramid (Washington, D.C.: International Food Information Council Foundation,
U.S. Department of Agriculture, Food Marketing Institute, 1995)

Okay, now stare at the original Food Guide Pyramid and the servings charts until they're burned into your brain. Then move on . . . to the spanking new version of the Food Guide Pyramid on a new interactive Web site, www.MyPyramid.gov.

The brand new 2005 USDA Food Guide Pyramid

By the time USDA/HHS got around to revising the *Dietary Guidelines for 2005*, it was pretty clear that the original food pyramid hadn't done its proposed job of teaching most Americans how to choose foods that provide sufficient nutrients without piling on the pounds.

What to do? What else? In a word, MyPyramid (see Figure 17-2).

Figure 17-2:
The
MyPyramid
image
promotes
both proper
diet and
exercise.

MyPyramid.gov
STEPS TO A HEALTHIER YOU

Courtesy of the United States Department of Agriculture (USDA)

Like the original Food Guide Pyramid, this new version is made up of sections representing the foods in your daily diet — from left to right, grains, vegetables, fruit, oils, milk, and meat/beans.

Like the building blocks on the original Food Guide Pyramid, the six bands on this one say "pick lots of different kinds of foods to build a better diet." The different sizes of the sections suggest that you should consume more of some foods than others. The steps going up the side of the pyramid say, "Physical activity matters, so get moving!"

And the MyPyramid slogan, "Steps to a Healthier You," tells you that you don't have to leap tall buildings in a single bound like Superman (or woman) to improve your nutrition. Even small steps can make a big difference.

But the big deal about MyPyramid is that you can personalize the diagram to meet your own special needs. For more information, visit www.mypyramid.gov.

Building your own pyramid

Okay, warm up your typing finger(s) and run this one over your keyboard: www.mypyramid.gov. This gets you to a Homepage with lots of special info buttons on the left side.

Click on the one labeled My Pyramid Plan, and up pops a set of boxes into which you type your age, gender, and activity level to get back a personalized plan for your very own body and lifestyle.

For example, Table 17-3 shows the recommended daily calorie totals and food amounts for a 27-year-old man or woman who exercises a moderate 30-to-60 minutes a day. (Yes, the number of times you walk back and forth across the floor at work or chase your 2-year-old around the living room counts as activity!) Table 17-4 shows the recommended weekly intake of various kinds of veggies.

Table 17-3	MyPyramid's Suggested Daily Amounts for a 27-Year-Old Who Exercises 30-60 Minutes a Day	
Food	*Male (2,600 Total Calories)*	*Female (2,000 Total Calories)*
Grains (including whole grains)	9 ounces	6 ounces
Whole grains*	4.5 ounces	3 ounces
Vegetables	3.5 cups	2.5 cups
Fruit	2 cups	2 cups
Milk	3 cups	3 cups
Meat/beans	6.5 ounces	5.5 ounces
Oils**	8 teaspoons	6 teaspoons
Extra calories (fats and sugars)	410 calories	265 calories

* Half the grains should be whole grains
** No more than this amount

Table 17-4	Varying the Veggies: Weekly Amounts for a 27-Year-Old Who Exercises 30-60 Minutes a Day	
Type of Vegetable	*Male*	*Female*
Dark green	3 cups	3 cups
Orange	2.5 cups	2 cups
Dry beans/peas	3.5 cups	3 cups
Starchy	7 cups	3 cups
Others	8.5 cups	6.5 cups

A word to the wise reader

Call me foolish. Call me old-fashioned. Call me a fan of the simplest solution. But when it comes to assembling a healthful diet, the original Food Guide Pyramid with its neat building blocks and list of ex-act-ly how many servings I need each day works best. Yes, interacting with MyPyramid is fun, sort of like a slot machine where you push in the nickels and get back a quarter. Or two. But what with meeting deadlines for my editors and making dinner for my husband and Katy the amiable cat, I'd rather use my fun time to read a good book than to calculate what constitutes 5.5 ounces of meat or a cup of veggies. MyPyramid.gov says your government promises to make the site even more glitzy in the future with cyber bells and whistles that'll enable you to assemble meals with specific servings of specific foods, like one baked apple or one ham sandwich or one glass of skim milk. Ex-*cuse* me, but you can do that yourself right now by checking the servings published along with the original Food Guide Pyramid and listed for your convenience a few pages back in this very chapter.

Better yet, the original Food Guide Pyramid is infinitely adaptable, offering a simple method for accommodating virtually any healthful eating plan. For example, look at how easy it is to use to original pyramid to follow the veggie-fruit-pasta-and-unsaturated-fat Mediterranean Diet:

Which proves — to me at least — that newer ain't always better. Ah, well.

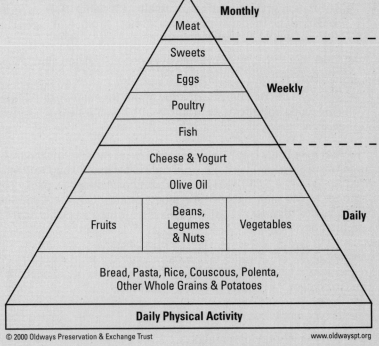

© 2000 Oldways Preservation & Exchange Trust   www.oldwayspt.org

Daily beverage recommendations: Drink six glasses of water.
If you drink wine, do so in moderation.

The other buttons on the page are interesting, too. My Pyramid Tracker enables you to compare your current diet and level of physical activity with the newest recommendations from the nutrition guides. Inside the Pyramid tells everything you ever wanted to know — maybe more — about the different food groups, including recommended daily amounts. For Professionals includes a downloadable worksheet that helps you track what you're really eating — as opposed to what you sorta remember you ate the day before yesterday.

Understanding the Nutrition Facts Labels

Once upon a time, the only reliable consumer information on a food label was the name of the food inside. The 1990 Nutrition Labeling and Education Act changed that forever with a spiffy new set of consumer-friendly food labels that include

- ✔ A mini-nutrition guide that shows the food's nutrient content and evaluates its place in a balanced diet

- ✔ Accurate ingredient listings, with all ingredients listed in order of their weight in the food; for example, the most prominent ingredient in a loaf of bread would be flour

- ✔ Clear identification of ingredients previously listed simply as *colorings* and *sweeteners*

- ✔ Scientifically reliable information about the relationship between specific foods and specific chronic health conditions, such as heart disease and cancer

The Nutrition Facts label is *required by law* for more than 90 percent of all processed, packaged foods, everything from canned soup to fresh pasteurized orange juice. Food sold in really small packages — a pack of gum, for example — can omit the nutrition label but must carry a telephone number or address so that an inquisitive consumer (you) can call or write for the information.

Just about the only processed foods exempted from the nutrition labeling regulations are those with no appreciable amounts of nutrients or those whose content varies from batch to batch:

- ✔ Plain (unflavored) coffee and tea

- ✔ Some spices and flavorings

- ✔ Deli and bakery items prepared fresh in the store where they're sold directly to the consumer, as well as food produced by small companies

- ✔ Food sold in restaurants, unless it makes a nutrition content or health claim (How do you eat well when eating out? Check out Chapter 18.)

Labels are voluntary for fresh raw meat, fish, or poultry and fresh fruits and vegetables, but many markets — perhaps under pressure from customers (Hint! Hint!) — put posters or brochures with generic nutrition information near the meat counter or produce bins.

Just the facts, ma'am

The star of the Nutrition Facts label is the Nutrition Facts panel on the back (or side) of the package. This panel features three important elements: serving sizes, amounts of nutrients per serving, and Percent Daily Value. (See Figure 17-3.)

Serving size

No need to stretch your brain trying to translate gram-servings or ounce-servings into real servings. This label does it for you, listing the servings in comprehensible kitchen terms such as one cup or one waffle or two pieces or one teaspoon. It also tells you how many servings are in the package.

Nutrition Facts

Serving Size 1 Cup (240mL)
Servings Per Container 2

Amount Per Serving	
Calories 120	Calories from Fat 45
	% Daily Value*
Total Fat 5g	**8%**
Saturated Fat 3.5g	**18%**
Trans Fat 0g	
Cholesterol 25mg	**8%**
Sodium 120mg	**5%**
Total Carbohydrate 11g	**4%**
Dietary Fiber 0g	**0%**
Sugars 11g	
Protein 8g	**16%**
Vitamin A 10% •	Vitamin C 2%
Calcium 30% • Iron 0% •	Vitamin D 25%

* Percent Daily Values are based on a 2,000 calorie diet. Your daily values may be higher or lower depending on your caloric needs.

Figure 17-3: A typical Nutrition Facts panel.

Serving size: This varies from package to package. Serving sizes don't always reflect the typical amount that an adult may eat. In some cases, the serving size may be a very small amount.

Calories: The calories contained in a single serving.

% daily values: The percentage of nutrients that one serving contributes to a 2,000-calorie diet. Parents or children may need more or less than 2,000 calories per day.

Nutrient amounts: The nutritional values of the most important, but not all, vitamins and other nutrients in the product.

The serving size is exactly the same for all products in a category. In other words, the Nutrition Facts chart enables you to compare at a glance the nutrient content for two different brands of yogurt, cheddar cheese, string beans, soft drinks, and so on.

When checking the labels, you may think the suggested serving sizes seem small (especially with so-called low-fat items). Think of these serving sizes as useful guides.

Amount per serving

The Nutrition Facts chart tells you the amount (per serving) for several important factors:

- ✔ Calories
- ✔ Calories from fat
- ✔ Total fat (in grams)
- ✔ Saturated fat (in grams)
- ✔ Trans fats (in grams)
- ✔ Cholesterol (in milligrams)
- ✔ Total carbohydrate (in grams)
- ✔ Dietary fiber (in grams)
- ✔ Sugars (in grams — total sugars, the ones occurring naturally in the food *and* the ones added during preparation)
- ✔ Protein (in grams)

Percent Daily Value

The Percent Daily Value enables you to judge whether a specific food is high, medium, or low in fat, cholesterol, sodium, carbohydrates, dietary fiber, sugar, protein, vitamin A, vitamin C, calcium, and iron.

The Percent Daily Value for vitamins and minerals is based on a set of recommendations called the *Reference Daily Intakes (RDI),* which are similar (but not identical) to the Recommended Dietary Allowances (RDAs) for vitamins and minerals discussed in Chapters 10 and 11.

RDIs are based on allowances set in 1973, so some RDIs now may not apply to all groups of people. For example, the Daily Value for calcium is 1,000 milligrams, but many studies — and two National Institutes of Health Conferences — suggest that postmenopausal women who are not using hormone replacement therapy need to consume 1,500 milligrams of calcium a day to reduce their risk of osteoporosis.

The Percent Daily Values for fats, carbohydrates, protein, sodium, and potassium are based on the *Daily Reference Values (DRV).* DRVs are standards for nutrients, such as fat and fiber, known to raise or lower the risk of certain health conditions, such as heart disease and cancer. For example, the *Dietary Guidelines for Americans 2005* says that no more than 30 percent of your daily calories should come from fat. That means a 2,000-calorie-per-day diet shouldn't have any more than 600 calories from fat. To translate fat calories to grams of fat (the units used in the DRVs), divide the number of calories from fat (600) by 9 (the number of calories in one gram of fat). The answer, 67, is slightly higher than the actual DRV. But it's close enough. For more about the evolving state of dietary recommendations, see Chapter 4. And — dare I say it? — your daily paper. Boy, is nutrition ever a work-in-progress!

Nutritionists use similar calculations to set the DRVs, such as

✔ Saturated fat — 10 percent of your calories/9 calories per gram

✔ Carbohydrates — 60 percent of your calories/4 calories per gram

✔ Dietary fiber — 11.5 percent of your calories/0 calories per gram

✔ Protein — 10 percent of your calories/4 calories per gram

Having set down this tidy list, I'm now compelled to tell you that the %DV (that's short for Percent Daily Value), as shown on the Nutrition Facts labels, are behind the times. New recommendations in the *Dietary Guidelines for Americans 2005* say

✔ Total fat calories should account for 20 to 35 percent of total daily calories.

✔ No safe level exists for saturated fats or trans fats, thus no %DV is provided for either one.

The total amount of saturated fat in the portion is the number of grams of sat fat plus the number of grams of trans fat. (Who else would tell you these things?)

✔ Calories from carbs should account for 45 to 65 percent of daily calories.

✔ Women younger than 50 need to consume 25 grams of dietary fiber a day; men younger than 50, 38 grams. After age 51, it's 21 grams for women and 30 grams for men.

✔ Calories from protein should account for 10 to 35 percent of total daily calories, an amount much higher than the current RDA for protein.

Will this change the numbers on the Nutrition Facts labels? The sensible answer is, sure it will . . . eventually. Are the current Nutrition Facts labels still useful? Absolutely.

Relying on labels: Health claims

Ever since man (and woman) came out of the caves, people have been making health claims for certain foods. These folk remedies may be comforting, but the evidence to support them is mostly anecdotal: "I had a cold. My mom gave me chicken soup, and here I am, all bright-eyed and bushy-tailed. Of course, it did take a week to get rid of the cold completely. . . ."

On the other hand, health claims approved by the USDA and the Food and Drug Administration (FDA) for inclusion on the new food labels are another matter entirely. If you see a statement suggesting that a particular food or nutrient plays a role in reducing your risk of a specific medical condition, you can be absolutely 100 percent sure that a real relationship exists between the food and the medical condition. You can also be sure that scientific evidence from well-designed studies supports the claim.

In other words, USDA/FDA-approved health claims are medically sound and scientifically specific. They highlight the known relationships between

- ✔ **Calcium and bone density:** A label describing a food as "high in calcium" may truthfully say: "A diet high in calcium helps women maintain healthy bones and may reduce the risk of osteoporosis later in life."

- ✔ **A diet high in fat, saturated fat, and cholesterol and a higher risk of heart disease:** A label describing a food as "low-fat, low cholesterol," or "no fat, no cholesterol" may truthfully say: "This food follows the recommendations of the American Heart Association's diet to lower the risk of heart disease."

- ✔ **A high-fiber diet and a lower risk of some kinds of cancer:** A label describing a food as "high-fiber" may truthfully say: "Foods high in dietary fiber may reduce the risk of certain types of cancer."

- ✔ **A high-fiber diet and a lower risk of heart attack:** A label describing a food as "high-fiber" may truthfully say: "Foods high in dietary fiber may help reduce the risk of coronary heart disease."

- ✔ **Sodium and hypertension (high blood pressure):** A label describing a food as "low-sodium" may truthfully say: "A diet low in sodium may reduce the risk of high blood pressure."

- ✔ **A fruit-and-vegetable-rich diet and a low risk of some kinds of cancer:** Labels on fruits and vegetables may truthfully say: "A diet high in fruits and vegetables may lower your risk of some kinds of cancer."

- ✔ **Folic acid (folate) and a lower risk of neural tube (spinal cord) birth defects such as spina bifida:** Labels on folate-rich foods may truthfully say: "A diet rich in folates during pregnancy lowers the risk of neural tube defects in the fetus."

Foods with more than 4 grams saturated fat and/or saturated fat plus trans fat per serving cannot have any health claims at all on their labels.

How high is high? How low is low?

Today, savvy consumers reach almost automatically for packages labeled "low fat" or "high fiber." But it's a dollars-to-doughnuts sure bet that hardly one shopper in a thousand knows what "low" and "high" actually mean.

Because these are potent terms that promise real health benefits, the new labeling law has created strict, science-based definitions:

- *High* means that one serving provides 20 percent or more of the Daily Value for a particular nutrient. Other ways to say "high" are "rich in" or "excellent source," as in "milk is an excellent source of calcium."

- *Good source* means one serving gives you 10 to 19 percent of the Daily Value for a particular nutrient.

- *Light* (sometimes written *lite*) is used in connection with calories, fat, or sodium. It means the product has one-third fewer calories or 50 percent less fat or 50 percent less sodium than usually is found in a particular type of product.

- *Low* means that the food contains an amount of a nutrient that enables you to eat several servings without going over the Daily Value for that nutrient.

  - *Low-calorie* means 40 calories or fewer per serving

  - *Low-fat* means 3 grams of fat or less

  - *Low saturated fat* means less than 0.5 grams trans fat per serving and 1 gram (or less) saturated fat.

  - *Low-cholesterol* means 20 milligrams or less

- *Reduced saturated fat* means that the amount of saturated fat plus trans fat has been reduced more than 25 percent from what's normal for in the given food product

- *Free* means "negligible" — not "none."

  - *Calorie-free* means fewer than 5 calories per serving

  - *Fat-free* means less than 0.5 grams of fat

- *Trans fat–free* means the food has less than 0.5 grams trans fat and 0.5 grams saturated fat per serving

- *Cholesterol-free* means less than 2 milligrams of cholesterol or 2 grams or less saturated fat

- *Sodium-free* or *salt-free* means less than 5 milligrams of sodium

- *Sugar-free* means less than 0.5 grams of sugar

Notice something missing? Right, there's no definition for "low sodium" per serving. On the other hand, a meal plan with less than 1,000 milligrams sodium per day is considered a low-sodium diet.

Organic — the not-quite-finished evolution of a label term

"Organic" (as in organic food) is a highly charged food word. But do you know what it means? Don't be embarrassed to say no. Until recently, neither did most health professionals.

To a chemist, *organic* means a substance that contains carbon, hydrogen, and oxygen. By this chemical standard, all foods — and all human beings — are organic.

Yet some people adopted the word *organic* to describe plant foods grown without pesticides or synthetic chemicals, or to describe the poultry, fish, beef, and lamb from animals raised on a diet with no antibiotics or other medicating chemicals to assure healthy and efficiently producing animals.

But these descriptions were not standards regulated by any federal agency. So USDA set out to create regulations that legally define the term:

- In December 1997, the USDA released its first proposal on new standards for organic foods.

- In May 1998, after receiving more than 280,000 comments from the public, food

growers, and food marketers, the agency announced that although bioengineered and irradiated foods are safe, they're not permitted to carry the organic label.

- In October 1998, the USDA issued three more proposals on how animals yielding organic food are to be treated and how the agency will certify producers of organic foods.

- In October 2002, the USDA implemented rules saying that foods carrying the organic label must be grown without pesticides or raised without non-organic feed.

Sounds simple, sounds good. Sounds . . . not quite final. Barely four months later, in February 2003, Congress passed legislation allowing organic livestock to be given non-organic feed at any time the price of organic feed reaches two times that of the regular stuff. As I write this book, the whole darn thing is in a state of flux. For the latest, check your local newspaper or visit www.usda.gov to see what you can dig up. Then, dig in. Maybe.

Listing what's inside

The extra added attraction on the Nutrition Facts label is the complete ingredient listing, in which every single ingredient is listed in order of its weight in the product, heaviest first, lightest last. In addition, the label must spell out the true identity of some classes of ingredients known to cause allergic reactions:

- ✔ Vegetable proteins (*hydrolyzed corn protein* rather than the old-fashioned *hydrolyzed vegetable protein*)

- ✔ Milk products (*nondairy* products such as coffee whiteners may contain the milk protein caseinate, which comes from milk)

- ✔ FD&C yellow No. 5, a full, formal chemical name instead of *coloring*

Naming the precise source of sweeteners (*corn sugar monohydrate* rather than just *sugar monohydrate*) is still voluntary, but as is true of information about raw meat, fish, and poultry, manufacturers and stores just may respond to consumer pressure. (Repeat advice: Hint! Hint!)

Choosing Foods with MyPyramid and the Nutrition Facts Label

The Food Guide Pyramid helps balance meals and snacks. In the kitchen, you can increase the nutritional value by thinking of individual dishes as mini–food pyramids. At snack time, you can use the Food Guide Pyramid to choose munchies that are a valuable part of your overall daily diet.

For example, although you know that fruits and veggies are good snacks, that doesn't mean that you're stuck with boring carrot sticks or an apple. The food pyramid says "fruits and vegetables," not raw fruits and raw vegetables. Yes, a fresh apple's fine. But so is a baked apple (100 calories), fragrant with cinnamon and decorated with no-fat sour cream (30–45 calories for two tablespoons). Carrot strips are okay. So are vegetarian baked beans — yes, baked beans (140 calories plus 26 grams of carbohydrates, 7 grams of protein, 7 grams of dietary fiber, and 2 grams of fat per ½ cup serving), which are considered both veggies *and* a member of the high-protein meat/beans group.

As for the Nutrition Facts label, you can use that to eat your cake and have it nutritiously by comparing products to choose the best alternatives.

Here's a good example: You find yourself irresistibly drawn to double dark chocolate ice cream (lots of fat, saturated fat, cholesterol, and a whopping 230 calories per ½ cup serving). But then, just as your hand is opening the freezer door, ready to reach for the ice cream, suddenly . . . out of the corner of your eye, you see the Nutrition Facts panel on the label of the no-fat but equally irresistible chocolate sorbet. It says, "No fat, no saturated fat, no cholesterol, and only 90 to 130 calories per serving." When you put the labels side-by-side, do you need to ask which one comes out the winner?

The Final Word on Diagrams and Stats

At the beginning of this chapter, I warned you that keeping track of all the facts may be difficult. But now I think that you can pretty much boil them all down to one nutritional Golden Rule exemplified by the food pyramids and the Nutrition Facts food label: *Keep things in proportion.*

Come to think of it, that's not a bad philosophy for life.

Chapter 18

Eating Smart When Eating Out

. . . .

In This Chapter

▶ Navigating a restaurant menu

▶ Ordering without overdoing

▶ Finding nutritious fast-food favorites

. . . .

*E*ating out is in. You don't have to cook, and somebody else washes the dishes. The challenge is to avoid letting luxury lull you into ceding responsibility for your food choices to some chef whose heart belongs to butter. This chapter lays out strategies for making your excellent adventure nutritionally sound. You find out how to edit a menu in a *white-tablecloth* restaurant (the food professional's description of an upscale eatery) to balance gustatory pleasure with common-sense nutrition. And you figure out how to juggle fast food so that it fits into a healthful diet. No cooking, no dishes, no guilt. Who could ask for anything more?

Interpreting a Restaurant Menu

Restaurants are businesses, and that means they respond to consumer demand. What consumers have demanded for years are rich foods and big portions, which means that the restaurant concept of a portion or of a healthy alternative is seriously out of whack with what the nutrition experts recommend. Does that mean you should stop eating out? Heck, no! But it does mean you need to use caution when navigating a menu.

Pinpointing portions

Restaurants don't make friends by serving up teensy little portions. In fact, tiny servings probably sank *nouvelle cuisine,* the 1980s fad that put one string bean, three garden peas, half an artichoke heart, and one sliced cherry tomato on a lettuce leaf and called it the salad course.

Reality dictates that the portions on restaurant plates rarely come within hailing distance of the official serving sizes issued by the U.S. Department of Agriculture. To protect yourself from humongous servings, you need to store real-life versions of the recommended portions in your memory banks. To do that, use an 8-ounce measuring cup and a kitchen scale to run through some basic practice drills at home:

✔ Broil a small steak or roast a chicken breast. Use a kitchen scale to weigh a 3-ounce portion. Does the steak look like a deck of cards? How about a small calculator? That's one serving.

✔ Boil some rice. After the rice is done, fill the measuring cup to the halfway mark. Take out the rice and roll it into a tennis ball or a billiard ball. Whatever. That's one serving.

✔ Shred some greens. Fill the measuring cup to the 8-ounce mark. Turn the greens out onto a salad plate. That's one serving.

✔ Open one can of beets or fruit cocktail. Fill the measuring cup to the halfway mark. Spoon the beets or fruit onto a plate. That's one serving.

✔ Open a can of soda. Pour it into the measuring cup, right up to the 8-ounce mark. Pour that into a glass. Add some ice. It's probably more than you get in an upscale restaurant, less than you get at the burger barn. No matter: It's still one certified USDA serving.

Now that you have a picture of a serving in your mind, you can slice away the extra from your restaurant plate — and take it home for lunch or dinner the next day. That's what *doggie bags* are for. (Now that I have my very first cat, after years and years of adaptable lovable dogs, I know that the sacks are called doggie bags because cats are too smart — okay, too finicky — to eat someone else's leftovers.)

Asking for proof

When the menu says, "Eat me! I'm healthy," ask for proof. The people who make and market processed foods are required by law to provide detailed ingredient labels on their packages. Restaurants ordinarily are exempt. They don't have to tell you exactly what's in the beef Stroganoff or vegetable stir-fry. The exception is a dish for which the restaurant makes a health claim.

The restaurant may write "low-fat" or "heart-healthy" next to the item on the menu or mark the entry with a little red heart to signify the same thing. When a restaurant does this, the Nutrition Education and Labeling Act says the restaurant has to back up that claim. The law is flexible; it doesn't require an ingredient listing on the menu, but it says that the restaurant can comply by making a notebook available that accomplishes at least one of the following tasks:

- ✔ The notebook can list the nutrient content of each labeled dish or show that the dish was made according to a recipe from an authoritative professional association or dietary group, such as the American Heart Association.

- ✔ The notebook can show that the nutritional values for the dish are based on a reliable nutrition guide, such as USDA's voluminous *Agriculture Handbook No. 8,* which is made up of several volumes with perhaps a thousand pages of nutritional analysis for all kinds of food. As with the new, improved labels on food packages, this policy is designed to make sure that any food that claims to be healthy actually is.

Making Smart Menu Choices

From a nutritional point of view, restaurant dining has three basic pitfalls:

- ✔ Serving sizes are too big.
- ✔ Garnishes and side dishes are too rich.
- ✔ Meals have too many courses.

Not to worry. Exercise a little care and caution, and you can order from any menu, secure in the knowledge that pleasing your palate doesn't mean tossing away all nutritional common sense. The following list of strategies can make any restaurant experience a joy.

Starting simple

Set the nutritional tone of dinner right off the bat with your choice of appetizer. You have two possible alternatives. The first is opting for a really rich, high-density food such as pâté de foie gras (literally: fat liver paste) and then coast downward, calorie-fat-and-cholesterol-wise, for the rest of the meal. A second alternative is choosing a tasty but low-calorie, low-fat appetizer such as clear soup, a salad with lemon juice dressing, or shellfish such as shrimp cocktail (10 to 30 calories a shrimp) with no-fat (catsup/horseradish) sauce. This choice allows you more food later on.

Elevating appetizers to entrees

For smaller portion sizes or to skip the calorie-laden sides that come with most entrees, order an appetizer as your main course. One of my favorite New York City restaurants, a Mediterranean fish house in the East 40s, serves an appetizer consisting of a really big (and I mean huge) bowl of maybe 30 steamed mussels in their shells in a low-oil fresh-tomato sauce with one crusty piece of French bread underneath to sop it up with. When I add a glass of cold, dry white wine and one more piece of bread, this appetizer becomes a meal in itself — with a lot fewer calories and less fat than most any entree on the menu. Less expensive, too.

Skipping the fat on the bread

Don't butter your bread. Don't oil it, either. Many chic and trendy restaurants now serve up a dish of flavored olive oil in place of butter. True, the olive oil has less saturated fat than butter, and it has no cholesterol, but the calorie count is exactly the same. All fats and oils (butter, margarine, vegetable oils) give you about 100 calories a tablespoon. *Note:* You may get even more calories from the oil if you do a lot of dipping.

Consumer alert: Don't assume that your bread is low-fat just because you didn't butter it. Many different types of breads come already buttered (or oiled). One example is foccacia, the thick squares of savory Italian bread. Others are popovers and muffins.

To test the fat content of your bread, pick up a piece or put it on your napkin. If your hand feels greasy or the bread leaves an oily spot on your napkin, you have your answer.

Going naked: Undressed veggies

Victorians boiled vegetables into a yucky muck — no color, no texture, no taste. Then came 20th century butter, cheese, and cream sauces, often burnished under the broiler to a browned crust. Now, smart restaurant cooks rely on herbs and spices, reduced (boiled down and thickened) fat-free bouillons, unusual salad combinations, and imaginative treatments such as purees and kabobs to make their vegetables tasty but trim. The result? Food heaven and nutrition joy. The vegetable flavors come through, and the calories stay very, very, very low.

You don't have to settle for that boring steamed stuff and definitely not veg-gies so raw they have no taste. The difference between raw cauliflower and cauliflower that's been steamed for 15 or 20 minutes and dusted with dill is so vast that people who insist on passing out the stuff cold should be charged with vegetable abuse.

To reap the low-calorie rewards, avoid veggie dishes labeled

- ✔ Au beurre (with butter)
- ✔ Au gratin (with cheese sauce)
- ✔ Batter-dipped (eggs, oil, fried)
- ✔ Breaded (breadcrumbs, oil, fried)
- ✔ Fritters (fried)
- ✔ Fritto (fried)
- ✔ Hollandaise (sauce with butter and egg yolks)
- ✔ Tempura (battered and fried)

Minimizing the main dish

I won't insult you by telling you to avoid fried foods. If you're reading this book, you already know that the best choice is something broiled, baked, or roasted — without added fat, and with the drippings siphoned off. But I can't avoid noting that you can lower the fat content of any main dish simply by wielding a mean knife and fork to cut away the vestiges of visible fat on your chops or steak or poultry.

Another approach is to order a main course meat dish without the "main" part. That is, order your meat, fish, or poultry as a small-serving appetizer, and then ask your waiter for a veggie entree. Or opt for all the nifty little extras that usually accompany the meat course, ordering the veggie side dishes à la carte instead of a veggie entree.

Demand tiny boiled onions. Baby peas with mint. Pickled beets and red cabbage. Sugared carrots. Sautéed spinach. Darling little boiled or baked potatoes with a crust of paprika or cumin. The more, the merrier. The result may not be entirely fat-free, but it almost certainly has fewer calories, less fat, more dietary fiber, and a wider variety of vitamins than plain meat or poultry.

Sidelining sauces

Dining out is a treat, so treat yourself — within reason. You can have your béarnaise (egg yolks, butter), béchamel (butter, flour, heavy cream), brown sauce (beef drippings, flour), and hollandaise (butter, egg yolks), as long as you have them in reasonable amounts.

Ask the waiter to bring the sauce on the side, take one tablespoonful (about a soup spoonful), and hand the rest back to the waiter. When ordering from an Italian menu, the general rule is to avoid the olive-oil-based sauces and choose the tomato-based red sauce. (If the chef where you're eating fattens up the tomato sauce with olive oil, forget this rule.) Many restaurants now make their red sauces skinny — all tomato, little or no oil.

Satisfying your sweet tooth

After a heavy meal, your body often craves something sweet. Lower your calories, fat, and so on by splitting a dessert with your dinner partner. Or opt for rich but fat-free sweetened coffees: espresso, Greek, and Turkish brews seem most satisfying. Hate coffee? Have a diet cola.

Discovering the Healthful Side of Fast Food

Fast food can be good food. By choosing carefully, you can enjoy burgers while still meeting recommended daily dietary allowances for all important vitamins and minerals. A fast-food burger on a bun, plus a salad and a small, low-fat milk shake, an 8-ounce cup of milk, a small cola, or plain old water may not sound like great nutrition, but the version served up in fast-food restaurants can actually be relatively low in fat and relatively high in valuable nutrients.

Choosing wisely at the drive-through

The greatest problem with fast food is *very* big servings. More food means more calories — and more you. Several people recently have filed lawsuits charging the fast-food restaurants made them overeat, which, in turn, made them overweight. At least one such suit was tossed out of court, but that doesn't mean another won't be filed down the road. So the question of the day becomes, does a smart cookie like you check your brains at the door when you enter a fast-food restaurant — or do you have the intelligence to choose wisely regardless of where you plunk yourself down for a meal?

Eating smart is a skill you can exercise in any location. For example, Table 18-1 compares the nutrient values of three basic McDonald's meals. All three meals derive about 30 percent of their calories from fat (although all three dish up about one-third the percent Daily Value for artery-clogging saturated fat). They're relatively low in cholesterol and provide plenty of vitamin A, vitamin C, and bone-building calcium. And the servings are reasonable:

- ✔ The burger is the basic, small, no-frills hamburger.

- ✔ The salad is a Caesar salad (no chicken) with one packet of Newman's Own low-fat balsamic vinaigrette dressing.

- ✔ The parfait is the Fruit 'n Yogurt without granola.

- ✔ The milk is an 8-ounce container of low-fat (1 percent) milk.

- ✔ The cola is a 16-ounce cup (small).

The initials DV stand for Daily Value, a nutritional guideline suggesting how much of each nutrient you need each day on a 2,000-calorie diet. For the complete skinny on the DV and how it's used on food labels, check out Chapter 17.

Stop! Before you bite into that burger, remember that the following chart is only a guide. Menus and ingredients may change, so check the nutrition brochure at your local burger haven, and do it every single time. You never know when something new will pop up on your plate.

Table 18-1	Nutritious Fast-Food Meals? Yes!		
Nutrient (% Daily Value)	**Burger, Salad, Milk (490 Calories)**	**Burger, Salad, Parfait (520 Calories)**	**Burger, Salad, Small Cola (540 Calories)**
Calories from fat	33%	30%	26%
Saturated fat	30.5%	34%	29%
Cholesterol	16%	15%	13%
Dietary fiber	31%	31%	31%
Vitamin A	132%	155%	122%
Vitamin C	60%	67%	56%
Calcium	65%	45%	35%

McDonald's Corporation, as of November 21, 2005

Trans fat: The Boooo! factor

Once upon a time, fast-food restaurants — indeed, most restaurants — fried up their foods in butter, which is loaded with the saturated fat and cholesterol that gum up your arteries and increase your risk of heart disease. Then, prodded by the Food Police, restaurants switched to vegetable fats, which are lower in saturated fat and have no cholesterol. Hooray? Well, not exactly. Instead of using heart-healthy vegetable oils, fast-food restaurants sometimes use solid vegetable shortenings, and that's a crucial difference. The shortenings are solid because they contain hydrogenated vegetable oils. Chapter 7 explains the chemistry of *hydrogenation* (adding hydrogen atoms to fats).

Hydrogenated vegetable oils are high in trans fatty acids, a form of fat that may clog your arteries as badly as saturated fats and cholesterol. With trans fats in the mix, an order of fries may have as much artery-hostile fat as a 4-ounce burger. Boooo!

Finding fast-food ingredient guides

Fast-food restaurants now make nutrition information available. McDonald's even puts its numbers on the food wrapper. If your local eatery doesn't have brochures on hand or post them on the wall, don't be shy: Write, call, or click for a copy. *Note:* Companies that don't give you a mailing address usually have a "write us" e-mail form on their Web sites.

Arby's
Consumer Affairs Department
1000 Corporate Dr.
Fort Lauderdale, FL 33334
Phone 800-487-2729
Web site www.arbys.com (Click on "Nutrition.")

Burger King Corporation
5505 Blue Lagoon Dr.
Miami, FL 33126
Phone 305-378-3535
Web site www.bk.com (Click on "Nutrition.")

Dunkin' Donuts
Consumer Care
130 Royall St.
Canton, MA 02021
Phone 800-859-5339
Web site www.dunkindonuts.com (Select "Nutrition" under "About Us.")

KFC (Kentucky Fried Chicken)
P.O. Box 725489
Atlanta, GA 31139
Phone 800-225-5532
Web site www.kfc.com (Click on "Nutrition.")

McDonald's
2111 McDonald's Dr.
Oak Brook, IL 60523
Phone 877-623-3663
Web site www.mcdonalds.com (Select your country and then click on "Food, Nutrition & Fitness.")

Pizza Hut
14841 Dallas Pkwy.
Dallas, TX 75254
Phone 800-948-8488
Web site www.pizzahut.com (Click on "Nutrition.")

Subway
325 Bic Dr.
Milford, CT 06460
Phone 800-888-4848 or 203-877-4281
Web site www.subway.com (Click on "Menu/Nutrition.")

Wendy's
Customer Service Department
4288 W. Dublin-Granville Rd.
Dublin, OH 43017
Phone: 614-764-3100
Web site www.wendys.com (Click on "Food.")

Fingers too fatigued to troll through the separate sites? Check out www.nutritiondata.com. Slide your mouse to the right side of the page and run it down the list of fast food restaurants. Choose one. Click. Choose your dish. Click. Up comes the most complete nutrition analysis known to man. Or woman. Yay NutritionData.com!

Part IV
Food Processing

"I substitute tofu for eye of newt in all my recipes now. It has twice the protein and doesn't wriggle around the cauldron."

In this part . . .

*H*ave you ever wondered why canned green beans aren't as green as fresh ones? Or why an originally translucent egg white turns white when you cook it? Or why frozen carrots are mushy when you defrost them? Or — modern technology at its most mysterious — why exposing food to radiation keeps it fresh longer? Wonder no more. Just shift your eyes to the right to find out what happens when you cook, freeze, dry, or zap food.

Chapter 19

What Is Food Processing?

. . . .

. . . .

Say "processed food," and most people think "cheese spread." They're right, of course. Cheese spread is, in fact, a processed food. But so are baked potatoes, canned tuna, frozen peas, skim milk, pasteurized orange juice, and scrambled eggs. In broad terms, food processing is any technique that alters the natural state of food — everything from cooking to freezing to pickling to drying and more and more and more.

In this chapter, you can read all about how each form of processing changes food from a living thing (animal or vegetable) into an integral component of your healthful diet — and at the same time

✔ Lengthens shelf life

✔ Reduces the risk of foodborne illnesses

✔ Maintains or improves a food's texture and flavor

✔ Upgrades the nutritional value of foods

What a set of bonuses!

Preserving Food: Five Methods of Processing

Where food is concerned, the term *natural* doesn't necessarily translate as "safe" or "good to eat." Food spoils (naturally) when microbes living (naturally) on the surface of meat, a carrot, a peach, or whatever reproduce (naturally) to a population level that overwhelms the food.

Sometimes you can see, feel, or smell when this is happening. You can see mold growing on cheese, feel how meat or chicken turns slippery, and smell when the milk turns sour. The mold on cheese, slippery slickness on the surface of the meat or chicken, and odor of the milk are caused by exploding populations of microorganisms. Don't even argue with them; just throw out the food.

All food processing is designed to prevent what happens to the chicken (or the cheese or the milk). It aims to preserve food and extend its *shelf life* (the period of time when it's safe to consume and nutritious) by stemming the natural tide of biological destruction. (But wait! Not all microbes are bad guys. We use "good" ones to ferment milk to yogurt or cheese and to produce wines and beers.)

Reducing or limiting the growth of food's natural microbe population not only lengthens its shelf life but also lowers the risk of foodborne illnesses. Increased food safety is a natural consequence of most processing that keep foods usable longer. This section discusses how food processing works.

For simplicity's sake, here's a list of the methods used to extend the shelf life of food. I explain each method in even more detail in Chapter 20, Chapter 21, or Chapter 22.

- ✔ Temperature methods
  - • Cooking
  - • Canning
  - • Refrigeration
  - • Freezing
- ✔ Air control
  - • Canning
  - • Vacuum-packaging
- ✔ Moisture control
  - • Dehydration
  - • Freeze-drying (a method that combines methods of controlling the temperature, air, and moisture)
- ✔ Chemical methods
  - • Acidification
  - • Mold inhibition
  - • Salting (dry salt or brine)
- ✔ Irradiation
- ✔ High-pressure processing

Tantalizing tidbit of food nomenclature

Central American Indians dried meat to produce *chaqui,* a name carried north by Spanish explorers who used it to describe the dried meats of the Southwestern Indians, which eventually became — you saw this coming, right? — jerky.

Temperature control

Exposing food to high heat for a sufficiently long period of time reduces the natural population of bacterial spoilers and kills microbes that otherwise may make you sick. For example, pasteurization (heating milk or other liquids such as fruit juice to 145 to 154.4 degrees Fahrenheit for 30 minutes) kills nearly all disease-causing and most other bacteria, as does high-temperature, short-time pasteurization (161 degrees Fahrenheit for 15 seconds).

Chilling also protects food. It works by slowing the rate of microbial reproduction. For example:

✔ Milk refrigerated at 50 degrees Fahrenheit or lower may stay fresh for almost a week because the cold prevents organisms that survived pasteurization from reproducing.

✔ Fresh chicken frozen to 0 degrees Fahrenheit or lower may remain safe for up to 12 months (whole) or 9 months (cut up).

Removing the water

Like all living things, the microbes on food need water to survive. Dehydrate the food, and the bugs won't reproduce, which means the food stays edible longer. That's the rationale behind raisins, prunes, and *pemmican,* a dried mix of meat, fat, and berries adapted from East Coast Native Americans and served to 18th- and 19th-century sailors of every national stripe. Dehydration (loss of water) occurs when food is

✔ Exposed to air and sunlight

✔ Heated for several hours in a very low (250 degrees Fahrenheit) oven or is smoked (the smokehouse acts as a very low oven)

Controlling the air flow

Just as microbes need water, most also need air. Reducing the air supply almost always reduces the bacterial population. The exception is anaerobes (microorganisms that can live without air), such as *botulinum* organisms, which thrive in the absence of air. Go figure!

Foods are protected from air by vacuum-packaging. A *vacuum* — from *vacuus,* the Latin word for "empty" — is a space with virtually no air. Vacuum-packaging is done on a container (generally a plastic bag or a glass jar) from which the air is removed before it's sealed. When you open a vacuum-packed container, you hear a sudden little pop as the vacuum is broken.

If there's no popping sound, the seal has already been broken, allowing air inside, and that means the food inside may be spoiled or may have been tampered with. Do not taste-test: Throw out the entire package, food and all.

Chemical warfare

About two dozen chemicals are used as *food additives* or *food preservatives* to prevent spoilage. (If the mere mention of chemicals or food additives makes the hair on the back of your neck rise, chill out with Chapter 22.) Here are the most common chemical preservatives:

- **Acidifiers:** Most microbes don't thrive in highly acidic settings, so a chemical that makes a food more acidic prevents spoilage. Wine and vinegar are acidifying chemicals, and so are *citric acid,* the natural preservative in citrus fruits, and *lactic acid,* the natural acid in yogurt.

- **Mold inhibitors:** Sodium benzoate, sodium propionate, and calcium propionate slow (but do not entirely stop) the growth of mold on bread. Sodium benzoate also is used to prevent the growth of molds in cheese, margarine, and syrups.

- **Bacteria-busters:** Salt is *hydrophilic* (hydro = water; phil = loving). When you cover fresh meat with salt, the salt draws water up and out of the meat — and up and out of the cells of bacteria living on the meat. Presto: The bacteria die; the meat dries. And you get to eat corned beef (which gets its name from the fact that large grains of salt were once called "corns").

Irradiation

Irradiation is a technique that exposes food to electron beams or to *gamma radiation,* a high-energy light stronger than the X-rays your doctor uses to make a picture of your insides. *Gamma rays* are ionizing radiation, the kind that kills living cells. As a result, irradiation prolongs the shelf life of food by

 ✔ Killing microbes and insects on plants (wheat, wheat powder, spices, dry vegetable seasonings)

 ✔ Preventing potatoes and onions from producing new sprouts at the eyes

 ✔ Slowing the rate at which some fruits ripen

 ✔ Killing disease-causing organisms such as *Trichinella, Salmonella, E. coli,* and *Listeria* (the organism responsible for a recent outbreak of food poisoning from packaged meats and cold cuts) on meat and poultry

In 1998, the U.S. Food and Drug Administration (FDA — which had already approved irradiation for plant foods, pork, and poultry) put its stamp of approval on irradiating fresh red meat products as a way to enhance, but not replace, the safe handling and storage of meat in the processing plant, supermarket, and your kitchen. As of 2005, there are also standards for irradiating fresh and frozen shellfish. And, no, irradiating food *does not make* the food radioactive. But you already knew that, right?

Making Food Better and Better for You

Some food processing really does make your food taste better; a well-broiled steak beats a raw one anytime. Processing also allows you to sample a wide variety of seasonal foods (mostly fruits and vegetables) all year long, and it enables food producers to improve the nutritional status of many basic foods, such as grains and milk, by enriching or altering them to meet the needs of modern consumers.

Intensifying flavor and aroma

One advantage of food processing is that it enables you to enjoy things never seen in nature, such as the ever-popular — and ever criticized — cheese spread. A more mundane benefit of food processing is that it intensifies aroma and flavor, almost always for the better. Here's how:

✔ **Drying concentrates flavor.** A prune has a different, darker, more intensely sweet flavor than a fresh plum. On the other hand, dried food can be hard and tough to chew (think beef jerky).

✔ **Heating heightens aroma by quickening the movement of aroma molecules.** In fact, your first tantalizing hint of dinner usually is the scent of cooking food. Chilling has the opposite effect: It slows the movement of the molecules. To sense the difference, sniff a plate of cold roast beef versus hot roast beef straight from the oven. Or sniff two glasses of vodka, one warm, one icy from the freezer. One comes up scent-free; the other has the olfactory allure of pure gasoline. Guess which is which. Or you can pass up the guessing and try for yourself. Nothing like firsthand experience!

✔ **Warming foods intensifies flavors.** This development is sometimes beneficial (warm roast beef is somehow more savory than cold roast beef), sometimes not (warm milk is definitely not as popular as the icy-cold version).

✔ **Changing the temperature also changes texture.** Heating softens some foods (butternut squash is a good example) and solidifies others (think eggs). Chilling keeps the fats in pâté firm so the stuff doesn't melt down into a puddle on the plate. Ditto for the gelatin that keeps dessert molds and dinner aspics standing upright.

Adding nutrients

The addition of vitamins and minerals to basic foods has helped eliminate many once-common nutritional deficiency diseases. The practice is so common that you take the following for granted:

✔ Breads, cereals, and grains are given extra B vitamins to replace the vitamins lost when whole grains are stripped of their nutrient-rich covering to make white flour or white rice or degermed cornmeal. Doing so reduces the risk of the B vitamin–deficiency diseases beriberi and pellagra.

✔ Breads, cereals, and grains also are given iron to replace what's lost in milling and to make it easier for American women to reach the RDA (Recommended Dietary Allowance) for this important mineral.

✔ All milk sold in the U.S. has added vitamin D to reduce the risk of the bone-deforming vitamin D–deficiency diseases rickets (among children) and osteomalacia (among adults).

✔ Added fat-free milk proteins turn *skim milk* — milk from which the fat has been removed — into a creamier liquid with more calcium but less fat and cholesterol than whole milk.

Combining benefits

Adding genes from one food (such as corn) to another food (such as toma-toes) may make the second food taste better and stay fresh longer. You can bet your bottom flapjack that this is one hot topic, so for more about genetic engineering at the dinner table, check out Chapter 22.

Faking It: Alternative Foods

In addition to its many other benefits, food processing offers you some totally fake but widely appreciated substitute fats and sweeteners. Actually, these may be just the tip of the iceberg, so to speak. Two years ago, the Brits sprang Quorn, food made from fungi (yes, fungi) on an unsuspecting U.S. public. Quorn seems to have slipped back into the nutritional netherworld, but as processing becomes more adventurous, who knows what strange and wonderful dishes lie just beyond the entrance to the Nutritional Twilight Zone? Dum-de-dum-dum . . .

Alternative foods No. 1: Fake fats

Fat carries desirable flavors and makes food "rich." But it's also high in calo-ries, and some fats (the saturated kind described in Chapter 7) can clog your arteries. One way to deal with this problem is to eliminate the fat from food (as in skim milk). Another way is to head for the food lab and create a no- or low-calorie, nonclogging substitute, such as Olestra/Olean or Simplesse.

Olestra/Olean

Olestra/Olean is a no-calorie compound made from sugar and vegetable oils. Olestra is indigestible, which means it adds no nutrients — such as fat or cholesterol — to food. Unfortunately, as it speeds through your intestinal tract, it's likely to pick up and swoosh along some fat-soluble nutrients such as vitamin A, vitamin D, and vitamin E. In addition, eating excess amounts of food made with Olestra may cause diarrhea.

In 1996, the FDA approved Olestra's use in snack foods such as potato chips. At the time, the agency-required label stated that Olestra may cause abdomi-nal cramping and loose stools. In the spring of 1998, an 18-member FDA food advisory committee reaffirmed the agency's original decision that Olestra is safe for use in snack foods. The committee concluded that the fat alterna-tive's gastrointestinal effects and its effects on your ability to absorb fat-soluble vitamins do not significantly affect public health. In August 2003, the FDA, after a scientific review of several studies conducted after foods with Olestra went on sale, concluded that the statement was no longer required.

But something's an ill wind — and a really bad food ingredient — that doesn't have at least some redeeming virtues. In 2004, researchers at the University of Cincinnati and the University of Western Australia treated a patient with chloracne (a skin condition caused by exposure to the toxic chemical dioxin) with a regimen of — get this — potato chips made with Olestra. The result? The patient's skin cleared up and his body level of dioxin went down. A-maz-ing.

For more information about the activities of the FDA's Center for Food Safety and Applied Nutrition, which conducted the tests evaluating Olestra, visit the Web site at `vm.cfsan.fda.gov`.

Simplesse

Simplesse is a low-calorie fat substitute used in processed foods. It is made by heating and blending proteins from egg whites and/or milk into extremely tiny round balls that taste like fat. Simplesse has 1 to 2 calories per gram versus 9 calories per gram for real fats or oils. Simplesse is not recommended for young children because they need essential fatty acids found in real fats, and its use may be problematic for people who are

- ✔ Sensitive to milk (the label on a food with Simplesse must carry the word "milk")
- ✔ Sensitive to eggs
- ✔ On low-protein diets (for example, kidney disease patients)

Alternative foods No. 2: Substitute sweeteners

Here's a scientific tidbit. Most substitute sweeteners were discovered by accident in laboratories where researchers touched a paper or a pencil, then stuck their fingers in their mouths to discover, "Eureka! It's sweet." As Harold McGee wrote in the first edition of his wonderful *On Food and Cooking* (Collier Books, 1988), "These stories make one wonder about the standards of laboratory hygiene."

Because substitute sweeteners are not absorbed by your body and don't provide any nutrients, scientists call them by their proper name: *non-nutritive sweeteners.* The best-known (listed in order of their discovery and/or FDA approval) are:

- ✔ **Saccharin (Sweet'N Low):** This synthetic sweetener was discovered by accident (the fingers-in-the-mouth syndrome) at Johns Hopkins in 1879. A ban on saccharin was proposed in 1977, after it was linked to bladder cancer in rats; however, it's still on the market, and diabetics who have used saccharin for years show no excess levels of bladder cancer. That aside, a warning label nevertheless may appear with saccharin-sweetened products, indicating that it is a mild rodent carcinogen. In December 1998, the executive committee of the National Toxicology Program (NTP) recommended that saccharin be taken off the list of suspected human carcinogens, but this step has not yet been taken. ***Note:*** Most people think saccharin is very sweet, but if you hate broccoli, you're likely to think saccharin's bitter. Check out Chapter 15 to see why.

✓ **Cyclamates:** These surfaced (on somebody's finger, of course) in 1937 at the University of Illinois. They were tied to cancer in laboratory animals and banned (1969) in the U.S. but not in Canada and many other countries. Never has any evidence of ill effects in human beings been attributed to cyclamates, which are available for use as a tabletop sweetener in Canada. In the U.S., the FDA is currently reconsidering its ban.

✓ **Aspartame (Equal, NutraSweet):** Another accidental discovery (1965), *aspartame* is a combination of two amino acids, aspartic acid and phenylalanine. The problem with aspartame is that during digestion, it breaks down into its constituent ingredients. The same thing happens when aspartame is exposed to heat. That's trouble for people born with a *phenylketonuria (PKU)*, a metabolic defect characterized by a lack of the enzyme needed to digest phenylalanine. The excess amino acid can pile up in brain and nerve tissue, leading to mental retardation in young children.

✓ **Sucralose (Splenda):** *Sucralose,* which was discovered in 1976, is a no-calorie sweetener made from sugar. But your body doesn't recognize it as a carbohydrate or a sugar, so it zips through your intestinal tract unchanged. More than 100 scientific studies conducted during a 20-year period attest to its safety, and the FDA has approved its use in a variety of foods, including baked goods, candies, substitute dairy products, and frozen desserts.

✓ **Acesulfame-K (Sunett):** The *K* is the chemical symbol for potassium, and this artificial sweetener, with a chemical structure similar to saccharin, is found in baked goods, chewing gum, and other food products. In 1998, the FDA approved its use in soft drinks, whose shelf life it seems to prolong.

✓ **Neotame:** This free-flowing, water-soluble sweetener is derived from amino acids (the building blocks of protein, the nutrient that stars in Chapter 6). In 2002, the FDA approved Neotame for use as a tabletop sweetener (the stuff you put in your coffee), as well as use in jams and jellies, syrups, puddings and gels, fruits, fruit juices, and non-alcohol beverages. To date, more than 113 animal and human studies have shown absolutely no adverse effects.

✓ **Tagatose (Naturlose, Shugr):** A white powder made from lactose, the sugar in milk. In 2003, FDA approved the use of tagatose in cereal, soft drinks, frozen desserts, candy, chewing gum, and cake frosting. Although tagatose may cause gastric upset (gas and diarrhea), it can also serve as an aid to digestion.

Table 19-1 compares the calorie content and sweetening power of sugar versus the substitute sweeteners. For comparison, sugar has 4 calories per gram.

Table 19-1	Comparing Substitute Sweeteners to Sugar	
Sweetener	*Calories Per Gram*	*Sweetness Relative to Sugar**
Sugar (sucrose)	4	
Saccharin	0	200–700 times sweeter than sugar
Cyclamates	0	30–60 times sweeter than sugar
Aspartame	4**	160–200 times sweeter than sugar
Sucralose	0	600 times sweeter than sugar
Acesulfame-K	0	150–200 times sweeter than sugar
Tagatose	1.5**	Similar to sugar
Neotame	0	7,000–13,000 times sweeter than sugar

* The range of sweetness reflects estimates from several sources.
** Aspartame has 4 calories per gram and tagatose 1.5, but you need so little to get a sweet flavor that you can count the calorie content as 0.

A Last Word: Follow That Bird

You can sum up the essence of food processing by following the trail of one chicken from the farm to your table. (Vegetarians are excused from this section.)

A chicken's first brush with processing comes right after slaughtering. It's plucked and shipped off to the food processor or the supermarket, packed in ice to slow the natural bacterial decomposition. In the food factory, your chicken may be boiled and canned whole, or boiled and cut up and canned in small portions like tuna fish, or boiled into chicken soup to be canned or dehydrated into bouillon cubes, or cooked with veggies and canned as chicken à la king, or fried and frozen in whole pieces, or roasted, sliced, and frozen into a chicken dinner, or . . . you get the picture (and if you don't, check out Figure 19-1).

When you buy a fresh (raw) chicken instead of a cooked one, you perform similar rituals in your own kitchen. First, the chicken goes to the refrigerator (or freezer), then to the stove for thorough cooking to make sure that no stray bacteria contaminate your dinner table (or you), and then back to the fridge for the leftovers. In the end, the chicken's been processed. And you have eaten. That's the point of this story.

Figure 19-1:
From the farm to your table: Chicken processing.

Chapter 20

Cooking and Nutrition

· ·

· ·

*Y*ou can bet that the first cooked dinner was an accident involving some poor wandering animal and a bolt of lightning that — zap! — charred the beast into medium sirloin. Then a caveman attracted by the aroma tore off a sizzled hunk and forthwith offered up the first restaurant rating: "Yum."

After that, it was but a hop, a skip, and a jump, anthropologically speaking, to gas ranges, electric broilers, and microwave ovens. This chapter explains how these handy technologies affect the safety, nutritional value, appearance, flavor, and aroma of the foods that you heat.

For more (much, much more) detail on what and how to cook, check out *Cooking Basics For Dummies,* 3rd Edition, (written by Bryan Miller, Marie Rama, Eve Adamson, and Wolfgang Puck), a compilation of the kind of no-nonsense, easy-to-follow instructions that you've come to expect from the big books with the yellow-and-black covers. If cutting fat and calories is your pleasure (or necessity), choose *Lowfat Cooking For Dummies,* by Lynn Fisher and W. Virgil Brown. Wiley publishes both books.

What's Cooking?

Ever since man discovered fire and how to control cooking — rather than having to wait for a passing thunderbolt — the human race has generally relied on three simple ways of heating food:

✔ **An open flame:** You hold the food directly over — or under — the flame or put the food on a griddle on top of the flame. The electric heating coil is a 20th-century variation on the open flame.

✔ **Hot air:** You put the food in a closed box (an oven) and heat the air in the oven to create high-temperature dry heat.

✔ **Hot liquid:** You submerge the food in hot liquid or suspend the food over the liquid so that it cooks in the steam escaping from the surface.

Cooking food in a wrapper such as aluminum foil combines two methods: open fire (the grill) or hot air (the oven) plus the steam from the food's own juices (hot liquid).

Here are the basic methods used to cook food with heat generated by fire or an electric coil:

Open Flame	*Hot Air*	*Hot Liquid*
Broiling	Baking	Boiling
Grilling	Roasting	Deep-frying
Toasting		Poaching
		Simmering
		Steaming
		Stewing

Cooking with electromagnetic waves

A gas or electric stove generates thermal energy (heat) that warms and cooks food. A microwave oven generates electromagnetic energy (microwaves) produced by a device called a magnetron (see Figure 20-1).

Figure 20-1:
Your typical microwave oven.

How hot is boiling water?

Water is a molecule (H2O) composed of three atoms: two hydrogen and one oxygen. When water is exposed to energy (heat), some of the water molecules *vaporize* (or separate into their gaseous components). These vapors collect in tiny pockets at the bottom of the vessel (pot) in which the water's contained. Continued heating energizes the vapors, and they begin to push up against the water.

To break through the water's surface, the vapors must acquire enough energy to equal the force (pressure) of the atmosphere (air) pushing down on the water. The temperature at which this happens is called the *boiling point*.

At sea level (elevation: 0 feet), the atmosphere is heavier (has more oxygen) than at higher elevations. That's why you breathe more easily in Miami, Florida, (elevation: 10 feet) than atop Mount McKinley in Alaska (elevation: 20,320 feet).

The heavier air at sea level exerts more pressure against the surface of the water in your pot, so making the water boil takes more energy (higher heat).

At sea level, the boiling point of water is 212 degrees Fahrenheit (100 degrees on the Celsius — C — scale). As a general rule, the boiling point of water drops one degree Fahrenheit for every 500-foot increase in altitude above sea level. In other words, at an altitude 500 feet above sea level, the boiling point for water is 211 degrees Fahrenheit (99.4 degrees Celsius); at 1,000 feet, it's 210 degrees Fahrenheit (98.9 degrees Celsius).

The following chart shows the approximate boiling points for water in specific American cities at specific altitudes.

Altitude	Place	Boiling Point °F	Boiling Point °C
Sea level	Atlantic City, NJ	212	100
500 feet	Austin, TX	211	99.4
5,000	Denver, CO	202	94.4
6,000	Cheyenne, WY	200	93.3
7,000	Santa Fe, NM	198	92.2

The World Almanac and Book of Facts 1994 (Mahwah, NJ: World Almanac, 1993)

Note: How fast the water is boiling does not affect the temperature; a slow boil (few bubbles) is as hot as a fast one (lots of bubbles).

Microwaves transmit energy that excites water molecules in food. The water molecules leap about like hyperactive 3-year-olds, producing friction, which then produces the heat that cooks the food. The dish holding food in a microwave oven generally stays cool because it has so few water molecules.

Cooking away contaminants

Many microorganisms that live naturally in food are harmless or even beneficial. For example:

- *Lactobacilli* (lacto = milk; bacilli = rod-shaped bacteria) are used to digest sugars in milk and convert the milk to yogurt.

- Nontoxic molds convert milk to blue cheese. The blue ribbons in the cheese are safe, edible mold.

Some organisms, however, carry the risk of food poisoning. For example:

- *Clostridium botulinum (C. botulinum),* a bad bug that thrives in the absence of air (as in low-acid, canned food), produces the potentially fatal toxin that causes botulism.

- *Campylobacter jejuni (C. jejuni),* which flourishes in raw meat and poultry and unpasteurized milk, has been linked to Guillain-Barré syndrome, a paralytic illness that sometimes follows flu infection.

Are you surprised to find out that, every year, several million Americans experience diarrhea and other more-serious symptoms of food poisoning after eating food contaminated with such an organism? Take a look at some of the incidences of food poisoning in the United States:

- In 2003 alone, the USDA estimated 1,341,873 cases of food poisoning due to *Salmonella.*

- Since 1995, the Food and Drug Administration has tracked at least 19 incidents, 409 cases of reported illness, and two deaths linked to fresh and freshly cut lettuce and leafy greens contaminated by disease-causing organisms that were transmitted by exposure to sewage and animal waste.

- In the winter of 1998–1999, Americans were reported to be suffering illness and death caused by consumption of packaged meats contaminated with *Listeria monocytogenes.*

  This incident was particularly troublesome, because the contaminated products (packaged meats) were made to be served cold. The only way to reduce the risk would have been to heat the cold cuts — unlikely except with hot dogs, which must be boiled or broiled (not microwaved) to reach a safe internal temperature of 165 degrees Fahrenheit.

  Note: During pregnancy, a fetus whose mother consumes *Listeria*-contaminated food may suffer damage or, in extreme cases, may die.

- Children and adults have died in this country following consumption of undercooked chopped meat containing *Escherichia coli 0157:H7* (sometimes called pathogenic *E. coli*).

Converting between Fahrenheit and Celsius

Pssst! Here's how to convert temperatures from Fahrenheit (F) to Celsius (C) and back again:

1. Degrees Celsius = $\dfrac{(\text{degrees F} - 32)}{9} \times 5$

   For example, to convert the Fahrenheit boiling point of water (212 degrees F) to the Celsius boiling point of water (100 degrees C):

   $$\dfrac{(212 - 32) \times 5}{9} = 100$$

2. Degrees Fahrenheit = $\dfrac{(\text{degrees C}) \times 9}{5} + 32$

   For example, to convert the Celsius boiling point of water (100 degrees C) to the Fahrenheit boiling point of water (212 degrees F):

   $$\dfrac{(100 \times 9)}{5} + 32 = 212$$

Although simply heating food to the temperatures shown in Table 20-2 is not a guaranteed protection against food-borne illness, cooking food thoroughly and keeping it hot (or chilling it quickly) after it has been cooked destroys many dangerous bugs or slows the rate at which they reproduce, thus reducing the risk. Table 20-1 lists some common *pathogens* (disease-causing organisms) linked to foodborne illnesses and notes the foods likely to harbor them; Table 20-2 shows the recommended safe cooking temperatures for various foods. Use a food thermometer to make sure you reach the recommended temps. Because some things are more complicated than they seem, read the directions that come with the thermometer to be sure you're doing it right. Really.

Two hours — and you're out!

Microorganisms thrive on food at temperatures between 40 and 140 degrees Fahrenheit (the cooking temperature that inactivates many — though not all — bad guys).

For maximum safety, follow the USDA/FDA Two-Hour Rule: After cooking the food to the proper temperature, never allow it to sit at temperatures between 40 degrees Fahrenheit and 140 degrees Fahrenheit for more than two hours.

More questions about food safety? Call or click:

- ✔ USDA Meat and Poultry Hotline
  Phone 800-535-4555
  E-mail mphotline.fsis@usda.gov

- ✔ FDA Seafood Hotline
  Phone 800-332-4010

- ✔ Food Safety and Information Service
  Web site www.fsis.usda.gov

- ✔ Food Safety Network at the University of Guelph (Canada)
  Phone 866-503-7638
  Web site (English) www.foodsafety network.ca/en/

Although pathogens (disease-causing organisms) in food are equal-opportunity bad guys — anyone who eats food carrying them may get sick — they are most dangerous for the very young, the very old, and those whose immune systems have been weakened by illness or medication.

Table 20-1	Disease-Causing Organisms in Food
The Bug	**Where You Find It**
Campylobacter jejuni	Raw meat and poultry, unpasteurized milk
Clostridium botulinum	Poorly processed canned low-acid foods or vacuum-packed smoked fish
Clostridium perfringens	Foods made from poultry or meat
E. coli	Raw beef
Listeria monocytogenes	Raw meat and seafood, raw milk, some raw cheeses
Salmonella bacteria	Poultry, meat, eggs, dried foods, dairy products
Staphylococcus aureus	Custards, salads (that is, egg, chicken, and tuna salads)

USDA Meat and Poultry Hotline

Table 20-2	How Hot Is Safe?
This Food . . .	**Is Done (Generally Safe to Eat) When Cooked to This Internal Temperature**
Eggs and Egg Dishes	
Eggs	Cook until yolk and white are firm
Egg dishes	160°F
Ground Meat and Meat Mixtures*	
Turkey, chicken	165°F
Veal, beef, lamb, pork	165°F
Fresh Beef*	
Medium rare	145°F
Medium	160°F
Well-done	170°F

This Food . . .	Is Done (Generally Safe to Eat) When Cooked to This Internal Temperature
Fresh Pork	
Medium	160°F
Well-done	170°F
Poultry	
Chicken, whole	180°F
Turkey, whole	180°F
Poultry breasts, roasts	170°F
Poultry thighs, wings	Cook until juices run clear
Stuffing (cooked in bird)	165°F on thermometer inserted into the center of the stuffing**
Duck and goose	180°F
Ham	
Fresh (raw)	160°F
Precooked (to reheat)	140°F

* Undercooked hamburger is a major source of the potentially lethal organism E. coli 0157:H7. To be safe, the internal temperature of the meat must read 165°F
** After the bird is cooked, the stuffing should be removed immediately and stored separately in the refrigerator.
USDA Food Safety and Inspection Service, "A Quick Consumer Guide to Safe Food Handling," Home and Garden Bulletin, No. 248 (August 1995)

Making Changes: How Cooking Affects Food

Cooking foods changes the way they feel, look, taste, and smell. In fact, the appetizing texture of food, its rich color, intense flavor, and fragrant aroma all are products of, yes, that's right: cooking.

Cook me tender: Changing texture

Exposure to heat alters the structures of proteins, fats, and carbohydrates, so it changes food's *texture* (the way food particles are linked to make the food feel hard or soft). In other words, cooking can turn crisp carrots mushy and soft steak to shoe leather.

Protein

Proteins are made of very long molecules that sometimes fold over into accordion-like structures (see Chapter 6 for details about proteins). Although heating food doesn't lower its protein value, it does

- Break protein molecules into smaller fragments
- Cause protein molecules to unfold and form new bonds to other protein molecules
- Make proteins clump together

Need an example? Consider the egg. When you cook one, the long protein molecules in the white unfold, form new connections to other protein molecules, and link up in a network that tightens to squeeze out moisture so that the egg white hardens and turns opaque. The same unfold-link-squeeze reaction turns translucent poultry firm and white and makes gelatin set. The longer you heat proteins, the stronger the network becomes, and the tougher, or more solid, the food will be.

To see this work, scramble two eggs — one beaten and cooked plain and one beaten with milk and then cooked. Adding liquid (milk) makes squeezing out all the moisture more difficult for the protein-network. So the egg with the added milk cooks up softer than the plain egg.

Fat

Heat melts fat, which can run off food, lowering the calorie count. In addition, cooking breaks down connective tissue — the supporting framework of the body, which includes some adipose (fatty) tissue — thus making the food softer and more pliable. You can see this most clearly when cooking fish. The fish flakes when it's done because its connective tissue has been destroyed.

When meat and poultry are stored after cooking, their fats continue to change, this time by picking up oxygen from the air. Oxidized fats have a slightly rancid taste more politely known as *warmed-over flavor.* You can slow — but not entirely prevent — this reaction by cooking and storing meat, fish, and poultry under a blanket of food rich in *antioxidants,* chemicals that prevent other chemicals from reacting with oxygen. Vitamin C is a natural antioxidant, so gravies and marinades made with tomatoes, citrus fruits, tart cherries, or blueberries slow the natural oxidation of fats in cooked or stored foods.

TECHNICAL STUFF

Grains: Split personality performers

In cooking, grains, such as corn, exhibit split personalities — part protein, part complex carbohydrates. When you boil an ear of corn, the protein molecules inside the kernels do the break-unfold-network dance (the molecules break their links, the protein unfolds, and the molecules form new links). At the same time, carbohydrate starch granules begin absorbing moisture and then soften.

The trick to boiling perfect corn is controlling this process, removing the corn from the water when starch granules have absorbed enough moisture to soften the kernels but before the protein network has tightened.

That's why cookbooks advise a short stay in the pot. But if you're a person who likes corn chewy, just let it boil away, 15 minutes, 30 minutes — you be the judge.

Carbohydrates

Cooking has different effects on simple carbohydrates and complex ones (if you're confused about carbohydrates, see Chapter 8). When heated

- ✔ Simple sugars — such as sucrose or the sugars on the surface of meat and poultry — caramelize, or melt and turn brown. (Think of crème caramel.)

- ✔ Starch, a complex carbohydrate, becomes more absorbent, which is why pasta expands and softens in boiling water.

- ✔ Some dietary fibers (gums, pectins, hemicellulose) dissolve, so vegetables and fruits soften when cooked.

The last two reactions — absorption and dissolved cell walls — can improve the nutritional value of foods by making the nutrients inside previously fiber-stiffened cells more available to your body.

A less-beneficial effect of heat on carbs surfaced early in 2002 when Swedish researchers set off a nutritional hoo-ha with the announcement that exposing starchy carbohydrate foods — such as potatoes and bread — to the high heat of baking or frying produces *acrylamides,* a family of chemicals known to cause cancer in rats. Then things got worse when scientists at the City of Hope Cancer Research Center (Los Angeles) said that acrylamides could trigger cell changes leading to cancer in human beings. But a 2003 analysis of data from a study of 987 cancer patients and 538 healthy "controls" conduc[ted] by researchers at Harvard School of Public Health and the Department[s of] Oncology-Pathology and Medical Epidemiology at Karolinska Instit[ute] Stockholm shows no evidence of an increased risk of bowel, bl[adder, or] kidney cancer among fans of fries and toast. And in June 20[0—] at the National Toxicology Program of the National Inst[itute]

Health Sciences said the level of acrylamides in a normal American diet — even one that includes baked and fried carbs — is too low to be carcinogenic. Fries on toast, anyone?

At a follow-up U.N.–sponsored meeting in Geneva, a group of really important international food scientists confirmed the Stockholm discovery of acrylamide in carbs but couldn't agree on what to do about it other than to call for another study, which showed up pretty quickly. By the end of the year, kitchen scientists agreed that moderate amounts of fries are safe. Nutritious, too. The most healthful potato, it's true, is one that hasn't been fried, but even when crisped to a fare-thee-well, one ounce of potato chips nevertheless may still deliver up to 12 percent of the RDA for vitamin C, up to 7 percent of the RDA for folate, up to 4 percent of the RDA for iron, and more than a gram of dietary fiber. In other words, as one part of a varied diet, the chip may still be okay to dip. The problem is: Are you sure you can have just one? Or two? Or . . .

Enhancing flavor and aroma

Heat degrades (breaks apart) flavor and aroma chemicals. As a result, most cooked food has a more intense flavor and aroma than raw food.

Cheeseburgers for your health: A hot story

When you heat fats, their molecules break apart into chemicals known as *free radicals*, molecule fragments that may hook up together to form potentially carcinogenic (cancer-causing) compounds. These ___nds are produced in higher ___ heats; the usual safe ___es Fahrenheit (right ___dial). Burned fat or ___more nasties than ___but not smoking.

___ warn against ___tely yummy ___ally burned ___ linked to a ___f course, ___ is true ___y may ___nce.

___lue

yes, cheeseburgers . . . grilled, fried, broiled, whatever — are rich in CLA (short for conjugated dienoic linoleic acid), a form of an essential fatty acid (a topic that I cover in Chapter 7).

In Belury's lab, CLA slowed or reversed skin, breast, and stomach cancers in mice at the three stages of tumor development: early, when the cell is first damaged; midway in the process, when precancerous cells multiply to form tumors; and late, when tumors begin to enlarge and spread to other organs.

Whether this benefit happens in people nobody knows, but it sure reminds me of the Woody Allen movie *Sleeper*, in which the hero wakes up at some point in the future to discover that corned beef sandwiches are health food. Hey, you can't make this stuff up!

A good example is the mustard oils that give cruciferous vegetables, such as cabbage and cauliflower, their distinctive (some may say offensive) odors. The longer you cook these vegetables, the worse they smell. On the other hand, heat destroys _diallyl disulfide,_ which is the chemical that gives raw garlic its bite and bark. So cooked garlic tastes and smells milder than the raw version.

Altering the palette: Food color

Carotenoids — the natural red and yellow pigments that make carrots and sweet potatoes orange and tomatoes red — are practically impervious to heat and the acidity or alkalinity of cooking liquids. No matter how you cook them or how long, carotenoids stay bright and sunny.

You can't say the same for the other pigments in food: The other pigments that make food naturally red, green, or white react — usually for the worse — to heat, acids (such as wine, vinegar, or tomato juice), and basic (alkaline) chemicals (such as mineral water or baking soda and water). Here's a brief rundown on the color changes that you can expect when you cook food:

- Red beets and cabbage get their colors from pigments called _anthocyanins_. Acids make these pigments redder. Alkaline solutions fade anthocyanins from red to bluish purple.

- Potatoes, cauliflower, rice, and white onions are white because they contain pigments called _anthoxanthins_. When anthoxanthins are exposed to alkaline chemicals (mineralized water or baking soda), they turn yellow or brownish. Acids prevent this reaction. Boil cauliflower florets in tomato juice, rinse off the juice, and you'll see — white cauliflower!

- Green veggies are colored by _chlorophyll_, a pigment that reacts with acids in cooking water (or in the vegetable itself) to form _pheophytin_, a brown pigment. The only way to short-circuit this reaction is to protect the vegetables from acids. Old-time cooks added alkaline baking soda, but that increases the loss of certain vitamins (see "Protecting the Nutrients in Cooked Foods" later in this chapter) and softens the vegetables. Fast cooking at high heat or cooking in lots of water (which dilutes acids) lessens these color changes.

- The natural red color of fresh meat comes from _myoglobin_ in the muscle tissue and _hemoglobin_ in blood. When meat is heated, the pigment molecules are _denatured,_ or broken into fragments. They lose oxygen and turn brown or — after long cooking — turn the really unappetizing gray characteristic of steam-table meats. This inevitable change is more noticeable in beef than in pork or veal because beef starts out naturally redder.

Red to blue and back again

The following experiment lets you see colors change right before your very eyes. Gather

- ✔ 1 small can sliced beets
- ✔ 1 saucepan
- ✔ 3 small glass bowls
- ✔ 1 cup water
- ✔ 1 teaspoon baking soda
- ✔ 3 tablespoons white vinegar

Line up the glass bowls on your kitchen counter. Open the can. Remove six slices of beets. Put two slices in the first glass bowl and four slices in the saucepan. Put the rest in a small container and refrigerate for dinner. No sense wasting good beets!

Mix the baking soda into the water and add this alkaline solution to the saucepan. Heat for 4 minutes; don't heat too high — the solution foams. Turn off the heat. Remove the beets from the pan. Put two slices each in the second and third glass bowls.

Ignore the second bowl. Add the vinegar (an acid) to the third bowl. Wait two minutes. Now look: The beets in the first bowl (straight from the can) should still be bright red. Alkaline compounds darken colors, so the beets in the second bowl, straight from the baking soda bath, should be almost navy blue. Acids reverse the reaction, so beets in the third bowl, with added vinegar, should be heading back to bright red. Not yet? Add another tablespoon of vinegar.

Ain't chemistry grand?

Choosing Cookware: How Pots and Pans Affect Food

A pot is a pot is a pot, right? No way! In fact, your choice of pots can affect the nutrient value of food by

- ✔ Adding nutrients to the food
- ✔ Slowing the natural loss of nutrients during cooking
- ✔ Actively increasing the loss of nutrients during cooking

In addition, some pots make the food's natural flavors and aromas more intense, which, in turn, can make the food more — or less — appetizing. Read on to find out how your pot can change your food. And vice versa.

Copper and egg whites: A chemical team

When you whip an egg white, its proteins unfold, form new bonds, and create a network that holds air in. That's why the runny white turns into stable foam.

You can certainly whip egg whites successfully in a glass or ceramic bowl — chilled, and absolutely free of any fat, including egg yolk, which would prevent the proteins from linking tightly. But the best choice is copper: the ions (particles) flaking off the surface bind with and stabilize the foam. (Aluminum ions stabilize but darken the whites.)

But wait. Isn't copper toxic? (See Chapter 11.) Yes, but the amount you get in an occasional batch of whites is so small it's insignificant, safetywise.

Aluminum

Aluminum is lightweight and conducts heat well. That's good. But the metal

- ✔ Makes some aroma chemicals smellier (particularly those in the cruciferous vegetables — cabbage, broccoli, Brussels sprouts, and so on)
- ✔ Flakes off, turning white foods (such as cauliflower or potatoes) yellow or brownish

Copper

Copper pots heat steadily and evenly. To take advantage of this property, many aluminum or stainless steel pots are made with a layer of copper sandwiched into the bottom. But naked copper is a potentially poisonous metal. That's why copper pots are lined with tin or stainless steel. Whenever you cook with copper, periodically check the lining of the pot. If it's damaged — meaning that you can see the orange copper peeking through the silvery lining — have the pot relined or throw it out.

Ceramics

The chief virtue of plain terra cotta (the orange clay that looks like red bricks) is its *porosity,* a fancy way of saying that terra cotta roasting and baking pans allow excess steam to escape while holding in just enough moisture to make bread so moist and chicken such tender pickings.

Decorated ceramic vessels are another matter. For one thing, the glaze makes the pot much less porous, so that meat or poultry cooked in a covered painted ceramic pan steams instead of roasts. The practical result: a soggy surface rather than a crisp one.

More importantly, some pigments used to paint or glaze the pots contain lead. To seal the decoration and prevent lead from leaching into food, the painted pots are *fired* (baked in an oven). If the pots are fired in an oven that isn't hot enough or if they aren't fired for a long enough period of time, lead will leach from ceramics when in contact with acidic foods, such as fruit juices or foods marinated in wine or vinegar.

Ceramics made in the United States, Japan, and Great Britain generally are considered safe, but for maximum protection, hedge your bets. Unless the pot comes with a tag or brochure that specifically says it's acid-safe, don't use it for cooking or storing foods. And always wash decorated ceramics by hand; repeated passes through the dishwasher can wear down the surface.

Enamelware

Enameled pots are made of metal covered with *porcelain,* a fine translucent china. Enamelware heats more slowly and less evenly than plain metal. A good-quality enameled surface resists discoloration and does not react with food. But it can chip, and it's easily marked or scratched by cooking utensils other than wood or hard plastic. If the surface chips and you can see the metal underneath, discard the pot lest metals flake into your food.

Glass

Glass is a neutral material that does not react with food. Two cautions with glass:

- ✔ Do not use a glass-and-metal pot in the microwave oven. The metal blocks microwaves. More importantly, it can cause *arcing* — a sudden electrical flare that may damage the oven and scare you out of your wits.
- ✔ Remember that glass breaks — sometimes all over the floor. Are you a person who often drops things? Pass on the glass.

Iron

Like aluminum, iron pots are a good news/bad news item. Iron conducts heat well and stays hot significantly longer than other pots. It's easy to clean. It lasts forever, and it releases iron ions into food, which may improve the nutritional value of dinner.

In 1985, nutrition researchers at Texas Tech University in Lubbock set out to measure the iron content of foods cooked in iron pots. Among their discoveries: Beef stew (0.7 milligrams of iron per 100 grams/3.5 ounces, raw) can end up with as much as 3.4 milligrams of iron per 100 grams after cooking slightly longer than an hour in an iron pot.

Alas! There's a downside. The iron that flakes off the pot may be a form of the mineral that your body can't absorb. Also, more iron is not necessarily better. It encourages oxidation (bad for your body) and can contribute to excess iron storage in people who have *hemochromatosis,* a condition that leads to iron buildup that may damage internal organs.

By the way, did I mention that pumping iron is not a bad way to describe the experience of cooking with iron pots? They're really, really heavy.

Nonstick

Nonstick surfaces are made of plastic (polytetrafluoroethylene to be exact; PTFE for short) plus hardeners — chemicals that make the surface, well, hard. As long as the surface is unscratched and intact, the nonstick surface does not react with food.

Nonstick pots are a dieter's delight. They enable you to cook without added fat, but using them may also lighten your wallet. They scratch easily. Unless you stick scrupulously to wooden or plastic spoons, your pot can end up looking like chickens have been stomping on the surface.

Note: Scratched nonstick pots and pans are not a health hazard. If you swallow tiny pieces of the nonstick coating, they pass through your body undigested.

However, when nonstick surfaces get very hot, they may

- Separate from the metal to which they're bound (the sides and bottom of the pot)
- Emit odorless fumes

    If the cooking area is not properly ventilated, you may experience *polymer fume fever* — flu-like symptoms with no known long-term effect. To prevent this, keep the stove flame moderate and the windows open.

Stainless steel

Stainless steel is an alloy, a substance composed of two or more metals. Its virtues are hardness and durability; its drawback is poor heat conduction. In addition, the alloy includes nickel, a metal to which many people are sensitive. Finally, stainless steel isn't *really* stainless. When exposed to high heat, stainless steel develops a characteristic multi-hued "rainbow" discoloration. Starchy foods, such as pasta and potatoes, may darken the pot. Undissolved salt can pit the surface. Sorry about that!

If your stainless steel pot is scratched deeply enough to expose the inner layer under the shiny surface, the metals in the alloy may flake into your food. So toss the pot.

Plastic and paper

Plastic melts and paper burns, so you obviously can't use plastic or paper containers in a stove with an open flame (gas) or heat source (electric). But can you use them in the microwave? You bet! As long as you pick a proper plastic.

When plastic dishes or plastic wrap are heated in a microwave oven, they may emit potentially carcinogenic compounds that can migrate into your food. To reduce your exposure to these compounds, the U.S. Department of Agriculture's Food Safety and Inspection Service (FSIS) says you need to choose only plastic containers labeled "for microwave oven use." Thin plastic storage bags, margarine tubs, and whipped topping bowls are convenient but way, way off-limits. The American Plastic Council also offers three common-sense tips for using the right kind of plastics in the microwave:

✔ Follow the directions on the plastic container or package. If it doesn't say "microwaveable," it isn't. For example, Styrofoam and other take-out food carriers rarely are microwaveable, so put the food you've ordered into a different container before reheating it.

✔ Trays for microwave meals are meant to be used only once; after you heat the food, toss the tray.

✔ When covering food to prevent splatters, use microwave-safe plastic wraps only.

Because the Food and Drug Administration requires microwave-safe plastics to meet strict safety standards, repeated studies show no ill effects from their minimal leakage. On the other hand, if even very small exposure makes you edgy, you can switch to glass or ceramic dishes that are made specifically to be used in microwave ovens. Splatter-proof the dish with wax paper, parchment paper, or white paper towels labeled safe for microwave use.

For more about plastics in the microwave, visit the USDA's Food Safety and Inspection Service (FSIS) Web site at www.fsis.usda.gov or the American Plastics Council at www.americanplasticscouncil.org (select Plastics & Food Storage Safety and then click on the link to the "Plastics: Revolutionizing American Mealtime" document — or simply type "microwave" in the Search box and follow the prompts).

Protecting the Nutrients in Cooked Foods

Myth: All raw foods are more nutritious than cooked ones.

Fact: Some foods (such as meat, poultry, and eggs) are positively dangerous when consumed raw (or undercooked). Other foods are less nutritious raw because they contain substances that destroy or disarm other nutrients. For example, raw dried beans contain enzyme inhibitors that interfere with the work of enzymes that enable your body to digest protein. Heating disarms the enzyme inhibitor.

But there's no denying that some nutrients are lost when foods are cooked. Simple strategies such as steaming food rather than boiling, or broiling rather than frying, can significantly reduce the loss of nutrients when you're cooking food.

Maintaining minerals

Virtually all minerals are unaffected by heat. Cooked or raw, food has the same amount of calcium, phosphorus, magnesium, iron, zinc, iodine, selenium, copper, manganese, chromium, and sodium. The single exception to this rule is potassium, which — although not affected by heat or air — escapes from foods into the cooking liquid.

Those volatile vitamins

With the exception of vitamin K and the B vitamin niacin, which are very stable in food, many vitamins are sensitive and are easily destroyed when exposed to heat, air, water, or fats (cooking oils). Table 20-3 shows which nutrients are sensitive to these influences.

Table 20-3	What Takes Nutrients Out of Food?			
Nutrient	*Heat*	*Air*	*Water*	*Fat*
Vitamin A	X			X
Vitamin D				X
Vitamin E	X	X		X
Vitamin C	X	X	X	
Thiamin	X			X

(continued)

Table 20-3 *(continued)*

Nutrient	Heat	Air	Water	Fat
Riboflavin			X	
Vitamin B6	X	X	X	
Folate	X	X		
Vitamin B12	X		X	
Biotin			X	
Pantothenic acid	X			
Potassium			X	

To avoid specific types of vitamin loss, keep in mind the following tips:

✔ **Vitamins A, E, and D:** To reduce the loss of fat-soluble vitamins A and E, cook with very little oil. For example, bake or broil vitamin A–rich liver oil-free instead of frying. Ditto for vitamin D–rich fish.

✔ **B vitamins:** Strategies that conserve protein in meat and poultry during cooking also work to conserve the B vitamins that leak out into cooking liquid or drippings: Use the cooking liquid in soup or sauce. *Caution:* Do not shorten cooking times or use lower temperatures to lessen the loss of heat-sensitive vitamin B12 from meat, fish, or poultry. These foods and their drippings must be thoroughly cooked to ensure that they're safe to eat.

Do not rinse grains (rice) before cooking unless the package advises you to do so (some rice does need to be rinsed). Washing rice once may take away as much as 25 percent of the thiamin (vitamin B1). Toast or bake cakes and breads only until the crust is light brown to preserve heat-sensitive Bs.

✔ **Vitamin C:** To reduce the loss of water-soluble, oxygen-sensitive vitamin C, cook fruits and vegetables in the least possible amount of water. For example, when you cook 1 cup of cabbage in 4 cups of water, the leaves lose as much as 90 percent of their vitamin C. Reverse the ratio — one cup water to 4 cups cabbage — and you hold on to more than 50 percent of the vitamin C.

Serve cooked vegetables quickly: After 24 hours in the fridge, vegetables lose one-fourth of their vitamin C; after two days, nearly half.

Root vegetables (carrots, potatoes, sweet potatoes) baked or boiled whole, in their skins, retain about 65 percent of their vitamin C.

Chapter 21

What Happens When Food Is Frozen, Canned, Dried, or Zapped

· ·

In This Chapter

▶ Freezing food safely

▶ Creating canned food

▶ Explaining the ancient art of drying food

▶ Using radiation to protect food

· ·

Cold air, hot air, no air, and radioactive rays — all can be used to make food safer for longer periods of time by reducing or eliminating damage from exposure to air or organisms (microbes) that live on food.

The methods described in this chapter all have one important thing in common: Used correctly, each process can dramatically lengthen food's shelf life. The downside? Nothing's perfect, so you still have to monitor your food to make sure that the preservation treatment has, well, preserved it. The following pages tell you how.

Cold Comfort: Chilling and Freezing

Keeping food cold, sometimes very cold, slows or suspends the activity of microbes bent on digesting your food before you do.

Unlike heat, which actually kills many of the microbes (see Chapter 20), chilling food (or freezing it) may not kill all the microbes, but the cold will reduce the microbial population to some degree depending on the microflora present and will sideline them for a while. For example, *mold spores* (hibernating mold organisms) snuggle inside frozen food to sleep quietly like so many comfy bears inside a wintry cave. When spring comes, the bears bounce back to life; thaw the food, and the mold does the same.

How long things stay safe in the refrigerator or freezer varies from food to food and to some extent on the packaging (better packaging, longer freezing time). Table 21-1 provides a handy guide to the limits of safe cool storage. These ranges depend on foods being fresh to start out and on the refrigerator/freezer maintaining a constant temperature. Whenever these conditions aren't met, food may spoil more quickly. Use your common sense: If food seems in any way questionable, *throw it out without tasting.* Or as the catchy saying goes: When in doubt, throw it out.

Table 21-1	How Long Foods Generally Stay Safe in Cold Storage	
Food	*Refrigerator (40°F)*	*Freezer (0°F)*
Eggs		
Fresh, in shell	3 weeks	Don't freeze
Raw yolks, whites	2–4 days	1 year
Hard cooked	1 week	Doesn't freeze well
Liquid pasteurized eggs or egg substitutes, opened	3 days	Doesn't freeze well
Liquid pasteurized eggs or egg substitutes, unopened	10 days	1 year
Mayonnaise, Commercial		
Open jar	2 months	Don't freeze
TV Dinners, Frozen Casseroles		
As originally packed, until ready to serve	Don't refrigerate: Keep frozen	3–4 months
Deli and Vacuum-Packed Products		
Prestuffed pork and lamb chops, chicken breasts stuffed with dressing	1 day	Doesn't freeze well
Store-cooked convenience meals	1–2 days	Doesn't freeze well
Commercial brand vacuum-packed dinners with USDA seal, unopened	2 weeks	Doesn't freeze well
Soups and Stews		
Vegetable or meat-added	3–4 days	2–3 months
Ground Meats and Stew Meats		
Hamburger and stew meats	1–2 days	3–4 months
Ground turkey, veal, pork, lamb, and mixtures of them	1–2 days	3–4 months

Food	Refrigerator (40°F)	Freezer (0°F)
Hot Dogs** and Lunch Meats*		
Hot dogs, opened	1 week	In freezer wrap, 1–2 months
Hot dogs, unopened	2 weeks	In freezer wrap, 1–2 months
Lunch meats, opened	3–5 days	In freezer wrap, 1–2 months
Lunch meats, unopened	2 weeks	In freezer wrap, 1–2 months
Bacon and Sausage		
Bacon*	7 days	1 month
Sausage, raw — pork, beef, turkey	1–2 days	1–2 months
Smoked breakfast links, patties	7 days	1–2 months
Hard sausage — pepperoni, jerky sticks	2–3 weeks	1–2 months
Ham, Corned Beef		
Corned beef in pouch with pickling juices*	5–7 days	Drained and wrapped, 1 month
Ham, canned, label says to keep refrigerated	6–9 months	Don't freeze
Ham, fully cooked — whole	7 days	1–2 months
Ham, fully cooked — half	3–5 days	1–2 months
Ham, fully cooked — slices	3–4 days	1–2 months
Fresh Meat		
Steaks — beef	3–5 days	6–12 months
Chops — pork	3–5 days	4–6 months
Chops — lamb	3–5 days	6–9 months
Roast — beef	3–5 days	6–12 months
Roast — lamb	3–5 days	6–9 months
Roasts — pork, veal	3–5 days	4–6 months
Variety meats — tongue, brain, kidneys, liver, heart, chitterlings	1–2 days	3–4 months

(continued)

Table 21-1 *(continued)*

Food	Refrigerator (40°F)	Freezer (0°F)
Meat Leftovers		
Cooked meat and meat dishes	3–4 days	2–3 months
Gravy and broth	1–2 days	2–3 months
Fresh Poultry		
Chicken or turkey, whole	1–2 days	1 year
Poultry pieces	1–2 days	2–3 months
Giblets	1–2 days	3–4 months
Cooked Poultry, Leftover		
Fried chicken	3–4 days	4 months
Cooked poultry dishes	3–4 days	4–6 months
Poultry pieces, plain	3–4 days	4 months
Poultry pieces covered with broth or gravy	1–2 days	6 months
Chicken nuggets, patties	1–2 days	1–3 months

*Follow date on package.
** Caution: Even when food is in date and has been properly refrigerated, always boil or broil hot dogs to an internal temperature of 165°F.
Food Safety and Inspection Service, "A Quick Consumer's Guide to Safe Food Handling," Home and Garden Bulletin, No. 248 (U.S. Department of Agriculture, August 1995)

How freezing affects the texture of food

When food freezes, the water inside each cell forms tiny crystals that can tear cell walls. When the food is thawed, the liquid inside the cell leaks out, leaving thawed food dryer than fresh food.

Beef that has been frozen, for example, is noticeably dryer than fresh beef. Dry cheeses, such as cheddar, turn crumbly. Bread dries, too. You can reduce the loss of moisture by thawing the food in its freezer wrap so that it has a chance to reabsorb the lost moisture that's still in the package.

You can't restore the crispness of vegetables that get their crunch from stiff, high-fiber cell walls. After ice crystals puncture the walls, the vegetable (carrots are a good example) turns mushy. The solution? Remove carrots and other crunchies, such as cabbage, before freezing the stew.

What's that brown spot on my burger?

Freezer burn is a dry brownish spot left when moisture evaporates from the surface of frozen food. Because freezer burn changes the composition of fats on the surface of foods such as meat and poultry, it may cause some change in flavor, as well.

To prevent freezer burn, wrap food securely in freezer paper or aluminum foil and put the item in a plastic bag. The more air you keep out, the fewer brown spots will develop.

Refreezing frozen food

The official word from the U.S. Department of Agriculture is that you can refreeze frozen food — as long as the food still has ice crystals or feels refrigerator-cold to the touch.

The personal, unofficial word from me is that I confess to feeling safer when I simply throw out partially thawed food that I'm not going to use right away. I'm particularly wary of sauced frozen food, such as frozen macaroni and cheese, because it seems to me that there just have to be hidden pockets of thawed food where the bacteria are whooping it up as we speak. Call me a worrywart, if you will, but for me, following this rule is just easier: Partial thaw? Out the door.

Canned Food: Keeping Out Contaminants

Food is canned by heating what goes into the container and then sealing the container to keep out air and microbes. It is then reheated after the can/jar is sealed. Like cooked food, canned food is subject to changes in appearance and nutritional content. Heating food often changes its color and texture (see Chapter 20). It also destroys some vitamin C. But canning effectively destroys a variety of pathogens, and it deactivates enzymes that might otherwise cause continued deterioration of the food.

A modern variation on canning is the sealed plastic or aluminum bag known as the *retort pouch*. Food sealed in the pouch is heated but for a shorter period than that required for canning. As a result, the pouch method does a better job of preserving flavor, appearance, and heat-sensitive vitamin C.

The sealed can or pouch also protects food from deterioration caused by light or air, so the seal must remain intact. When the seal is broken, air seeps into the can or pouch, spoiling the food.

The essence of canned food

The technique of canning food in glass containers was discovered (depending on your source) either in 1809 or 1810 by Nicholas Appert, a Frenchman who noted that if he sealed food in a container while it was heating, the food stayed edible longer — much longer — than fresh food. According to Harold McGee, author of *On Food and Cooking: The Science and Lore of the Kitchen,* a wonderful guide to food technology, a tin of 114-year-old canned meat once was eaten without making anyone sick. To be fair, I must note that nobody cried, "Oh, wow, this is good," either.

According to Joseph Nathan Kane's *Famous First Facts* (H. W. Wilson Company), the first food canned in tin — salmon, oysters, and lobsters — was introduced in 1819 by New Yorkers Ezra Daggett and Thomas Kensett. Four years later, Daggett and Kensett took out a patent to "preserve animal substances in tin." New York inventor J. Osterhoudt later patented the first can with a key opener on October 2, 1866. (For the most part, keys have been replaced by pull tabs.) The first beer in cans (from the Gottfried Krueger Brewing Company of Newark, New Jersey) went on sale on January 24, 1935, in Richmond, Virginia. Pop!

A more serious hazard associated with canned food is *botulism,* a potentially fatal form of food poisoning caused by the failure to heat the food to high-enough temperatures or for a long-enough time to kill all *Clostridium botulinum* (or *C. botulinum*) bacteria. Canning is based on temperatures and times necessary to destroy *C. bot* spores. *C. botulinum* is an *anaerobic* (an = without; aerobic = air) organism that thrives in the absence of oxygen, a condition nicely fulfilled by a sealed can. *Botulinum* spores not destroyed by high heat during the canning process may produce a toxin that can kill by paralyzing your heart muscles and the muscles that enable you to breathe.

To avoid potentially hazardous canned food do not buy, store, or use any can that is

- ✔ Swollen, which indicates that bacteria are growing inside and producing gas

✔ Damaged, rusted, or deeply dented along the seam, because a break in the can permits air to enter and may promote the growth of organisms (other than *botulinum*)

Consumer alert: Never, never, *never* taste any food from a swollen or damaged can "just to see if it's all right." **Remember:** When in doubt, throw it out.

Dried Food: No Life without Water

Drying protects food by removing the moisture that bacteria, yeasts, and molds need to live. Drying is an ancient technique, used to produce the famous dates of the desert and the dried meat of the American plains.

Drying food the low-tech way means putting it out in the sun and waiting for it to dry on its own. Drying food the high-tech, modern way means putting food out on racks and employing fans to quick-dry the food at a low temperature under vacuum pressure.

Another form of drying is spray drying. *Spray drying* is a technique used to dry liquids, such as milk, by blowing the liquids (in very small droplets) into a heated chamber where the droplets dry into a powder that can be reconstituted (made back into a liquid) by adding water. Instant coffee is a spray-dried product. So are instant teas and all the various instant fruit beverages.

How drying affects food's nutritional value

As always, exposure to heat and/or air (oxygen) reduces a food's vitamin C content, so dried foods have less vitamin C than fresh foods.

One good example is the plum versus the prune (a dried plum):

✔ One fresh, medium-size plum, weighing 66 grams (a bit more than 2 ounces) without the pit, has 6 milligrams vitamin C, 7 to 8 percent of the Recommended Dietary Allowance for a healthy adult.

✔ An equivalent amount of uncooked dried (low-moisture) prunes (66 grams) has only 1.3 milligrams vitamin C.

But wait! Before you leap to the conclusion that fresh is always more nutritious than dried, feed these facts into your memory banks: Dried fruit has less water than fresh fruit. That means its weight reflects more solid fruit. Although drying destroys some vitamin C, removing water concentrates what's left, along with other nutrients, jamming more calories, dietary fiber, and/or air-resistant vitamins and minerals into a smaller space.

As a result, dried food often has surprisingly more nutritional bounce to the ounce than fresh food. Once again, consider the plum and the prune:

✔ A medium-size, pit-free plum weighing slightly more than 2 ounces provides 35 calories, 0.1 milligram iron, and 670 IU (67 RE) vitamin A. (What's IU? What's RE? Check out Chapter 4.)

✔ Two ounces of uncooked, low-moisture prunes have about 193 calories, 2 milligrams iron, and 952 IU (72 RE) vitamin A. In other words, if you're trying to lose weight, you need to be aware that although dried fruit is low in fat and rich in nutrients, it's also high in calories.

When dried fruit may be hazardous to your health

Many fruits contain an enzyme (polyphenoloxidase) that darkens the fruit flesh when the fruit is exposed to air. To prevent the fruits from darkening when dried, the fruits are treated with sulfur compounds known as sulfites. The sulfites — sulfur dioxide, sodium bisulfite, sodium metabisulfite — can cause potentially serious allergic reactions in sensitive individuals. For more about sulfites, see Chapter 22.

Irradiation: A Hot Topic

Irradiation is a technique that exposes food to electron beams or gamma radiation, a high-energy light stronger than the X-rays your doctor uses to make a picture of your insides. Gamma rays are ionizing radiation, the kind of radiation that kills living cells. Ionizing radiation can sterilize food or at least prolong its shelf life by

✔ Killing microbes and insects on plants (wheat, wheat powder, spices, dry vegetable seasonings)

✔ Killing disease-causing organisms on pork *(Trichinella),* poultry *(Salmonella),* and ground beef (pathogenic *E. coli*)

✔ Preventing potatoes and onions from sprouting during storage

✔ Slowing the rate at which some fruits ripen

Irradiation does not change the way food looks or tastes. It does not change food texture. It does not make food radioactive. It does, however, alter the structure of some chemicals in foods, breaking molecules apart to form new substances called *radiolytic products* (radio = radiation; lytic = break).

Are irradiated foods harmful?

Many scientific organizations, including the 27,000-member Institute of Food Technologists and an international Expert Committee on the Wholesomeness of Irradiated Foods (which includes representatives from the United Nations, the International Atomic Energy Agency, and the World Health Organization), believe that irradiation is a safe and important weapon in the fight against food poisoning caused by microbial and parasitic contamination.

The Food and Drug Administration has been approving various uses of food irradiation since 1963. In addition, irradiation is approved for more than 40 food products in more than 37 countries around the world.

Some consumers, however, remain leery of irradiation, fearful that it may expose them to radiation (it can't; no radioactive residues are present in irradiated food) or that URPs (unique radiolytic products) — compounds produced only when foods are irradiated — may eventually turn out to be harmful. For now, irradiated food seems safe, but it's fair to point out that the story of irradiating foods is still unfolding, a situation that makes many people uneasy. For example, the

FDA's 2003 decision to allow irradiated ground beef into the National School Lunch Program has triggered debates in many school districts; several — including Los Angeles and the District of Columbia — have simply banned irradiated foods from their menus.

Around the world, all irradiated food is identified with this international symbol. Just in case that isn't enough to get the message across, the package must also carry the words "treated by irradiation" or "treated with irradiation." The only exception is commercially produced food that contains some irradiated ingredients, such as spices. The symbol and/or wording isn't required, for example, on the packaging for a frozen pizza that's seasoned with irradiated oregano.

About 90 percent of all compounds identified as radiolytic products (RP) also are found in raw, heated, and/or stored foods that have not been deliberately exposed to ionizing radiation. A few compounds, called *unique radiolytic products* (URPs), are found only in irradiated foods.

You can get answers online to the most commonly asked questions about food irradiation at the Web site maintained by the Centers for Disease Control (CDC): www.cdc.gov/ncidod/dbmd/diseaseinfo/food irradiation.htm.

Table 21-2 tells you when certain irradiated foods were deemed safe in the U.S.

Table 21-2	Foods Approved for Irradiation in the U.S.
Food	*Approval date*
Wheat, wheat flour	1963
White potatoes	1964
Pork	1986
Fruit and vegetables (fresh)	1986
Herbs, spices, vegetable seasonings	1986
Poultry (fresh, frozen)	1990 (FDA), 1992 (USDA)*
Animal/pet food	1995
Meat (uncooked, chilled, frozen)	1997 (FDA), 2000 (USDA)*
Mollusks/seafood (fresh, frozen)	1999**
Ready-to-eat, unrefrigerated meat/poultry products	1999**
Fresh eggs (in shell)	2000
Seeds for sprouting	2000

* Both the FDA and the USDA must approve treatment of meat and poultry
** Application awaiting FDA approval
Federal Centers for Disease Control

Is that food still good to eat? Understanding the dates on food labels

The following terms can help you figure out whether you should check whether your food's still good or whether you should just pitch it:

✔ **Sell-by:** The last date on which the food can be offered for sale. If stored properly, most perishable foods such as milk, cheese, and packaged meats are safe for a few days past the "sell by" date.

✔ **Best if used by or Use by:** Refers to the food's flavor and quality, not its safety; the manufacturer's recommendation of the last date on which the food is likely to taste best.

✔ **Expires or Do not use after:** The last date on which a product either provides the highest nutritional value or works best (for instance, the last date on which yeast or baking powder is likely to make your bread or cake rise).

✔ **Packing date:** Used on eggs from USDA-inspected facilities to show the date on which the eggs were packed. The date is written as a number from 1 (January 1) to 365 (December 31 — except in a leap year, naturally). Eggs from USDA-inspected plants may also carry an expiration date.

Chapter 22

Better Eating through Chemistry

- -

In This Chapter

▶ Understanding food additives

▶ Regulating food additives

▶ Considering additives that cause health problems

▶ Creating new foods with biotechnology

- -

*I*f the title of this chapter turns you off, you're not alone. More people than you can shake a stick — heck, a whole oak tree — at think that when you're talking food, natural's good and chemical's bad. Period. But it ain't necessarily so.

This chapter is about the natural *and* synthetic ingredients and the technological processes that help make food more nutritious; enhance its appearance, flavor, and texture; and keep it fresh on the shelf longer. More to the point, this chapter explains that without these products and processes, human beings would still have to gather (or kill) dinner fresh each day to serve it up fast before it spoils.

And, yes, this chapter talks about new and unusual processes, such as genetic engineering (which is discussed in the section "Looking Beyond Additives: Foods Nature Never Made" at the end of this chapter). Try it. You may like it.

Exploring the Nature (and Science) of Food Additives

What are food additives? Here's a really simple definition: *Food additives* are substances added to food. The list of common food additives includes

✔ Nutrients

✔ Coloring agents

✔ Flavors and flavor enhancers

✔ Preservatives

Food additives may be natural or synthetic. For example, vitamin C is a natural preservative. Butylated hydroxyanisole (BHA) and butylated hydroxy-toluene (BHT) are synthetic preservatives. Many people think natural additives are safer than synthetic ingredients, probably because "synthetic" seems synonymous with "chemical," a sort of scary word. Besides, synthetic additives often have names no one can pronounce, much less translate, which makes them even more forbidding.

In fact, every single thing in the world is made of chemicals: your body, the air you breathe, the paper on which this book is printed, and the glasses through which you read it, not to mention every single bite of food you eat and every ounce of beverage you drink.

To ensure your safety, the natural *and* synthetic food additives used in the United States come only from the group of substances known as the *Generally Recognized as Safe (GRAS)* list.

All additives on the GRAS list

✔ Are approved by the Food and Drug Administration (FDA), meaning that agency is satisfied that the additive is safe and effective

✔ Must be used only in specifically limited amounts

✔ Must be used to satisfy a specific need in food products, such as protection against molds

✔ Must be effective, meaning that they must actually maintain freshness and safety

✔ Must be listed accurately on the label

Adding nutrients

One example of a clearly beneficial food additive is vitamin D, which is added to virtually all milk sold in the United States. Most bread and grain products are fortified with added B vitamins, plus iron and other essential minerals to replace what's lost when whole grains are milled into white flour for white bread. Some people say that we'd be better off simply sticking to whole grains. But adding vitamins and minerals to white flours enhances a product that many people just plain like better. Another example of a nutrient used as a food additive is the calcium found in some commercially prepared orange juices.

Some nutrients also are useful preservatives. For example, vitamin C is an antioxidant that slows food spoilage and prevents destructive chemical reactions. Manufacturers must add a form of vitamin C *(isoascorbic acid)* to bacon to prevent the formation of potentially cancer-causing compounds.

Adding colors and flavors

Colors, flavoring agents, and flavor enhancers make food look and taste better. Like other food additives, these three may be either natural or synthetic.

Colors

Coloring agents make food look better. An example of a natural coloring agent is *beta carotene,* the natural yellow pigment in many fruits and vegetables. Beta carotene is used to make margarine (which is naturally white) look like creamy yellow butter. Other natural coloring agents are *annatto,* a yellow-to-pink pigment from a tropical tree; *chlorophyll,* the green pigment in green plants; *carmine,* a reddish extract of *cochineal* (a pigment from crushed beetles); *saffron,* a yellow herb; and *turmeric,* a yellow spice.

An example of a synthetic coloring agent is FD&C Blue No. 1, a bright blue pigment made from coal tar and used in soft drinks, gelatin, hair dyes, and face powders, among other things. And, yes, as scientists have discovered more about the effects of coal-tar dyes, including the fact that some are carcinogenic, many of these coloring agents have been banned from use in food but are still allowed in cosmetics.

To avoid these dyes entirely, read the label and choose foods made with only natural colors.

Flavors and flavor enhancers

Every cook worth his or her spice cabinet knows about natural flavor ingredients, especially the most basic natural ones: salt, sugar, vinegar, wine, and fruit juices.

Artificial flavoring agents reproduce natural flavors. For example, a teaspoon of fresh lemon juice in the batter lends cheesecake a certain *je ne sais quoi* (French for "I don't know what" — a little something special), but artificial lemon flavoring works just as well. You can sweeten your morning coffee with natural sugar or with the artificial sweetener saccharin. (For more about substitute sweeteners, see Chapter 19.)

Flavor enhancers are a slightly different kettle of fish. They intensify a food's natural flavor instead of adding a new one. The best-known flavor enhancer is *monosodium glutamate (MSG),* which is widely used in Asian foods. MSG may trigger headaches and other symptoms in people sensitive to the seasoning.

Alphabet soup: Understanding artificial colors

When you read the label on a food, drug, or cosmetic product containing artificial colors, you may see the letters *F, D,* and *C* — as in FD&C Yellow No. 5. The *F* stands for food. The *D* stands for drugs. The *C* stands for cosmetics. An additive whose name includes all three letters can be used in food, drugs, and cosmetics. An additive without the *F* is restricted to use in drugs and cosmetics or is for external use only (translation: You don't take them by mouth). For example, D&C Green No. 6 is a blue-green coloring agent used in hair oils and pomades. FD&C Blue No. 2 is a bright blue coloring agent used in hair rinses, as well as mint jellies, candies, and cereals.

Adding preservatives

Food spoilage is a totally natural phenomenon. Milk sours. Bread sprouts mold. Meat and poultry rot. Vegetables lose moisture and wilt. Fats turn rancid. The first three kinds of spoilage are caused by *microbes* (bacteria, mold, and yeasts). The last two happen when food is exposed to *oxygen* (air).

All preservative techniques — cooking, chilling, canning, freezing, drying — prevent spoilage either by slowing the growth of the organisms that live on food or by protecting the food from the effects of oxygen. Chemical preservatives do essentially the same thing:

✔ *Antimicrobials* are natural or synthetic preservatives that protect food by slowing the growth of bacteria, molds, and yeasts.

✔ *Antioxidants* are natural or synthetic preservatives that protect food by preventing food molecules from combining with oxygen (air).

Table 22-1 is a representative list of some common preservative chemicals and the foods in which they're found.

Table 22-1	Preservatives in Food
Preservative	*Found in . . .*
Ascorbic acid	Sausages, luncheon meats
Benzoic acid	Beverages (soft drinks), ice cream, baked goods
BHA (butylated hydroxyanisole)	Potato chips and other foods
BHT (butylated hydroxytoluene)	Potato chips and other foods
Calcium propionate	Breads, processed cheese

Preservative	Found in . . .
Isoascorbate	Luncheon meats and other foods
Sodium ascorbate	Luncheon meats and other foods
Sodium benzoate	Margarine, soft drinks

Ruth Winter, *A Consumer's Dictionary of Cosmetic Ingredients* (New York: Crown, 1996)

Naming some other additives in food

Food chemists use a variety of the following types of natural and chemical additives to improve the texture of food, to keep it smooth, or to prevent mixtures from separating:

- ✔ *Emulsifiers,* such as lecithin and polysorbate, keep liquid-plus-solids such as chocolate pudding from separating into, well, liquid and solids. They can also keep two unfriendly liquids, such as oil and water, from divorcing so that our salad dressing stays smooth.

- ✔ *Stabilizers,* such as the alginates (alginic acid) derived from seaweed, make food such as ice cream feel smoother, richer, or creamier in your mouth.

- ✔ *Thickeners* are natural gums and starches, such as apple pectin or cornstarch, that add body to foods.

- ✔ *Texturizers,* such as calcium chloride, keep foods such as canned apples, tomatoes, or potatoes from turning mushy.

Although many of these additives are derived from foods, their real benefit is aesthetic (the food looks and tastes better), not nutritional.

Determining the Safety of Food Additives

The safety of any chemical approved for use as a food additive is based on whether it is

- ✔ Toxic
- ✔ Carcinogenic
- ✔ Allergenic

The nitrate/nitrite conundrum

Some preservatives are double-edged — good and not-so-good at the same time. For example, nitrates and nitrites are effective preservatives that prevent the growth of disease-bearing organisms in cured meat. But when they reach your stomach, nitrates and nitrites react with natural ammonia compounds called *amines* to form *nitrosamines,* substances known to cause cancer in animals fed amounts of nitrosamines much higher than found in any human food.

But guess what? Avoiding foods with added nitrates and nitrites won't prevent your having to cope with nitrosamines. Beets, celery, eggplant, lettuce, radishes, spinach, and turnip greens all contain naturally occurring nitrates and nitrites. When their nitrates and nitrates shake hands in your stomach they make — you got it! — nitrosamines.

To take the sting out of added nitrates and nitrites in foods such as cured meats, USDA, which regulates meat, fish and poultry, sensibly requires manufacturers to add an antioxidant vitamin C compound such as sodium ascorbate or an antioxidant vitamin E compound (a tocopherol). The antioxidant vitamins prevent the formation of nitrosamines while boosting the antimicrobial powers of the nitrates and nitrites.

Defining toxins

A *toxin* is a poison. Some chemicals, such as cyanide, are toxic (poisonous) in very, very small doses. Others, such as sodium ascorbate (a form of vitamin C), are nontoxic even in very large doses. All chemicals on the GRAS (Generally Recognized as Safe) list are considered nontoxic in the amounts that are permitted in food. By the way, did you realize that both examples — cyanide and vitamin C — are *natural* chemicals?

Explaining carcinogens

A *carcinogen* is a substance that causes cancer. In 1958, New York Congressman James Delaney proposed, and Congress enacted into law, an amendment to the Food, Drug, and Cosmetic Act that banned from food any synthetic chemical known to cause cancer (in animals or human beings) when ingested in any amount.

Since then, the only exception to the Delaney clause has been saccharin, which was exempted in 1970. Although ingesting very large amounts of the artificial sweetener is known to cause bladder cancer in animals, no similar link can be found to human cancers. In addition, saccharin provides clear benefits for people who cannot use sugar. Note: In 1977, Congress required all products containing saccharin to carry a warning statement: *Use of this product may be hazardous to your health. This product contains saccharin, which has been determined to cause cancer in laboratory animals.* This requirement was lifted in 2000; the warning is no more.

As of this writing, the Delaney clause is still in effect, even though many scientists, including cancer specialists, consider it to be outmoded because it imposes an impossible standard — zero risk — and applies only to synthetic chemicals. The Delaney clause does not apply to natural chemicals, even those known to cause cancer, such as aflatoxins, poisons produced by molds that grow on peanuts.

Listing allergens

Allergens are substances that trigger allergic reactions. Some foods, such as peanuts, contain natural allergens that can provoke fatal allergic reactions.

The best-known example of an allergenic food additive is sulfites, a group of preservatives that

- ✔ Keep light-colored fruits and vegetables (apples, potatoes) from browning when exposed to air
- ✔ Prevent shellfish (shrimp and lobster) from developing black spots
- ✔ Reduce the growth of bacteria in fermenting wine and beer
- ✔ Bleach food starches
- ✔ Make dough easier to handle

The following is a list of foods that may contain sulfites. (Also see Figure 22-1.)

- ✔ Beer
- ✔ Maraschino cherries
- ✔ Cakes, cookies, pies
- ✔ Molasses
- ✔ Cider (hard)
- ✔ Potatoes (dehydrated, pre-cut, peeled fresh)
- ✔ Condiments
- ✔ Shrimp
- ✔ Dried fruit
- ✔ Soup mixes
- ✔ Fruit juices
- ✔ Tea
- ✔ Jams and jellies
- ✔ Vegetables (canned)
- ✔ Gravy
- ✔ Vegetable juices
- ✔ Wine

Ruth Papazian, "Sulfites" (FDA Consumer, December 1996)

Sulfites are safe for most people but not for all. In fact, the FDA estimates that one out of every 100 people is sensitive to these chemicals; among people with asthma, the number rises to five out of every 100. For people sensitive to sulfites, even infinitesimally small amounts may trigger a serious allergic reaction, and asthmatics may develop breathing problems by simply inhaling fumes from sulfite-treated foods.

The FDA tried banning sulfites from food but lost in a court case brought by food manufacturers who wanted to use the additive. To protect sulfite-sensitive people, the FDA created rules for safe use of the preservatives. The rules called for a total ban on sulfites in food at salad bars and a requirement that sulfites be listed on the label of any food or beverage product with more than ten parts sulfites to every million parts food (10 ppm). These rules, plus plenty of press information about the risks of sulfites, have led to a dramatic decrease in the number of sulfite reactions.

Figure 22-1: Where the sulfites may be!

Looking Beyond Additives: Foods Nature Never Made

Genetically engineered foods, also known as bioengineered foods, are foods with extra genes added artificially through special laboratory processes. Like preservatives, flavor enhancers, and other chemical boosters used in food, the genes — which may come from plants, animals, or microorganisms such as bacteria — are used to make foods

- ✔ More nutritious
- ✔ Better tasting
- ✔ More resistant to disease and insects

Genetic engineering may also help plants and animals grow faster and larger, thus increasing the food supply. And it may enable us to produce foods with medicines bred right into the food itself. (Check out Chapter 26.)

The Big Question is: Are genetically engineered foods safe? Boy, oh boy, can you get a fight going over that one! The best answer may be that only time can tell. As you can imagine, many ordinary people don't want to wait to find out. For them, genetically engineered foods are simply unacceptable, characterized dismissively as "frankenfoods" (as in Dr. Frankenstein's monster).

To permit consumers to make a clear choice — "Yes, I'll take that biotech food" or "No, I won't" — the European Union requires food labels to specifically state the presence of any genetically altered ingredients. In the United States, the FDA currently requires wording on labels to alert consumers to genetic engineering only when it results in an unexpected allergen, such as corn genes in tomatoes, or changes the nutritional content of a food.

Whether the wording on the label matters to most consumers or whether most consumers are willing to accept genetically altered foods seems to depend on whom you ask. The International Food Information Council (IFIC), a trade group for the food industry, accepts the current label wording rules. The Center for Science in the Public Interest (CSPI), a Washington-based consumer advocacy group, wants to see the words "genetically altered" on all foods that have been, well, genetically altered. CSPI also wants the FDA to finalize a rule requiring food marketers to notify the agency in advance when introducing a new altered food or plant, a policy that's already in place for foods from genetically altered animals.

Naturally, each organization has conducted a survey to bolster its point of view. For example, IFIC's survey says that nearly two-thirds (61 percent) of Americans expect food technology to serve up better-quality, better-tasting food. CSPI's competing survey says, "Not so fast." The difference lies in the questions. The IFIC's survey questions emphasize the benefits of biotech; CSPI's survey questions lean more heavily on the drawbacks. Here are a couple of comparable questions from the CSPI and IFIC surveys:

1. **Question**

   CSPI Version: Should food labels tell you if a food has been genetically altered in any way? 70 percent (Yes)

   IFIC Version: Would you say you support or oppose FDA's [current labeling] policy? 59 percent (Support)

2. **Question**

   CSPI Version: Would you buy food labeled "genetically engineered"? 43 percent (Yes)

   IFIC Version: Would you buy a food if it had been modified by biotechnology to taste better or fresher? Or stay fresher? 54 percent (Yes)

In other words, despite a slight wariness about exploring new nutritional ground, Americans seem intrigued by the promise of food innovations and are willing to give the whole idea a try. After that, the proof will be in the — genetically engineered — pudding.

To read the CSPI survey, click on www.cspinet.org, choose Reports, and scroll down to "National Opinion Poll on Labeling of Genetically Engineered Foods." To read the IFIC survey, type this into your Search bar: ific.nisgroup.com/research/upload/2005BiotechSurvey.pdf

Part V
Food and Medicine

"Doctor, I'm feeling nauseous and disoriented. Do you think I'm having a reaction to something I ate?"

In this part . . .

*H*ow come a civilization (yours) that has antibiotics, analgesics, and decongestants still serves up chicken soup for a cold, coffee for a headache, and chocolate for a broken heart? Because they work!

Food and medicine are natural partners. Sometimes they fight (the technical term is *food/drug interactions*), but more often — as you find out in this part — they go hand in hand on the road to keeping your body in tiptop shape.

Chapter 23

When Food Gives You Hives

According to the Food Allergy & Anaphylaxis Network (FAAN), at least 11.4 million Americans have true *food allergies* (also known as *food hypersensitivity*); this number includes more children than adults because many childhood allergies seem to fade with age.

So, you may ask, if allergies are likely to disappear, why do I need a whole chapter about them? Good question. I have two good answers. First, food allergies that don't disappear can trigger reactions ranging from the trivial (a stuffy nose the day after you eat the food) to the truly dangerous (immediate respiratory failure). Second, a person with food allergies is likely to be allergic to other things, such as dust, pollen, or the family cat. And forewarned (about food allergies) is forearmed (against the rest), right? Right.

Finding Out More about Food Allergies

Your immune system is designed to protect your body from harmful invaders, such as bacteria. Sometimes, however, the system responds to substances normally considered harmless. The substance that provokes the attack is called an *allergen;* the substances that attack the allergen are called *antibodies.*

A food allergy can provoke such a response as your body releases antibodies to attack specific proteins in food. When this happens, some of the physical reactions include

✔ Hives

✔ Itching

✔ Swelling of the face, tongue, lips, eyelids, hands, and feet

✔ Rashes

✔ Headaches, migraines

✔ Nausea and/or vomiting

✔ Diarrhea, sometimes bloody

✔ Sneezing, coughing

✔ Asthma

✔ Breathing difficulties caused by *tightening* (swelling) of tissues in the throat

✔ Loss of consciousness (from anaphylactic shock)

If you're sensitive to a specific food, you may not have to eat the food to have the reaction. For example, people sensitive to peanuts may break out in hives just from touching a peanut or peanut butter and may suffer a potentially fatal reaction after simply tasting chocolate that has touched factory machinery that previously touched peanuts. People sensitive to seafood — fin fish and shellfish — have been known to develop breathing problems after simply inhaling the vapors or steam produced by cooking the fish.

Understanding how an allergic reaction occurs

When you eat a food containing a protein to which you're sensitive, your immune system releases antibodies that hitch a ride on white blood cells called *basophils.* The basophils circulate through your entire body, giving the antibodies the chance to hop off and bind to immune system cells called *mast cells.*

Basophils and mast cells produce, store, and release *histamine,* a natural body chemical that causes the symptoms — itching, swelling, hives — associated with allergic reactions. Yes, that's why some allergy pills are called antihistamines. When the antibodies carried by the basophils and mast cells come in contact with food allergens, boom! You have an allergic reaction.

Investigating two kinds of allergic reactions

Your body may react to an allergen in one of two ways — immediately or later on:

- Immediate reactions are more dangerous because they involve a fast swelling of tissue, sometimes within seconds after contact with the offending food.

- Delayed reactions, which may occur as long as 24 to 48 hours after you've been exposed to the offending food, are usually much milder, perhaps a slight cough or nasal congestion caused by swollen tissues.

NUTRITION SPEAK

Allergy lingo

So you think you have allergies. Now you need to know about the lingo of allergies. These words and definitions (an allergy glossary, if you will) can help you understand what's going on with allergies:

allergen: Any substance that sets off an allergic reaction (see "antigen" in this sidebar)

anaphylaxis: A potentially life-threatening allergic reaction that involves many body systems, creating a cascade of adverse effects beginning with sudden, severe itching and moving on to tissue swelling in the air passages that can lead to breathing difficulties, falling blood pressure, unconsciousness, and death

antibody: A protein in your blood that reacts to an antigen by trying to render it harmless

antigen: A substance that stimulates a response from the immune system; an allergen is a specific type of antigen

basophil: A white blood cell that carries IgE and releases histamine

ELISA: Short for *enzyme-linked immunosorbent assay,* a test used to determine the presence of

antibodies in your blood, including antibodies to specific allergens

histamine: The substance released by the immune system (specifically by basophils and mast cells) that produces the symptoms of an allergic reaction such as itching and swelling

intolerance: A nonallergic adverse reaction to food

IgE: An abbreviation for *immunoglobulin E,* the antibody that reacts to allergens

mast cell: A cell in body tissue that releases histamine

RAST: An abbreviation for *radioallergosorbent test,* a blood test used to determine whether you're allergic to certain foods

urticaria: The medical name for hives

American Academy of Allergy & Immunology, International Food Information Council Foundation, "Understanding Food Allergy" (April 1995)

Most allergic reactions to food are unpleasant but essentially mild. However, as many as 150 to 200 people die every year in the United States from a severe reaction to a food allergy.

Call 911 immediately if you — or a friend or relative — show any signs of an allergic reaction — including an allergic reaction to food — that affects breathing.

It's all in the family: Inheriting food allergies

A tendency toward allergies (although not the particular allergy itself) is inherited. If one of your parents has a food allergy, your risk of having the same problem is two times higher than if neither of your parents were allergic to foods. If both your mother and your father have food allergies, your risk is four times higher.

Considering Foods Most Likely to Cause Allergic Reactions

Here's something to chew on: More than 90 percent of all allergic reactions to foods are caused by just eight foods (see Figure 23-1):

- ✔ Milk
- ✔ Eggs
- ✔ Peanuts
- ✔ Tree nuts
- ✔ Soybean-based foods
- ✔ Wheat
- ✔ Fish
- ✔ Shellfish

Allergenic Foods

Eggs

Fish (aaachoo!)

Nuts

Milk

Shellfish

TOFU SOY MILK

Peanuts

Soy Foods

Wheat

Figure 23-1:
These foods
can set off
an allergic
reaction.

Bill it (peanut-free), and they will come

In the real world, having a peanut allergy may affect your ability to enjoy simple pleasures, such as a baseball game where peanuts are sold. So imagine the delight of parents in New Britain, Connecticut, when the local Eastern League team (the Rock Cats) decided to set aside a special 138-seat food-free section during its 2002 season for baseball-crazy but peanut-allergic kids and their families at a game between the Rock Cats and the New Haven Ravens.

The Rock Cats and the Food Allergy & Anaphylaxis Network, a national consumer advocacy group with 250 members in the Hartford area, cooked up the idea because, as Rock Cats assistant general manager John Willi

has said, "No child should be deprived of the Rock Cats experience."

Other minor league teams, such as the North Carolina Hickory Crawdads, the West Michigan Whitecaps, and the St. Paul (Minnesota) Saints have all had peanut-free sections for at least one game during the 2001, 2002, 2003, 2004, and 2005 seasons.

But with the exception of the Texas Rangers, who have experimented with a peanut-free section at one game per season, the big leagues are still striking out on this one. Write or e-mail your local clubs to urge them to join the anti-allergy team. Go. Now. Batter up!

Elimination diets

Because different people are sensitive to different foods, more than one elimination diet exists. The three listed here eliminate broad groups of foods known to cause allergic reactions in many people. Your doctor will pick the one that seems most useful for you.

Diet No. 1: No beef, pork, poultry, milk, rye, or corn

Diet No. 2: No beef, lamb, rice, or milk

Diet No. 3: No lamb, poultry, rye, rice, corn, or milk

The Merck Manual, 16th ed. (Rahway, N.J.: Merck Research Laboratories, 1992)

Testing, Testing: Identifying Food Allergies

To identify the culprit causing your food allergy, your doctor may suggest an *elimination diet.* This regimen removes from your diet foods known to cause allergic reactions in many people. Then, one at a time, the foods are added back. If you react to one, bingo! That's a clue to what triggers your immune response.

To be absolutely certain, your doctor may challenge your immune system by introducing foods in a form (maybe a capsule) that neither you nor he can identify as a specific food. Doing so rules out any possibility that your reaction has been triggered by emotional stimuli — that is, seeing, tasting, or smelling the food.

Two more-sophisticated tests — *ELISA* (enzyme-linked immunosorbent assay) and *RAST* (radioallergosorbent test) — can identify antibodies to specific allergens in your blood. But these two tests are rarely required.

Coping with Food Allergies

After you know that you're allergic to a food, the best way to avoid an allergic reaction is to avoid the food. Unfortunately, that task may be harder than it sounds because the offending ingredient may be hidden — peanuts in the chili or caviar ("fish eggs") in the dip.

Sometimes the "hidden" ingredient is hidden in plain sight on a food label that uses chemical code names for allergens. Example? How about "whey" or "casein" or "lactoglobulin" for "milk." Happily, in the summer of 2004, Congress passed and the President signed into law the Food Allergen Labeling and Consumer Protection Act. As of January 1, 2006, all food labels must use plain English words for the eight most-common food allergens. Goodbye "whey," "casein," and "lactoglobulin." Hello, *milk.* About time, I say.

If you're someone with a potentially life-threatening allergy to food (or another allergen, such as wasp venom), your doctor may suggest that you carry a syringe prefilled with *epinephrine,* a drug that counteracts the reactions. You may also want to wear a tag that identifies you as a person with a serious allergic problem. One company that provides these tags is Medic-Alert Foundation International, a 40+-year-old firm located in Turlock, California. The 24/7 telephone number for Medic-Alert is 888-633-4298 (in the U.S.) and 209-668-3333 (from outside the U.S.)

The food industry takes food allergies so seriously that the National Restaurant Association has joined forces with the American Academy of Allergy, Asthma, & Immunology; the Food Allergy & Anaphylaxis Network; and the International Food Information Council Foundation (IFIC) to produce a poster that shows allergenic foods and gives directions on how to assist in an allergy emergency. The poster is made to be hung in restaurant kitchens. For your very own $2.50 copy, go to the IFIC home page at www.ific.org, type "allergy poster" in the Search box, click on Food Allergy Poster for Food Service Workers, and follow the prompts.

You may want to visit the following Web sites for more details on food allergies:

✔ The American Academy of Allergy, Asthma, & Immunology (www.aaaai.org)

✔ The Food Allergy & Anaphylaxis Network (www.foodallergy.org)

Recognizing Other Body Reactions to Food

Allergic reactions aren't the only way your body registers a protest against certain foods.

Food intolerance is a term used to describe reactions that are common, natural, and definitely not allergic, which means that these reactions do not involve production of antibodies by the immune system. Some common food intolerance reactions are

 ✔ **A metabolic food reaction:** This response is an inability to digest certain foods, such as fat or lactose (the naturally occurring sugar in milk). Metabolic food reactions can produce gas, diarrhea, or other signs of gastric revolt and are an inherited trait.

 ✔ **A physical reaction to a specific chemical:** Your body may react to things such as the laxative substance in prunes or monosodium glutamate (MSG), the flavor enhancer commonly found in Asian food. Although some people are more sensitive than others to these chemicals, their reaction is a physical one that doesn't involve the immune system.

 ✔ **A body response to psychological triggers:** When you're very fearful or very anxious or very excited, your body moves into hyperdrive, secreting hormones that pump up your heartbeat and respiration, speed the passage of food through your gut, and cause you to empty your bowels and bladder. The entire process, called the *fight-or-flight response,* prepares your body to defend itself by either fighting or running. On a more prosaic level, a strong reaction to your food may cause diarrhea. It isn't an allergy; it's your hormones.

 ✔ **A change in mood and/or behavior.** Some foods, such as coffee, contain chemicals, such as caffeine, that have a real effect on mood and behavior, but that's the subject of Chapter 24. Turn the page, and it's yours.

Chapter 24

Food and Mood

*D*raw the curtains. Turn down the lights. Come a little closer. We're going to talk about something nutritionists never seem to write about: Food can make you feel good. And I don't mean the simple warm good feelings that follow a fine meal. I mean the pick-me-up-when-I'm-low, calm-me-down-when-I'm-hyper kind of good you usually associate with serious mood-altering drugs.

Why do most nutrition books ignore this subject? Frankly, I haven't a clue. But the nice thing about writing this book is that it gives me the opportunity to pass along a bunch of information that you may otherwise never see.

So here's a chapter on mood and food. The chapter names some of the common, naturally occurring, mood-alerting chemicals in food; explains how these chemicals work; and presents some simple strategies for increasing their effectiveness. Sit back, open a box of chocolates, pour a glass of wine, brew up the espresso — and enjoy.

How Chemicals Alter Mood

A *mood* is a feeling, an internal emotional state that can affect how you see the world. For example, if your team wins the World Series, your happiness may last for days, making you feel so mellow that you simply shrug off minor annoyances such as finding a ticket on your windshield because your parking meter expired while you were having lunch. On the other hand, if you feel sad because the project you spent six months setting up didn't work out, your disappointment can linger long enough to make your work seem temporarily unrewarding or your favorite television show unfunny.

Most of the time, after shifting one way or the other, your mood swings back to center fairly soon. You come down from your high or recover from your disappointment, and life resumes its normal pace — some good stuff here, some bad news there, but all in all, a relatively level field.

Occasionally, however, your mood may go haywire. Your happiness over your team's victory escalates to the point where you find yourself rushing from store to store buying things you can't afford, or your sadness over your failure at work deepens into a gloom that steals joy from everything else. This unpleasant state of affairs — a mood out of control — is called a *mood disorder.*

About one in every four human beings (women more often than men) experiences some form of mood disturbance during his or her lifetime. Eight or nine out of every 100 people experience a *clinical mood disorder,* a mood disorder serious enough to be diagnosed as a disease.

The two most common moods are happiness and sadness. The two most common mood disorders are *clinical depression,* an elongated period of overly intense sadness, and *clinical mania,* an elongated period of overly intense elation. Clinical depression alone is called a *unipolar* (one-part) *disorder;* clinical depression plus clinical mania is a *bipolar* (two-part) *disorder.*

Today, scientists have identified naturally occurring brain chemicals that affect mood and play a role in mood disorders. Your body makes a group of substances called *neurotransmitters,* which are chemicals that enable brain cells to send messages back and forth. Three important neurotransmitters are

- ✔ Dopamine *(DOE-pa-meen)*
- ✔ Norepinephrine *(NOR-e-pe-NEF-rin)*
- ✔ Serotonin *(ser-a-TOE-nin)*

Dopamine and *norepinephrine* are chemicals that make you feel alert and energized. *Serotonin* is a chemical that can make you feel smooth and mellow.

Some forms of clinical depression and mania appear to be malfunctions of the body's ability to handle these chemicals. Drugs known as antidepressants adjust mood by making neurotransmitters more available to your brain or enabling your brain to use them more efficiently. Medications used to treat mood disorders include

- ✔ **Tricyclic antidepressants:** These drugs are named for their chemical structure: three ring–shaped groups of atoms (tri = three; cyclic = ring). They relieve symptoms by increasing the availability of serotonin. One well-known tricyclic is amitriptyline (Elavil).

- ✔ **Selective serotonin reuptake inhibitors (SSRIs):** These medicines slow your body's reabsorption of serotonin so that more of that chemical is available to your brain. SSRIs are reported to have fewer side effects than the tricyclics. Two well-known SSRIs are fluoxetine (Prozac) and paroxetine (Paxil).

✔ **Monoamine oxidase inhibitors (MAO inhibitors):** These drugs slow your body's natural destruction of dopamine and other neurotransmitters so that they remain available for your brain. Phenelzine (Nardil) and tranylcypromine (Parnate) are MAO inhibitors.

✔ **Lithium:** This drug's precise actions remain unknown, but it may increase the availability of serotonin and lower the availability of norepinephrine.

✔ **A number of chemicals unrelated to each other or to other groups of antidepressants:** Some are known to regulate the availability of serotonin; others work in ways that have not yet been identified. This group includes bupropion (Wellbutrin, Zyban) and sertraline (Zoloft).

How Food Affects Mood

Good morning! Time to wake up, roll out of bed, and sleepwalk into the kitchen for a cup of coffee.

Good afternoon! Time for a moderate glass of whiskey or wine to soothe away the tensions of the day.

Good grief! Your lover has left. Time for chocolate, lots of chocolate, to soothe the pain.

Good night! Time for milk and cookies to ease your way to Dreamland.

For centuries, millions of people have used these foods in these situations, secure in the knowledge that each food will work its mood magic. Today, modern science knows why. Having discovered that your emotions are linked to your production or use of certain brain chemicals, nutrition scientists have been able to identify the natural chemicals in food that change the way you feel by

✔ Influencing the production of neurotransmitters

✔ Hooking onto brain cells and changing the way the cells behave

✔ Opening pathways to brain cells so that other mood-altering chemicals can come on board

The following sections describe chemicals in food most commonly known to affect mood.

Alcohol

Alcohol is the most widely used natural relaxant. Contrary to common belief, alcohol is a depressant, not a mood elevator. If you feel loosey-goosey and exuberant after one drink, the reason isn't that the alcohol is speeding up your brain; it's that alcohol relaxes your *controls,* the brain signals that normally tell you not to put a lampshade on your head or take off your clothes in public.

For more about alcohol's effects on virtually every body organ and system, turn to Chapter 9. Here in this chapter, it's enough to say that many people find that, taken with food and in moderation — defined as one drink a day for a woman and two for a man — alcohol can comfortably change one's mood from tense to mellow.

Anandamide

Anandamide is a *cannabinoid,* a chemical that hooks up to the same brain receptors that catch similar ingredients in marijuana smoke. Your brain produces some anandamide naturally, but you also get very small amounts of the chemical from (what else?) chocolate. In addition, chocolate contains two chemicals similar to anandamide that slow the breakdown of the anandamide produced in your brain, thus intensifying its effects. Maybe that's why eating chocolate makes you feel very mildly mellow. Not mellow enough to get you hauled off to the hoosegow (jail) or to bring in the Feds to confiscate your candy; just enough to wipe away the tears of lost love. (Don't worry; you'd need to eat at least 25 pounds of chocolate at one time to get any marijuana-like effect.)

Caffeine

I don't think that I have to tell you that caffeine is a mild stimulant that

- ✔ Raises your blood pressure
- ✔ Speeds up your heartbeat
- ✔ Makes you burn calories faster
- ✔ Makes you urinate more frequently
- ✔ Causes your intestinal tract to move food more quickly through your body

Nor do I have to tell you that caffeine is a mood elevator. Although it increases the level of serotonin, the calming neurotransmitter, it also hooks up at specific receptors (sites on the surface of brain cells) normally reserved for another naturally occurring tranquilizer, adenosine *(a-DEN-o-seen)*. When caffeine latches on in place of adenosine, brain cells become more reactive to stimulants such as noise and light, making you talk faster and think faster. Lately, athletes who take coffee before an event have reported that it also improves performance in some endurance events.

However, how people react to caffeine is a highly individual affair. Some can drink seven cups of regular ("with caffeine") coffee and still stay calm all day and sleep like a baby at night. Others — me, for instance — tend to hop about on decaf. Or as my husband often says, "What was the blur that just went through the living room?" Perhaps those who stay calm have enough brain receptors to accommodate both adenosine and caffeine, or perhaps they're more sensitive to the adenosine that manages to hook up to brain cells. Nobody really knows.

Either way, caffeine's bouncy effects may last anywhere from one to seven hours. I know that I can count on missing a night's sleep when I have real (as opposed to decaffeinated) coffee after 5 p.m. Espresso at dinner? I'll still be awake when the birds get up the next morning. Table 24-1 lists some common food sources of caffeine.

Table 24-1	Foods That Give You Caffeine
Food	*Amount of Caffeine (mg)*
5-ounce cups	
Coffee, regular, drip	80–150
Coffee, regular, instant	40–108
Coffee, decaffeinated	1–6
Tea	20–110
Tea, instant	25–60
Cocoa	2–50
12-ounce can	
Soft drinks	30–72
8-ounce container	
Chocolate milk	2–7

(continued)

Table 24-1 *(continued)*	
Food	*Amount of Caffeine (mg)*
1-ounce serving	
Milk chocolate	1–15
Semisweet chocolate	5–35
Bitter (baker's) chocolate	26

George M. Briggs and Doris Howes Callaway, Nutrition and Physical Fitness, 11th ed. (New York: Holt, Rinehart and Winston, 1984); Current Medical Diagnosis and Treatment, 36th ed. (Stamford, CT: Appleton and Lange, 1997)

Tryptophan and glucose

Tryptophan is one of the *amino acids,* a group of chemicals commonly called the building blocks of protein (see Chapter 6). Glucose, the end product of carbohydrate metabolism, is the sugar that circulates in your blood, the basic fuel on which your body runs (see Chapter 8). Milk and cookies, a classic calming combo, owe their power to the tryptophan/glucose team.

Start with the fact that neurotransmitters dopamine, norepinephrine, and serotonin are made from the amino acids tyrosine and tryptophan, which are found in protein foods (like milk). *Tyrosine* is the most important ingredient in dopamine and norepinephrine, the alertness neurotransmitters. *Tryptophan* is the most important ingredient in serotonin, the calming neurotransmitter.

All amino acids ride into your brain like little trains on tiny chemical railroads. But Mother Nature — clearly a party animal! — has arranged the switches so that your brain makes way for the bouncy tyrosine train first and the soothing tryptophan train last. That's why a high-protein meal heightens your alertness.

To move the tryptophan train up the track, you need glucose, and that means you need carbohydrate foods (like those cookies). When you eat carbs, your pancreas releases *insulin,* a hormone that enables you to metabolize the carbs and produce glucose. The insulin also keeps tyrosine and other amino acids circulating in your blood so that tryptophan trains can travel on plenty of open tracks to the brain. With more tryptophan coming in, your brain can increase its production of soothing serotonin. That's why a meal of starchy pasta (starch is composed of chains of glucose molecules, as explained in Chapter 8) makes you calm, cool, and kind of groovy.

The effects of simple sugars such as sucrose (table sugar) are more complicated. If you eat simple sugars on an empty stomach, the sugars are absorbed rapidly, triggering an equally rapid increase in the secretion of insulin, a hormone needed to digest carbohydrates. The result is a rapid decrease in the amount of sugar circulating in your blood, a condition known as *hypoglycemia* (hypo = low; glycemia = sugar in the blood) that can make you feel temporarily jumpy rather than calm. However, when eaten on a full stomach — dessert after a full meal — simple sugars are absorbed more slowly and may exert the calming effect usually linked to complex carbohydrates (starchy foods).

So some foods, such as meat, fish, and poultry, make you more alert. Others, such as pasta, bread, potatoes, rice and other grains, calm you down. The effect of the food depends on its ability to alter the amount of serotonin available to your brain. (See Figure 24-1.)

Figure 24-1: Some foods may calm you, and some foods may make you more alert.

Phenylethylamine (PEA)

Phenylethylamine — sometimes abbreviated PEA — is a natural chemical that your body releases when you're in love, making you feel, well, good all over. A big splash occurred in the late 1980s when researchers discovered that chocolate, the food of lovers, is a fine source of PEA.

In fact, many people think that PEA has a lot to do with chocolate's reputation as the food of love and consolation. Of course, to be fair about it, chocolate also contains the mood-elevator caffeine, the muscle stimulant theobromine, and the cannabinoid anandamide (see the discussion on anandamide earlier in this chapter).What is there to say other than, "Hey, can you please pass that box of chocolates down to this end of the table?

Using Food to Manage Mood

No food will change your personality or alter the course of a mood disorder. But some may add a little lift or a small moment of calm to your day, increase your effectiveness at certain tasks, make you more alert, or give you a neat little push over the finish line.

Caution! Medicine at work

Some of the mood-altering chemicals in food interact with medicines. As you may have guessed, the two most notable examples are caffeine and alcohol.

✔ Caffeine makes painkillers such as aspirin and acetaminophen more effective. On the other hand, many over-the-counter (OTC) painkillers and cold medicines already contain caffeine. If you take the pill with a cup of java, you may increase your caffeine intake past the jitters stage.

✔ Alcohol is a no-no with most medicines because it increases the sedative or depressant effects of some drugs, such as antihistamines and painkillers, and alters the rate at which you absorb or excrete others.

Always ask your pharmacist about food/drug interactions (you can read more about this in Chapter 25) when you fill a prescription. For OTC products, read the label very carefully.

The watchword is balance:

✔ One cup of coffee in the a.m. is a pleasant push into alertness. Seven cups of coffee a day can make your hands shake.

✔ One alcohol drink is generally a safe way to relax. Three may be a disaster.

✔ A grilled chicken breast (white meat, no skin) for breakfast — yes, breakfast — on a day when you have to be on your toes before lunch can help make you sharp as a tack.

✔ Got an important lunch meeting? Order starches without fats or oils: pasta with fresh tomatoes and basil, no oil, no cheese; rice with veggies; rice with fruit. Your aim is to get the calming carbs without the high-fat food that slows thinking and makes you feel sleepy.

In this, as in other aspects of a healthy life, the point is to make sure that you use the tool (in this case, food), not the other way around.

Chapter 25

Food and Drug Interactions

. . . .

. . . .

*F*oods nourish your body. Medicines cure (or relieve) what ails you. You'd think the two would work together in perfect harmony to protect your body. Sometimes they do. Occasionally, however, foods and drugs square off like boxers slugging it out in the ring. The drug keeps your body from absorbing or using the nutrients in food, or the food (or nutrient) prevents you from getting the benefits of certain medicines.

The medical phrase for this sad state of affairs is *adverse interaction*. This chapter describes several adverse interactions and lays out some simple strategies that enable you to short-circuit them.

How a Food and Drug Interaction Happens

When you eat, food moves from your mouth to your stomach to your small intestine, where the nutrients that keep you strong and healthy are absorbed into your bloodstream and distributed throughout your body. Take medicine by mouth, and it follows pretty much the same path from your mouth to your stomach, where it's dissolved and passed along to the small intestine for absorption. Nothing is unusual about that.

The problem, however, arises when a food or drug brings the process to a screeching halt by behaving in a way that stops your body from using either the drug or the food (see Figure 25-1). Many possibilities exist:

✔ Some drugs or foods change the natural acidity of your digestive tract so that you absorb nutrients less efficiently. For example, your body absorbs iron best when your stomach is acidic. Taking antacids reduces stomach acidity — and iron absorption.

✔ Some drugs or foods change the rate at which food moves through your digestive tract, which means that you absorb more (or less) of a particular nutrient or drug. For example, eating prunes (a laxative food) or taking a laxative drug speeds things up so that foods (and drugs) move more quickly through your body and you have less time to absorb medicine or nutrients.

✔ Some drugs and nutrients *bond* (link up with each other) to form insoluble compounds that your body can't break apart. As a result, you get less of the drug and less of the nutrient. The best-known example: Calcium (in dairy foods) bonds to the antibiotic tetracycline so that both zip right out of your body.

✔ Some drugs and nutrients have similar chemical structures. Taking them at the same time fools your body into absorbing or using the nutrient rather than the drug. One good example is warfarin (a drug that keeps blood from clotting) and vitamin K (a nutrient that makes blood clot). Eating lots of vitamin K-rich leafy greens counteracts the intended effect of taking warfarin.

✔ Some foods contain chemicals that either lessen or intensify the natural side effects of certain drugs. For example, the caffeine in coffee, tea, and cola drinks reduces the sedative effects of antihistamines and some antidepressant drugs but increases the nervousness, insomnia, and shakiness common with some diet pills and cold medications containing caffeine or a *decongestant* (an ingredient that temporarily clears a stuffy nose).

Figure 25-1:
Some foods may affect the way your body interacts with drugs.

Food Fights: Drugs versus Nutrients versus Drugs

Sometimes the combinations of interacting foods and drugs are positively astounding. Or, as the next paragraph suggests, breathtaking.

Here's a prime example. Everyone knows that people with asthma may find it hard to take a deep breath around the barbecue. The culprit's the smoke, right? Yes. And no. True: Breathing in smoke irritates air passages. But the kicker is that eating charcoal-broiled food speeds the body's elimination of theophylline, a widely used asthma drug, reducing the drug's ability to protect against wheezing. Take the drug, eat the food, and end up wheezing. Yipes.

Another potential troublemaker is fruit juice. Acidic beverages (colas as well as fruit juice) can send the antibiotics erythromycin, ampicillin, and penicillin down for the count.

Grapefruit juice is another acidic actor. In the mid-1990s, researchers tracking the effects of alcohol beverages on the blood pressure drug felodipine (Plendil) tripped across the *Grapefruit Effect,* a dramatic reduction in your ability to metabolize and eliminate certain drugs. Grapefruit juice contains substances that suppress the effectiveness of CYP 3A4, an intestinal enzyme required to convert many drugs to water-soluble substances you can flush out of your body; without the enzyme, you can't get rid of the drug. The result may be an equally dramatic rise in the amount of medication in your body, leading to unpleasant side effects. The list of drugs that interact with grapefruit juice has now expanded beyond felodipine to include a second blood pressure med, nifedipine (Adalat, Procardia), plus — among others — the cholesterol-lowering drugs lovastatin (Mevacor), pravastatin (Pravachol), and simvastatin (Zocor); the antihistamine loratadine (Claritin); the immunosuppressant drug cyclosporine; and saquinavir (Invirase), a protease (enzyme) inhibitor used to treat HIV. By the way, if you feel particularly wired after drinking grapefruit juice with your a.m. coffee or tea, maybe it's because the juice also interacts with caffeine. Who knew?

Water pills, more properly known as *diuretics,* make you urinate more often and more copiously, thus increasing your elimination of the mineral potassium. To make up what you lose, experts suggest adding potatoes, bananas, oranges, spinach, corn, and tomatoes to your diet. Consuming less sodium (salt) while you're using water pills makes the water pills more effective and decreases your loss of potassium.

Oral contraceptives seem to reduce the ability to absorb B vitamins, including folate. Taking lots of aspirin or other NSAIDs (nonsteroidal anti-inflammatory drugs) such as ibuprofen can trigger a painless, slow but steady loss of small amounts of blood from the lining of your stomach that may lead to iron-deficiency anemia.

Persistent use of antacids made with aluminum compounds may lead to loss of the bone-building mineral phosphorus, which binds to aluminum and rides right out of the body. Laxatives increase the loss of minerals (calcium and others) in feces.

The antiulcer drugs cimetidine (Tagamet) and ranitidine (Zantac) can make you positively giddy. These drugs reduce stomach acidity, which means the body absorbs alcohol more efficiently. According to experts at the Mayo Clinic, taking ulcer medication with alcohol leads to twice the wallop, like drinking one beer and feeling the effects of two.

The point, of course, is to read the label and definitely check with your doctor or pharmacist for any potential food and drug interactions whenever you take medication.

Finally, consider nutritional supplements. The vitamins and minerals in nutritional supplements are simply food reduced to its basic nutrients, so interactions between drugs and supplements aren't a surprise. Table 25-1 lists some common vitamin/mineral and drug interactions. (For more information on supplements, see Chapter 5.)

Table 25-1	Battling Nutrients and Medications
You Absorb Less	*When You Take*
Vitamin A	Aluminum antacids Bisacodyl (laxative) Cholestyramine (lower cholesterol) Fenfluramine (diet pill) Mineral oil (laxative) Neomycin (antibiotic)
Vitamin D	Bisacodyl (laxative) Cholestyramine (lowers cholesterol) Mineral oil (laxative) Neomycin (antibiotic)
Vitamin K	Bisacodyl (laxative) Cholestyramine (lowers cholesterol) Mineral oil (laxative) Neomycin (antibiotic)
Vitamin C	Aspirin Barbiturates (sleeping pills) Cortisone and related steroid drugs
Thiamin	Antacids (calcium) Aspirin Cortisone and related steroid drugs
Riboflavin	Birth control pills

You Absorb Less	When You Take
Folate	Aspirin Cholestyramine (lowers cholesterol) Penicillin Phenobarbital, primidone, phenothiazines (antiseizure drugs) Sulfa drugs
Vitamin B12	Cholestyramine (lowers cholesterol) Neomycin (antibiotic)
Calcium	Cortisone and related steroid drugs Diuretics (water pills) Magnesium antacids Neomycin (antibiotic) Phosphorus laxatives Tetracycline (antibiotic)
Phosphorus	Aluminum antacids
Magnesium	Amphotericin B (antibiotic) Diuretics (water pills) Tetracycline (antibiotic)
Iron	Aspirin and other nonsteroidal anti-inflammatory drugs Calcium antacids Calcium supplements (with meals) Cholestyramine (lowers cholesterol) Neomycin (antibiotic) Penicillin (antibiotic) Tetracycline (antibiotic)
Zinc	Diuretics (water pills)

James J. Rybacki, The Essential Guide to Prescription Drugs 2002 (New York: Harper Collins, 2001);
Brian L. G. Morgan, The Food and Drug Interaction Guide (New York: Simon and Schuster, 1986);
Eleanor Noss Whitney, Corinne Balog Cataldo, and Sharon Rady Rolfes, Understanding Normal
and Clinical Nutrition, 4th ed. (Minneapolis/St. Paul: West Publishing, 1994)

Avoiding Adverse Food and Drug Interactions

When you pick up an over-the-counter drug or get a new prescription, *read the label.* Let me repeat that: Read. The. Label. Warnings and interactions often are right there on the package. If they're not, ask your doctor or pharmacist whether you need to avoid any specific foods while you're taking the drug. Go on, now — ask.

Or you can plunk down a few bucks for your very own copy of *The Essential Guide to Prescription Drugs 2006* (New York: Harper Collins, 2006), the latest edition of the book listed as one of the sources for the tables in this chapter. The book is affordable, readable, and reliable. Go for it.

Using Food to Improve a Drug's Performance

Not every food and drug interaction is an adverse one. Sometimes a drug works better or is less likely to cause side effects when you take it on a full stomach. For example, aspirin is less likely to upset your stomach if you take the painkiller with food, and eating stimulates the release of stomach juices that improve your ability to absorb griseofulvin, an antifungus drug.

Table 25-2 lists some drugs that may work better when your stomach is full.

Table 25-2	Drugs That Work Better on a Full Stomach
Purpose	*Drug*
Analgesics (painkillers)	Acetaminophen
	Aspirin
	Codeine
	Ibuprofen
	Indomethacin
	Mefenamic acid
	Metronidazole
	Naproxen/naproxen sodium
Antibiotics, Antivirals, Antifungals	Ethambutol
	Griseofulvin
	Isoniazid
	Ketoconazole
	Pyrimethamine
Antidiabetic Agents	Glipizide
	Glyburide

Purpose	Drug
	Tolazamide
	Tolbutamide
Cholesterol-Lowering Agents	Cholestyramine
	Colestipol
	Lovastatin
	Probucol
Gastric Medications	Cimetidine
	Ranitidine

James J. Rybacki, The Essential Guide to Prescription Drugs 2002 (New York: Harper Collins, 2001)

Don't guess about drugs and food. Every time you take a pill, read the package label or check with your doctor/pharmacist to find out whether taking the medicine with food improves or reduces its ability to make you better. Or thumb through your brand-new copy of *The Essential Guide to Prescription Drugs.*

With this medicine, who can eat?

Interactions aren't the only drug reactions that keep you from getting nutrients from food. Some drugs have side effects that also reduce the value of food. For example, a drug may

✔ Sharply reduce your appetite so that you simply don't eat much. The best-known example may be the amphetamine and amphetamine-like drugs such as fenfluramine used (surprise!) as diet pills.

✔ Make food taste or smell bad or steal away your senses of taste or smell so that eating isn't pleasurable. One example is the antidepressant drug amitriptyline (Elavil), which can leave a peculiar taste in your mouth.

✔ Cause nausea, vomiting, or diarrhea so that you either can't eat or do not retain nutrients from the food you do eat. Examples include the antibiotic erythromycin and many drugs used to treat cancer.

✔ Irritate the lining of your gut so that even if you do eat, your body has a hard time absorbing nutrients from food. One example of a drug that causes this side effect is cyclophosphamide, an antitumor medication.

The moderately good news is that new medications appear to make some drugs (including anticancer drugs) less likely to cause nausea and vomiting. The best news is that many drugs are less likely to upset your stomach or irritate your gut if you take them with food (see Table 25-2). For example, taking aspirin and other nonprescription painkillers such as ibuprofen with food or a full glass of water may reduce their natural tendency to irritate the lining of your stomach.

Chapter 26

Using Food as Medicine

In This Chapter

▶ Discovering diets for special medical conditions

▶ Using food to ease annoying but relatively minor health problems

▶ Eating to prevent disease

▶ Serving up meds in food

▶ Knowing when food is not your best medicine

A healthful diet gives you the nutrients you need to keep your body in top-flight condition. In addition, evidence suggests that eating well may prevent or minimize the risk of a long list of serious medical conditions, including heart disease, high blood pressure, and cancer.

This chapter describes what nutritionists know right now about how to use food to prevent, alleviate, or cure what ails you — with a couple of hints about what's to come in the evolving world of medical nutrition.

Defining Food as Medicine

Start with a definition. A food that acts like a medicine is one that increases or reduces your risk of a specific medical condition or cures or alleviates the effects of a medical condition. For example:

✔ Eating foods with lots of beta carotene (the natural chemical in deep yellow and dark green fruits and veggies that your body converts to vitamin A) — along with vitamin C, vitamin E, and zinc — protects your vision by reducing the risk of age-related degeneration of the macula, the organ at the back of your eye that enables you to perceive light.

✔ Eating foods, such as wheat bran, that are high in insoluble dietary fiber (the kind of fiber that doesn't dissolve in your gut) moves food more quickly through your intestinal tract and produces soft, bulky stool that reduces your risk of constipation.

✔ Eating foods such as beans that are high in soluble dietary fiber (fiber that dissolves in your intestinal tract) seems to help your body mop up the cholesterol circulating in your bloodstream, preventing it from sticking to the walls of your arteries. This reduces your risk of heart disease.

✔ Eating sufficient amounts of calcium-rich foods ensures the growth of strong bones early in life and protects bone density later on.

✔ Eating very spicy foods, such as chili, makes the membrane lining your nose and throat weep a watery fluid that makes blowing your nose or coughing up mucus easier when you have a cold.

✔ Eating (or drinking) foods (or beverages) with mood-altering substances such as caffeine, alcohol, and phenylethylamine (PEA) may lend a lift when you're feeling down or help you chill when you're tense.

The joy of food-as-medicine is that it's cheaper and much more pleasant than managing illness with drugs. Given the choice, who wouldn't opt to control cholesterol levels with oats or chili (all those yummy beans packed with soluble dietary fiber) than with a drug whose possible side effects include kidney failure and liver damage?

Examining Diets with Absolutely, Positively Beneficial Medical Effects

Some foods and some diet plans are so obviously good for your body that no one questions their ability to keep you healthy or make you feel better when you're ill. For example, if you've ever had abdominal surgery, you know all about liquid diets — the water-gelatin–clear broth regimen your doctor prescribed right after the operation to enable you to take some nourishment by mouth without upsetting your gut.

Or if you have type 1 diabetes (an inherited inability to produce the insulin needed to process carbohydrates), you know that your ability to balance the carbohydrates, fats, and proteins in your daily diet is important to stabilizing your illness.

Other proven diet regimens include

✔ **The low-cholesterol, low-saturated-fat diet:** The basic version, known as the Stage 1 Diet, is used as a first step in lowering a person's cholesterol level. The diet limits cholesterol consumption to no more than 300 milligrams a day and total fat intake to no more than 30 percent of your total daily calories (see Chapter 16).

A nifty bonus to this diet is that it's a relatively painless way of losing weight.

✔ **The high-fiber diet:** A high-fiber diet quickens the passage of food through the digestive tract. This diet is used to prevent constipation. If you have *diverticula* (outpouchings) in the wall of your colon, a high-fiber diet may reduce the possibility of an infection. It can also alleviate the discomfort of irritable bowel syndrome (sometimes called a nervous stomach). Extra bonus: A diet high in soluble fiber also lowers cholesterol (see the preceding section, "Defining Food as Medicine").

✔ **The sodium-restricted diet:** Sodium is hydrophilic (hydro = water; philic = loving). It increases the amount of water held in body tissues. A diet low in salt often lowers water retention, which can be useful in treating high blood pressure, congestive heart failure, and long-term liver disease.

By the way, not all the sodium in your diet comes from table salt. Check out Chapter 16 for a list of the sodium compounds used in food.

✔ **The extra-potassium diet:** People use this diet to counteract the loss of potassium caused by *diuretics* (drugs that make you urinate more frequently and more copiously, causing you to lose excess amounts of potassium in urine). Some evidence also suggests that the high-potassium diet may lower blood pressure a bit.

✔ **The low-protein diet:** This diet is prescribed for people with chronic liver or kidney disease or an inherited inability to metabolize amino acids, the building blocks of proteins. The low-protein regimen reduces the amount of protein waste products in body tissues, thus reducing the possibility of tissue damage.

Using Food to Prevent Disease

Using food as a general preventive is an intriguing subject. True, much anecdotal evidence ("I did this, and that happened") suggests that eating some foods and avoiding others can raise or lower your risk of some serious diseases. But anecdotes aren't science. The more important indicator is the evidence from scientific studies tracking groups of people on different diets to see how things such as eating or avoiding fat, fiber, meat, dairy foods, salt, and other foods affect their risk of specific diseases.

Sometimes, the studies show a strange effect (meat fat increases the risk of colon cancer, high-fat dairy foods lower the risk). Sometimes studies show no effect at all. And sometimes — I like this category best — they turn up results nobody expected. For example, in 1996, a study was designed to see whether a diet high in selenium would reduce the risk of skin cancer. After four years, the answer was "Not so you'd notice." But then researchers noticed — by accident — that people who ate lots of high-selenium foods had a lower risk of lung, breast, and prostate cancers. Naturally, researchers immediately set up another study, which happily confirmed the unexpected results of the first.

Foods that serve up a health benefit in addition to basic good nutrition have been christened "functional foods." Fruits and veggies rich in vitamin A are naturally functional foods that prevent night blindness (the inability to see clearly in low light) along with their low-calorie, low-fat goodness. A second kind of functional food is one created to produce a specific medical result, such as a food that can actually deliver a vaccine (which you can read more about later in this chapter).

Battling deficiency diseases

The simplest example of food's ability to act as preventive medicine is its ability to ward off a *deficiency disease,* a condition that occurs when you don't get sufficient amounts of a specific nutrient. For example, people deprived of vitamin C develop scurvy, the vitamin C–deficiency disease. The identifying characteristic of a deficiency disease is that simply adding the missing nutrient to your diet can cure it; scurvy disappears when people eat foods such as citrus fruits that are high in vitamin C.

Fighting off cancer with food

Is there really an anticancer diet? Right now, the answer seems to be a definite maybe. The problem is that cancer isn't one disease; it's many. Some foods seem to protect against some specific cancers, but none seem to protect against all. For example:

- **Fruits and vegetables:** Plants contain some potential anticancer substances, such as antioxidants (chemicals that prevent molecular fragments called free radicals from hooking up to form cancer-causing compounds); hormone-like compounds that displace natural and synthetic estrogens; and sulfur compounds that interfere with biochemical reactions leading to the birth and growth of cancer cells. (For more about these protective substances in plant foods, see Chapter 12.)

- **Foods high in dietary fiber:** Human beings can't digest dietary fiber, but friendly bacteria living in your gut can. Chomping away on the fiber, the bacteria excrete fatty acids that appear to keep cells from turning cancerous. In addition, fiber helps speed food through your body, reducing the formation of carcinogenic compounds.

  For more than 30 years, doctors have assumed that eating lots of dietary fiber reduces the risk of colon cancer, but in 1999, data from the long-running Nurses' Health Study at Boston's Brigham and Women's Hospital and Harvard's School of Public Health threw this into question. By 2005, several very large studies — one with more than 350,000 people! — confirmed that dietary fiber has no protective effect against colon cancer. But even if dietary fiber doesn't fight cancer, it does prevent constipation. One out of two ain't bad.

✔ **Low-fat foods:** Dietary fat appears to increase the proliferation of various types of body cells, a situation that may lead to the out-of-control reproduction of cells known as cancer. But all fats may not be equally guilty. In several studies, fat from meat seems linked to an increased risk of colon cancer, but fat from dairy foods comes up clean. In the end, the link between dietary fat and cancer remains up in the nutritional air . . . so to speak.

The American Cancer Society Advisory Committee on Diet, Nutrition, and Cancer Prevention issued a set of nutrition guidelines that shows how to use food to reduce the risk of cancer. These are the American Cancer Society's recommendations:

✔ **Choose most of the foods you eat from plant sources.** Eat five or more servings of fruits and vegetables every day. Eat other foods from plant sources, such as breads, cereals, grain products, rice, pasta, or beans, several times a day.

✔ **Limit your intake of high-fat foods, particularly from animal sources.** Choose foods low in fat; limit consumption of meats, especially high-fat meats.

✔ **Be physically active.** Achieve and maintain a healthy weight. Be at least moderately active for 30 minutes or more on most days of the week. Stay within your healthy weight range.

✔ **If you drink alcohol, drink in moderation.** Chapter 9 lays it out: Moderate consumption means no more than one drink a day for a woman, two for a man.

CA-A Cancer Journal for Clinicians, *November/December 1996*

DASHing to healthy blood pressure

More than 50 million Americans have high blood pressure (also referred to as hypertension), a major risk factor for heart disease, stroke, and heart or kidney failure.

As you can read in *High Blood Pressure For Dummies* (published by Wiley), the traditional treatment for hypertension has included drugs (some with unpleasant side effects), reduced sodium intake, weight reduction, alcohol only in moderation, and regular exercise. Recent data from a National Heart, Lung, and Blood Institute (NHLBI) study, "Dietary Approaches to Stop Hypertension" — DASH, for short — offer strong evidence that the diet that protects your heart and reduces your risk of some forms of cancer may also help control blood pressure.

Three degrees of vegetarianism

Vegetarianism isn't one diet; it's three, each one distinguished by what's allowed in addition to fruits, grains and, yup, veggies.

✔ Variation #1 is a plant-based diet for people who don't eat meat but do eat fish and poultry or just fish. (Fairness dictates that I add that many strict vegetarians don't consider people who eat fish or poultry to be vegetarians.)

✔ Variation #2 is a plant-based diet for people who don't eat meat, fish, or poultry but do eat other animal products such as eggs and dairy products. Vegetarians who follow this regimen are called *ovo-lacto vegetarians* (ovo = egg; lacto = milk).

✔ Variation #3 is a diet for people who eat absolutely no foods of animal origin. Vegetarians who eat only plant foods are called *vegans*.

The DASH diet is rich in fruits and vegetables, plus low-fat dairy products. No surprise there. But the diet is lower in fat than the ordinary low-fat diet. The USDA/U.S. Department of Health and Human Services Dietary Guidelines for Americans 2005 (see Chapter 16) recommend that you get no more than 35 percent of your total calories from fat. DASH says to aim for no more than 27 percent.

The difference seems to make a difference. Your blood pressure is measured in two numbers that look something like this: 130/80. The first number is your *systolic pressure,* the force exerted against artery walls when your heart beats and pushes blood out into your blood vessels. The second, lower number is the *diastolic pressure,* the force exerted between beats.

When male and female volunteers with high blood pressure followed the DASH diet during clinical trials at medical centers in Boston, Massachusetts; Durham, North Carolina; Baltimore, Maryland; and Baton Rouge, Louisiana, their systolic blood pressures dropped an average 11.4 points and their diastolic pressures an average 5.5 points. And unlike medication, the diet produced no unpleasant side effects — except, of course, for that occasional dream of chocolate ice cream with real whipped cream, pound cake . . . Oh well, nothing's perfect.

Conquering the common cold

This section is not about chicken soup. That issue has been settled, and Dr. Mom was right. In the 1980s, Dr. Marvin Sackler of Mount Sinai Medical Center in Miami, Florida, published the first serious study showing that cold sufferers who got hot chicken soup felt better faster than those who got plain hot water, and dozens of studies since have said, man, he's right. Nobody really knows why it works, but who cares? It works.

So let's move on to other foods that make you feel better when you have the sniffles — for example, sweet foods. Scientists do know why sweeteners — white sugar, brown sugar, honey, molasses — soothe a sore throat. All sugars are *demulcents,* substances that coat and soothe the irritated mucous membranes. Lemons aren't sweet, and they have less vitamin C than orange juice, but their popularity in the form of *hot lemonade* (tea with lemon and sugar) and sour lemon drops is unmatched. Why? Because a lemon's sharp flavor cuts through to your taste buds and makes the sugary stuff more palatable. In addition, the sour taste makes saliva flow, and that also soothes your throat.

Hot stuff — such as peppers, horseradish (freshly grated is definitely the most potent), and onions — contain mustard oils that irritate the membranes lining your nose and mouth and even make your eyes water. As a result, it's easier to blow your nose or cough up mucus.

Food and sex: What do these foods have in common?

Oysters, celery, onions, asparagus, mushrooms, truffles, chocolate, honey, caviar, bird's nest soup, and alcohol beverages. No, that's not a menu for the very, very picky. It's a partial list of foods long reputed to be *aphrodisiacs,* substances that rev up the libido and improve sexual performance. Take a second look and you'll see why each is on the list.

Two (celery, asparagus) are shaped something like a male sex organ. Three (oysters, mushrooms, and truffles) are said to arouse emotion because they resemble parts of the female anatomy. (Oysters are also high in zinc, the mineral that keeps the prostate gland healthy and ensures a steady production of the male hormone testosterone. A 3-ounce serving of Pacific oysters gives you 9 milligrams of zinc, about 82 percent of the 11 milligrams a day recommended for adult men.)

Caviar (fish eggs) and bird's nest soup are symbols of fertility. Onions — and *Spanish fly* (cantharides) — contain chemicals that produce a mild burning sensation when eliminated in urine; some people, masochists to be sure, may confuse this with arousal. Honey is the quintessential sweetener: The Bible's Song of Solomon compares it to the lips of the beloved. Alcohol beverages relax the inhibitions (but overindulgence reduces sexual performance, especially in men). As for chocolate, well, it's a veritable lover's cocktail, with stimulants (caffeine, theobromine), a marijuana-like compound called anandamide, and phenylethylamine, a chemical produced in the bodies of people in love.

So do these foods actually make you feel sexy? Yes and no. An aphrodisiac isn't a food that sends you in search of a lover as soon as you eat it. No, it's one that makes you feel so good that you can follow through on your natural instincts. Which is as fine a description as you're likely to get of oysters, celery, onions, asparagus, mushrooms, truffles, chocolate, honey, caviar, bird's nest soup, and wine.

Finally, there's coffee, a real boon to snifflers. When you're sick, your body piles up *cytokines,* chemicals that carry messages among immune system cells that fight infection. When cytokines pile up in brain tissue, you get sleepy, which may explain why you're so drowsy when you have a cold. True, rest can help to boost your immune system and fight off the cold, but once in a while you have to get up. Like to go to work.

The caffeine in even a single cup of regular coffee (or one cup of decaf if, like me, you don't ordinarily drink regular coffee) can make you more alert. Caffeine is also a mood elevator (see Chapter 24) and a *vasoconstrictor* (a chemical that helps shrink swollen, throbbing blood vessels in your head.) That's why it may help relieve a headache. When I have a cold, one cup of espresso with tons of sugar can make life bearable. But nothing's perfect: Drinking coffee may intensify the side effects of OTC (over-the-counter) cold remedies containing decongestants and/or caffeine that make some people feel jittery.

Check the label warnings and directions before using coffee with your cold medicine. Vasoconstrictors reduce the diameter of certain blood vessels and may restrict proper circulation. Couldn't hurt to check with your doctor, too, if you're taking meds for a chronic condition such as high blood pressure.

Eating for a Better Body (and Brain)

Citrus fruits are rich in vitamin C, an antioxidant vitamin that seems to slow the development of cataracts. Bran cereals provide fiber that can rev up your intestinal tract, countering the natural tendency of the contractions that move food through your gut to slow a bit as you grow older (which is why older people are more likely to be constipated). Getting enough calories to maintain a healthy weight helps protect against wrinkles. And although a diet with adequate amounts of fat doesn't totally prevent dry skin, it does give you a measure of protection. That's one reason why virtually all sensible diet gurus, including the American Heart Association and the Dietary Guidelines, recommend some fat or oil every day.

And now for a word about memory. Actually, two words: varied diet. A study of 250 healthy adults, ages 60 to 94, at the University of New Mexico School of Medicine in 1983 showed that the people who ate a wide range of nutritious foods performed best on memory and thinking tests. According to researcher Philip J. Garry, Ph.D., professor of pathology at New Mexico School of Medicine, overall good food habits seemed to be more important than any one food or vitamin. Maybe people with good memory are just more likely to remember that they need a good diet.

Or maybe it's really the food. In 1997, another survey, this time at Complutense University (Madrid, Spain), showed that men and women ages 60 to 90 who eat foods rich in vitamin E, vitamin C, folic acid, dietary fiber, and complex carbohydrates do better on cognitive tests. Is it the antioxidant vitamins? Does a low-fat diet protect the brain? No one knows for sure right now, but it may turn out that sticking with this same-old, same-old low-fat, high-fiber diet as you grow older may help you to remember to stick to the same-old low-fat, high-fiber diet — for years and years and years.

Delivering Meds with Dinner

If an adventurous band of plant biologists have their way, the world's children — and their needle-phobic parents — will someday get their vaccine inoculations with dinner rather than from a sharp stick in the arm.

Vaccines protect by introducing a substance called an antigen into your body. The *antigen* — a live or killed microbe particle — provokes an immune response in which you make antibodies to fight the antigen. This reaction inoculates you by teaching your body how to fight a specific infectious agent, such as the flu virus. If you're exposed later on, you're ready to beat the bug.

Most modern vaccines are injected. Some, like the polio vaccine, may be delivered on a sugar cube. Others can be inhaled. But for 15 years, Charles Arntzen, founder of Arizona State University's Biodesign Institute at Arizona State University, and his fellows across the country have been working toward creating "edible vaccines" — vaccines created via genetic engineering, by inserting the antigen, a viral gene, into food.

Not just any food, mind you. Heat destroys vaccines, so to get the benefits, you'd have to eat the food raw. To date, researchers have concentrated on potatoes, tomatoes, and bananas, with the emphasis on the latter two because — let's face it — raw potatoes are no treat.

The primary target for the vaccines is diarrheal disease such as cholera and E. coli, which kill more than 2.5 million children under the age of 5 every year. Other possibilities include the Norwalk virus that's played havoc with cruise liner vacations, hepatitis B, and HIV, the virus that causes AIDS.

In trials with cows, mice, rabbits, and mink, antigen-containing tobacco leaves, alfalfa, tomatoes, and lettuce leaves have been able to trigger immune reactions to diseases as varied as anthrax and the common cold. In a handful of FDA-approved human studies at the National Vaccine Testing Center, the University of Maryland, and Roswell Park Cancer Centre in Buffalo, New York, human volunteers who ate about 100 grams (3.5 ounces) of raw potatoes containing anti-diarrheal or hepatitis vaccines showed an immune response similar to what you might expect from an injected vaccine.

Most researchers expect edible vaccines for animals to show up before edible vaccines for human beings. When the human versions do arrive, the plant scientists say they'll be cheap, administered without a needle and without a doctor.

Just don't expect to toss some seeds in the window box and grow your own. For one thing, fresh food has a relatively short shelf life. You can't stick your vaccine-laden banana in the fridge and use it sometime in the next six months. Second, unless the food is grown in controlled conditions, you can't be sure it has the correct amount of protective antigen. Finally, nobody wants these genetically modified foods to somehow slip into the general food supply.

In the end, the plant guys say, the banana, tomato, potato, or other vaccine-toting food will probably be sliced and diced, frozen, or ground to powder and pressed into chips or tucked into a pill to make a stable med that can be produced with basic agricultural and food-processing technologies available virtually anywhere around the globe.

No needles, no doctors, no fuss. Now that's a med any mother could love.

The Last Word on Food versus Medicine

Sometimes, a person with a life-threatening illness is frightened by the side effects or the lack of certainty in standard medical treatment. In desperation, he may turn down medicine and turn to diet therapy. Alas, doing this may be hazardous to his already-compromised health.

No reputable doctor denies the benefits of a healthful diet for any patient at any stage of any illness. Food not only sustains the body but also can lift the spirit. But although food and diet may enhance the effects of many common drugs, no one has found them to be an adequate, effective substitute for (among other medicines)

✔ Antibiotics and other drugs used to fight infections

✔ Vaccines or immunizations used to prevent communicable diseases

✔ Anticancer drugs

If your doctor suggests altering your diet to make your treatment more effective, your brain will tell you, *Hey, that makes sense.* But if someone suggests chucking your doctor and tossing away your medicine in favor of food therapy alone, heed the natural warning in your head. You know there's no free lunch and — as yet — no truly magical food, either.

Part VI
The Part of Tens

The 5th Wave   By Rich Tennant

"Gordon's always had trouble controlling his appetite at restaurants. I had to explain to him that you're not supposed to pull your chair up to the salad bar."

In this part . . .

If you've ever read a *For Dummies* book, you know what to expect here — nifty lists of useful factoids that make great conversation starters and help you wind your way through the subject at hand.

In this book, that means ten great Web sites, ten superstar foods, and ten easy ways to cut the calories without eliminating tasty food. What a bargain!

Chapter 27

Ten Nutrition Web Sites

*T*he ten nutrition-oriented sites listed in this chapter give you reliable, accurate, balanced information: nutritional guidelines, medical news, interactive sites, directories, and more. And these sites are only a start. If Wiley Publishing had called this part of the book The Part of Hundreds rather than The Part of Tens, I could've included many more super sources, but alas, I don't have room for them here.

Nevertheless, here's a sampling: the USDA National Agricultural Library at www. nal.usda.gov, and the American Diabetes Association at www.diabetes. org, and the Mayo Clinic at www.mayo.edu, and . . . well, you get the picture.

Click!

U.S. Department of Agriculture Nutrient Database

www.nal.usda.gov/fnic/foodcomp/search

The USDA Nutrient Database is the ultimate food info chart, with nutrient data for more than 5,000 foods in several serving sizes and different preparations. Each entry is a snapshot of a specific food serving (for example, a raw apple with skin) that lists the amount of

▶ Water (by weight)

▶ Food energy (calories)

▶ Protein

✔ Total fat

✔ Carbohydrates

✔ Dietary fiber

✔ Minerals: Calcium, iron, magnesium, phosphorus, potassium, sodium, and more

✔ Vitamins: Vitamin C, thiamin (vitamin B1), riboflavin (vitamin B2), niacin, vitamin B6, folate, vitamin B12, vitamin A, and more

✔ Lipids: Saturated, monounsaturated, and polyunsaturated fat, as well as cholesterol

✔ Amino acids

✔ Other substances, such as caffeine, alcohol, and beta carotene

When you visit this site, the first page that comes up is headlined "Search the USDA National Nutrient Database for Standard Reference." To find the food you're looking for, type its name — "apple," for example — into the empty box below, and then click on Submit. That brings up a list of possibilities, such as "Babyfood, juice, apple and grape" or "Babyfood, dinner, apples and chicken, strained." Ignore the fancy stuff and scroll down to something basic, such as "Apples, raw, with skin." Click on the circle next to that entry and click on Submit, and a new screen lists various forms of raw apple, such as "100 grams" or "1 cup, quartered or chopped" or "1 large (3-¼" dia) (approx 2 per lb)." Choose the box in front of the serving you prefer, click on the button marked Submit, and — bingo! There you are — calories and nutrients for one large apple. Neat!

To access a list of foods showing the content of a single nutrient such as protein or calories or vitamin C or calcium or beta-carotene, click on the button marked Nutrient Lists from the main page. Then follow directions to get the list you want, with the foods arranged either in alphabetical order or by the amount of the nutrient in the food. The lists are displayed as PDF (portable document format) files; to read these files, you need Adobe Acrobat Reader, a program available free at www.adobe.com/products/acrobat/readermain.html.

USDA Food and Nutrition Information Center (FNIC)

www.nal.usda.gov/fnic

Have you worked your way through every single one of the several thousand listings on the USDA Nutrient Database in the previous section? Then come on over to FNIC, which is part of the USDA National Agricultural Library.

To access its info, slide your mouse over to the box on the left side of the homepage and pick a subject. For me, the best are FNIC Resource Lists and Food Composition.

The first offers, well, resource lists. The second provides pathways to such nuggets of nutritional data as a report on "Isoflavone Content of Foods." (Don't know what an isoflavone is? Stick a pencil in this page and turn back, right now, to Chapter 12.) Yeah, some of the things pasted here may be much more than you ever wanted to know about, well, the isoflavone content of foods, but for the adventurous, this is a su-pah site. Take a flyer and try it.

U.S. Food and Drug Administration

www.fda.gov

Entering the FDA Web site is like opening the door to the world's biggest nutritional-information toy store. So much stuff is on the (virtual) shelves that you hardly know which item to grab first. Luckily, in this store, all the toys are free, and plenty of links to other helpful information mean you can linger here happily for days. Weeks. Years. Maybe forever.

FDA's charter includes drugs as well as food, so on the left of the homepage, you can click on links to information on medicines for people and pets, poisons and side effects, medical devices (think pacemakers), and products that give off radiation. The links under Let Us Hear from You, near the center of the page, let activists report on adverse events ("I took that antibiotic and got hives!") or allow you to contact the FDA with your questions and comments. For *foodies* (people who want to know ab-so-lute-ly everything about different kinds of food and food preparation), though, the main event is, well, food.

On the FDA homepage, scroll down the left side and click on Food. Doing so takes you to a page headed "Center for Food Safety and Applied Nutrition" (CFSAN) (www.cfsan.fda.gov), which is more fun than a barrel of, oh, M&M's.

The main page of the food section is devoted to Recent News, Program Areas, National Food Safety Programs, Special Interest Areas, and the ever popular Other Sources of Information. On the left side of the page are links to FDA Documents and sites, phone numbers, and e-mail addresses where you can interact with CFSAN.

Only my editor's insistence that we keep this book to fewer than 1,000 pages prevents me from telling you what's listed under each main headline and then what's listed under the subheads, and then . . . see? Try it. You'll love it.

American Dietetic Association

www.eatright.org

This site features nutrition recommendations, tips, guidelines, research, policy, and stats from the world's largest membership association of nutrition professionals, primarily registered dietitians. (For a quick rundown on who's who in nutrition science, see Chapter 1.)

The ADA homepage features links to categories (such as Professional Development) that are clearly meant to appeal to association members. But the site also has tidbits for consumers, such as daily nutrition tips, a monthly feature, nutrition position papers, and an online store where you can find, yes, *Dieting For Dummies* (Wiley).

The niftiest feature on the homepage is the link to Find a Nutrition Professional. Click on this link and you gain access to the ADA's Nationwide Nutrition Network, a referral service that links consumers, doctors, food companies, and restaurant people with dietetic professionals. ADA's mission is to serve the public by promoting nutrition, health, and well-being. If you can bend your brain around the much-too-adorable net address ("eatright"? Give me a break!), you'll discover this site is a true treasure trove. And golly gee, who wouldn't love having a personal dietitian to lead the way through the maze of conflicting nutritional advice?

The American Heart Association

www.americanheart.org

This site tells you everything you ever wanted to know about diet and heart disease. Starting at the homepage, run your mouse down the left side to Healthy Lifestyle. Click on it — and then click on Diet & Nutrition. Up pops a page with features such as the American Heart Association No-Fad Diet, Delicious Decisions (heart healthy yummies), Nutrition Facts, Dietary Recommendations, and Shopping Made Simple.

The indisputable link between diet and heart disease risk, not to mention the AHA site's user-friendly approach, makes this a must-stop on your nutritional tour of the Web.

The American Cancer Society

www.cancer.org

The ACS Web site is dedicated primarily to information about cancer: definitions, treatments, research, and support services. True, most of the nutrition news you find here is available elsewhere, but this site's defined focus provides easy access to other cancer-related topics.

On the ACS homepage, type "diet" into the Search box at top. Bingo! You've opened a grab bag of ACS press releases, guidelines, and the most common questions people ask about food and cancer (with answers). More-targeted searches — such as "high-fiber food" — yield more-specific responses, such as information on whether dietary fiber is related to a lower risk of colon cancer.

Until now, the American Cancer Society was barely a blip on the screen of nutrition sources. Today, with a growing number of well-designed studies to demonstrate that some foods and diet regimens may reduce your risk of certain types of cancer while others put you in harm's way, the ACS Web site offers solid reporting on this area of nutritional research.

The Food Allergy and Anaphylaxis Network

www.foodallergy.org

The Food Allergy and Anaphylaxis Network (FAAN) is a nonprofit membership organization (membership fee: $30/year for individuals) whose participants include families, doctors, dietitians, nurses, support groups, and food manufacturers in the U.S., Canada, and Europe. The group provides education about food allergies in addition to support and coping strategies for people who are allergic to specific foods.

From FAAN's homepage, you can link to updates, daily tips, newsletter excerpts, and all the usual service-oriented goodies. The site's best feature — an e-mail alert system — is free. Click the link under Special Allergy Alerts, fill out the form, and submit it to the site. You're now connected to an early warning system with allergy-linked news and information about recalls of troublesome products, such as 2-ounce bags of cashews that may mistakenly contain peanuts.

This no-nonsense, highly accessible site is required reading for people with food allergies. Others, such as families and friends, can also benefit from its solid information and support services.

International Food Information Council (IFIC)

ific.org

The International Food Information Council (IFIC), created in 1985, is a non-profit organization dedicated to improving the relationship between the nutrition community — scientists, food manufacturers, health professionals, government officials — and the news media. Although the council's membership includes corporations that make and sell food products, IFIC plays no role in marketing products or promoting its members. Its aim is to make sure that consumers get accurate information about diet and health.

The IFIC homepage allows you to access features in English or Spanish. Consumers can bypass the professional stuff and head for links under Nutrition and Food Safety Information or click on the "Food Insight Newsletter" or the terrific Glossary of Food-Related Terms.

The site also offers articles on basic nutrition topics, such as functional foods, oral health, dietary fats and fat replacers, and additional resources. The writing is accessible, the information impeccable.

IFIC is a trade group, so purists may complain about some IFIC positions, such as its endorsement of some food additives, but the site's intelligent approach to complex and emotional issues allows you to make up your own mind.

American Council on Science and Health (ACSH) and the Center for Science in the Public Interest (CSPI)

www.acsh.org

www.cspinet.org

The American Council on Science and Health and the Center for Science in the Public Interest are two nonprofit consumer-friendly organizations that usually sit on opposite sides of any nutritional issue. ACSH is cool and calm; CSPI is a hot-button advocate.

For example, CSPI believes many additives are hazardous to your health; ACSH says some additives are useful in some foods for some people. This kind of disagreement ensures that if you punch up the same search word or phrase on both sites, you'll find out about the pros and cons of an issue. Neat.

Both sites feature news releases, position papers, online membership enrollment, order forms for publications, and links to other sites.

Which site you prefer is pretty much a matter of personality, but you can't go wrong with either one if you're looking for highly reliable information about nutrition issues and how food and diet affect your health.

Tufts University Nutrition Navigator

The Tufts University Nutrition Navigator is (or was) the mother of all nutrition guides, a site that evaluated several hundred other Web sites on a 25-point scale measuring content and reliability — for ratings ranging from Among the Best (22–25 points) down to Not Recommended (below 12 points).

The site should be included in this list, but when I went to check it out for this edition of *Nutrition For Dummies,* this message popped up: "*Tufts University Nutrition Navigator* (`navigator.tufts.edu`) is not available at this time. We thank all of you who have visited the site over the past seven years."

Horrors! An e-mail and call to Tufts elicited the information that the University is looking for funding and expects to have the Navigator back online sooner or later. So keep clicking on the address. Sooner (or later) I hope the Navigator returns to help you set a reliable course through the gazillions of nutrition sites.

Chapter 28

Ten (Well, Okay, Twelve) Superstar Foods

• •

In This Chapter

▶ Investigating why bison beats beef

▶ Experiencing the joy of chocolate

▶ Waking up with a few mood-elevators in your cup

▶ Examining other foods that raise your mood and keep you healthy

▶ Listing foods that may cause problems

• •

*E*ver since Eve pulled that apple (really a pomegranate) off the tree of knowledge in the Garden of Eden, people have been attributing special powers to one food or another.

This chapter is by no means the complete A+ list. For example, I haven't included chicken soup, because what more can anyone say about this universal panacea? Ditto for garlic and onions, both now honored as probably heart-healthy. Winnowing down the list was hard, but somebody had to do it! So here are my nominations for the Top Ten (actually, the Top Twelve, but who's counting?), plus a bonus list of baddies assembled by *Men's Health* magazine.

Alcohol

Alcohol beverages play such an important part in human culinary and nutrition history that they have their very own chapter earlier in this book. Simply listing alcohol's natural properties tells you right off why ancient peoples called it a "gift of the gods" or the "water of life." It's an effective antiseptic, sedative, and analgesic.

Moderate alcohol consumption relaxes muscles and mood, expands blood vessels to lower blood pressure temporarily, and appears to lower the risk of heart disease, either by reducing the stickiness of *blood platelets* (small particles that can clump together to form a blood clot) or by relaxing blood vessels (making them temporarily larger) or by increasing the amount of HDLs ("good cholesterol") in your blood. Although some forms of alcohol, such as red wines, have gotten more press attention with regard to these effects, the truth is that controlled studies show similar effects with all forms of alcohol beverages — wine, beer, and spirits.

Common wisdom to the contrary, alcohol sometimes may also be beneficial to the brain. Yes, drinking can make you fuzzy, which is why — really — you should never drink and drive. However, recent studies from the Institute of Preventive Medicine at Kommunehospitalet in Copenhagen, Denmark, and Johns Hopkins University in Maryland hint that regular consumption of moderate amounts of wine may keep minds sharp into older age. (Check it out in Chapter 9.) Next time you lift a glass and say, "To your health," consider yourself right on the money.

Beans

Modern science says that beans lower cholesterol levels with *gums* and *pectin,* soluble dietary fibers that mop up fats and prevent their being absorbed by your body. Oats, which also are rich in gums, particularly a gum called *beta glucan,* produce the same effect.

Beans are also valuable for people with diabetes. Because beans are digested very slowly, eating them produces only a gradual increase in the level of sugar circulating in your blood. As a result, metabolizing beans requires less insulin than eating other types of high-carb foods such as pasta and potatoes. In one well-known study at the University of Kentucky, a diet rich in beans made it possible for people with Type 1 diabetes (their bodies produce virtually no insulin) to reduce their daily insulin intake by nearly 40 percent. Patients with Type 2 diabetes (their bodies produce some insulin) were able to reduce insulin intake by 98 percent.

Just about the only drawback to a diet rich in beans is gas resulting from the natural human inability to digest some dietary fiber and complex sugars such as *raffinose* and *stachyose,* which sit in your gut as fodder for the resident friendly bacteria that digest the carbs and then release carbon dioxide and (ugh) methane, a smelly gas.

One way to reduce intestinal gas production is to reduce the complex sugar content of the beans before you eat them. Here's how: Bring a pot of water to a boil. Turn off the heat. Add the beans. Let them soak for several hours. The sugars leach out into the water, which means you can discard the sugars by draining the beans and adding fresh water to cook in. If that doesn't do the job, try two heat-and-soak sessions before cooking.

Berries

"Cholesterol buster" is easy to say. "Pterostilbene" (ter-o-STILL-bean) is a tongue twister. But USDA researchers at the Natural Products Utilization Research Unit in Oxford, Mississippi, think they may be synonyms. Pterostilbene, an antioxidant found primarily in blueberries (as well as cranberries, lingonberries, and huckleberries), appears to step up the activity of cells in your liver that reduce the production of cholesterol and other artery-clogging fats. In fact, the USDA people hint that pterostilbene could be extracted from blueberries to make commercial anticholesterol meds with fewer side effects than those currently on the market. Until human tests are run, nobody will know how many blueberries you have to eat to lower your cholesterol, but some nutrition studies suggest that ounce for ounce, blueberries have one of the highest antioxidant contents in the whole wide vegetable and fruit world. So enjoy.

Bison

Bison is back. The really big _bovid ruminant_ (translation: an animal related to a cow) is no longer an endangered species. In fact, according to the 2,500-member National Bison Association, the current bison herd is up to a whopping 350,000 animals to be shipped to your table as _the other red meat_ — translation: beef.

Ounce for ounce, bison has less fat, less sat fat, less cholesterol, fewer calories, and more protein than you-know-what. It's pretty tasty, too, with a rich meaty flavor that survives broiling and grilling but may, alas, turn dry when roasted. Not to worry: Most Americans get their first taste of bison as the broiled burger now popping up on coffee shop menus all across the country. While you're waiting to be served, take a gander at the widely distributed four-color table tent, which lists relative amounts of nutrients in 3.5-ounce (100-gram) servings of bison, beef, pork, and chicken. As you may expect, the bison wins.

One more thing: Never say "buffalo" when you mean "bison." The scientific name for American bison is — no kidding — _Bison bison._ The word _buffalo_ comes from French explorers who called bison "boeuf" (meaning beef). English changed that to "buff." Common usage smoothed that out to "buffle" and eventually "buffalo." Actual buffalo are native to Asia and Africa.

Breast Milk

Human breast milk is more nutritious than cow's milk for human babies. It has a higher percentage of easily digested, high-energy fats and carbohydrates. Its proteins stimulate an infant's immune system, encouraging his or her white blood cells to produce plenty infection-fighting antibodies, including those that go after viruses linked to infant diarrhea, which accounts for 23 percent of all deaths among children younger than 5. And get this: In 2004, a report in the British Medical Journal *Lancet* said that feeding a baby breast milk rather than formula for the first month of life may lower the child's cholesterol levels later in life, reduce the child's eventual risk of high blood pressure, and keep a person slimmer as he or she grows older.

All in all, a pretty good way to start off in life, doncha think?

Chocolate

Westerners have been fools for chocolate ever since the Spanish conquistadors discovered it at Montezuma's Mexican court. And why not? The cocoa bean is a good source of energy, fiber, protein, carbohydrates, B vitamins, and minerals (one ounce of dark sweet chocolate has 12 percent of the iron and 33 percent of the magnesium a healthy woman needs each day).

Nutritionwise, the rap on chocolate is that cocoa butter (the fat in chocolate) is 59 percent saturated fat, primarily stearic acid. But nobody seems to have told stearic acid that it's a villain. Unlike other saturated fats, stearic acid neither increases LDLs ("bad cholesterol") nor lowers HDLs ("good cholesterol"). In addition, stearic acid makes blood platelets less likely to clump together into a blood clot, thus lowering you risk of heart attack or stroke.

And don't forget the *phytosterols,* steroidlike compounds in plants that sop up cholesterol in your gut and zip it out of your body before it reaches your bloodstream. Phytosterols, the heart-healthy ingredients in Take Control and Benecol margarines, are found in cocoa beans and chocolate, leading canny researchers at the University of California-Berkeley Division of Cardiovascular Medicine and the Department of Nutrition to investigate whether drinking a cocoa beverage once a day or eating a chocolate chew twice a day can lower cholesterol levels in postmenopausal women.

In addition, a study published in the *Proceedings of the National Academy of Sciences* in January 2006 credits the cocoa compound (–)epicatechin (translation: *minus epicatechin*) with the ability to help blood vessels relax. And as we all know, relaxing your blood vessels means lowering your blood pressure — and your risk of heart attack.

Does all this mean chocolate is a bona fide health food? Not yet. But is chocolate healthful as part of a balanced diet? You bet. Especially because it's a veritable happiness cocktail containing *caffeine* (a mood elevator and central nervous system stimulant), *theobromine* (a muscle stimulant), *phenylethylamine* (another mood elevator), and *anandamide,* a chemical that stimulates the same areas of the brain that marijuana does. No, eating chocolate won't get you high. You'd have to consume 25 pounds or more at one sitting to get the smallest marijuana-like effect. Nonetheless, I think chocolate was Montezuma's way of making up for his, ahem, "revenge."

Coffee

For years, there was nothing but bad news about coffee. Pancreatic cancer. Cystic breasts. High cholesterol. Heart disease. Stroke. Birth defects. Heartburn and reflux. But the worm — okay, the coffee bean — has turned: Later studies show no link at all between drinking coffee and an increased risk of any of these conditions. True, coffee may upset your stomach and keep you up at night, but as *Heartburn & Reflux For Dummies* (published by Wiley) explains, for most people, these effects are almost always linked to excess consumption. (How much is "excess"? The amount varies from person to person, but when you hit your limit, you'll definitely know. Trust me.)

In the end, the simple fact is that taken in moderation, regular coffee definitely qualifies for anybody's list of super foods. Its most active ingredient, caffeine, elevates your mood and increases your ability to concentrate; may improve your athletic performance; can help shrink the swollen, throbbing blood vessels that make your head ache; and boosts the effect of painkillers, which is why caffeine is often included in over-the-counter analgesic (pain-relieving) products. Which is also why, time after time, the java really does the job.

Fish

Did your great-grandmother call fish "brain food"? If so, it was because fish is rich in iodine, the mineral that allows your thyroid gland to churn out thyroid hormones vital to your ability to think and move. Once upon a time, back in great-granny's day, people living far from the ocean (our best natural source of iodine) were often sluggish, sometimes even mentally retarded, because they were lacking iodine.

But this condition became rare in the U.S. after the introduction of iodized salt in the 1920s. Fish's modern reputation for medical magic comes from its ability to reduce the risk of heart disease and stroke, in large part, because of its omega-3 fatty acids. These unsaturated fats make blood less sticky, thus reducing the incidence of clots. They also knock down levels of bad cholesterol.

You want proof? Here's proof: In 2002, data from the long-running Harvard Health Professionals Study indicated that people who eat 3 to 5 ounces of fish just once a month have a 40 percent lower risk of *ischemic stroke,* a stroke caused by a blood clot in a cranial artery. The Harvard study did not include women. But a report on women and stroke published in the *Journal of the American Medical Association* in 2000 says women who eat about 4 ounces of fish — think one small can of tuna — two to four times a week appear to cut their risk of stroke by a similar 40 percent. And in 2005, the *American Journal of Preventive Medicine* published several reports from the Harvard Center for Risk Analysis project concluding that "any fish consumption confers substantial relative risk reduction compared to no fish consumption, with the possibility that additional consumption confers incremental benefits," including a "17% reduction in death from heart attack, with each additional serving per week associated with a further reduction in this risk of 3.9%."

Of course, there are catches to this catch. First, some fish are high in mercury, a metal that can damage a developing fetus, but small amounts of fish, say two 3-ounce servings a week, seem to be safe for everyone else. Second, frequent servings of fish may increase the risk of a stroke caused by bleeding in the brain. This situation is common among Native Alaskans who eat lots of fish and have a higher than normal incidence of hemorrhagic, or bleeding, strokes. The Harvard study found no significant link between fish consumption and bleeding strokes, but the researchers say more studies are needed to nail down the relationship or lack thereof.

While we're waiting, pass the chips. Sat fat– and trans fat–free, of course.

Nuts

Pass up the pretzels. Skip the chips. At snack time, reach for the almonds. Although nuts are technically a high-fat food, a series of studies including several at California's Loma Linda University say that adding moderate amounts of nuts to a cholesterol-lowering diet or substituting nuts for other high-fat foods such as meats may cut normal to moderately high levels of total cholesterol and LDLs ("bad cholesterol") as much as 12 percent.

These guys should know. A while back, they made headlines with a walnut study in which volunteers were given one of two diets, both based on National Cholesterol Education Program (NCEP) recommendations. People on Diet #1 got 20 percent of their calories from fats in oils and fatty foods such as meat. Folks on Diet #2 got 20 percent of their calories from high-fat nuts instead of meat, but both controlled-fat diets appeared to lower cholesterol levels.

The take-home message here is that although nuts are high in fat, their fats are polyunsaturated and monounsaturated cholesterol busters (more about them in Chapter 7). And let us not forget that nuts also provide other heart-healthy nutrients such as arginine (an amino acid your body uses to make a clot-blocking compound called nitric oxide), folate (a B vitamin that lowers blood levels of homocysteine, a risk factor for heart disease), vitamin E, and dietary fiber.

So feel free to go (sensibly) nuts for nuts. Crunch.

White Tea

Black and green? So 20th century. The hot new color in tea is white. The leaves for all three teas come from one plant, *Camellia sinensis.* But those leaves meant for black and green teas are rolled and fermented before drying, while those destined for white teas — which actually brew up pale yellow-red — aren't. Nutritionwise, this small change makes a big difference.

Flavonoids are natural chemicals credited with tea's ability to lower cholesterol, reduce the risk of some kinds of cancer, and protect your teeth from cavity-causing bacteria. Fresh tea leaves are rich in flavonoids called catechins, but processing the leaves to make black and green teas releases enzymes that enable individual catechins to hook up with others, forming new flavor and coloring agents called polyphenols (poly = many) that give flavor and color to black and green teas. Because white tea leaves are neither rolled nor fermented, fewer of their catechins marry into polyphenols. According to researchers at the Linus Pauling Institute (LPI) at Oregon State University, the plain catechin content of white tea is three times that of green tea. Black tea comes in a distant third.

Why should you care about this? Because all those catechins seem to be good for living bodies. For example, when LPI researchers tested white tea's ability to inhibit cell mutations in bacteria and slow down cell changes leading to colon cancer in rats, the white tea beat green tea, the former health champ. And when scientists at University Hospitals of Cleveland and Case Western Reserve University applied creams containing white-tea extract to human skin (on volunteers) and exposed the volunteers to artificial sunlight, the creamed skin developed fewer pre-cancerous changes. To be fair, green tea preparations were also protective, but white tea has less caffeine than either green or black tea, which makes it the perfect brew for a recovering caffeine fiend. Sip.

Whole Grains

If you're a man who plans to live forever, a team of nutrition scientists at Harvard/Brigham and Women's Hospital in Boston have three words for you: whole grain cereal. When the investigators took a look at the health stats for a one-year period in the lives of the 86,190 male doctors in the long-running Physicians' Health Study, they found 3,114 deaths among the study volunteers, including 1,381 deaths from heart attack and stroke. Then they looked a little closer and discovered that eating habits count. Men who ate at least one serving of whole grain cereal a day were 27 percent less likely to die than were men who ate refined grain products. The whole-grain group was also as much as 28 percent less likely to succumb to a heart attack, regardless of how much they weighed, whether they smoked or drank alcohol or took vitamins pills or had a history of high blood pressure and high cholesterol.

Nobody yet knows exactly why this should be so. But they do know that whole grains are a treasure trove of dietary fiber, vitamins, minerals, and other phytochemicals (plant compounds such as antioxidants) that protect by lowering blood pressure and cholesterol while improving the body's ability to process nutrients, particularly carbohydrates.

The question is, how much cereal must you eat to benefit? The studies say more is better, but one serving a day is better than none at all. To find the right cereal, haul out your magnifying glass or bifocals to check the Nutrition Facts label. If whole grain is the first ingredient and there's at least 2 grams dietary fiber per serving, you've found breakfast. For those who absolutely, positively hate cereal, try whole-grain bread. And, yes, whole grains are an equal opportunity dish. Earlier studies suggest that women, too, may come out ahead by adding whole grain to their daily diets.

Yogurt

Yogurt is milk with added friendly bacteria that digest milk sugar (lactose) to produce lactic acid, a natural preservative that gives the flavor of yogurt its pleasant bite. Yogurt is definitely magical for people who are *lactase deficient* (meaning they don't produce enough lactase to digest milk sugar so that they get gassy whenever they drink milk).

Tracking the terrible ten

In 2003, while others whistled a happy tune about good foods, the worrywarts at *Men's Health* magazine compiled a list of the ten foods most likely to make you feel absolutely awful — mostly due to their tendency to harbor organisms that can seriously upset your intestinal tract. The top troublemakers are undercooked chicken, ground beef, ground turkey, oysters, and eggs, followed by unheated cold cuts, raw scallions, peaches, cantaloupe, and packaged salad greens. Luckily, thorough cooking (or reheating) can make the first seven safe to eat. As for peaches, the guys say, peel 'em to eliminate pesticides stuck in the fuzz. Scrub your bumpy cantaloupe before slicing to dislodge bacteria in the rind that may otherwise be transferred to the fruit. And rinse your packaged salad greens. Then rinse again. Even if the packaged says "washed." Splash.

But there's no evidence to show that yogurt is a longevity tonic, a claim traced back to Ilya Ilyich Metchnikoff, a Russian Nobel Prize winner (1908; Physiology/Medicine) who believed that people die prematurely entirely because of the action of "putrefying bacteria" in the intestines. Searching for a way to disarm the putrefiers, Metchnikoff ended up in Bulgaria, a place where many people lived past 50 and a significant percentage made it into their late 80s.

Historians may argue that the only way to live that long in Bulgaria was to avoid Bulgarian politics, but Metchnikoff credited the organisms used to make Bulgarian cultured milk. He was wrong. The bugs, christened *L. bulgaricus,* make nice yogurt but don't take up residence in the human gut. This hardly mattered to Metchnikoff, who died in Paris in 1916, at the relatively young age of 71. His faith in yogurt, however, continues to cycle in and out of fashion.

Chapter 29

Ten Easy Ways to Cut Calories

*L*osing weight is simple math. If you cut 3,500 calories out of your diet in the course of a week without reducing your daily activity, you can say goodbye to one whole pound of fat.

Yes, I know reading that sentence is easier than actually doing it, so I'm ready to give you two tricks to make the job easier. First, cut your calories in small increments — 50 here, 100 there — rather than in one big lump. Second, instead of giving up foods you really love (and feeling deprived), switch to low-fat versions.

This chapter tells you how to accomplish both. I've included some brand-name products just so that you can compare different versions made by the same companies.

Switching to Low-Fat or No-Fat Dairy Products

Milk and milk products are the best source for the calcium that keeps bones strong. But these same products may also be high in cholesterol, saturated fat, and calories. You can reduce all three by choosing a low- or no-fat milk product.

For example, a cup of whole milk has 150 calories, but a cup of skim milk has only 85. One slice of regular Kraft American cheese has 60 calories, but one slice of Kraft Free American cheese has only 30. A sandwich made with three slices of cheese is 90 calories lighter if the cheese is "free."

Substituting Sugar Substitutes

Coffee has no calories, but every teaspoon of sugar you stir into your cup has 15 big ones. Multiply that by four (1 teaspoon each in four cups of coffee), and your naturally no-cal beverage can add 60 calories a day to your diet. Sixty calories a day times seven days a week, and yipes, that's 420 calories! That's about as much as you'd get from four or five medium slices of unbuttered toast or five medium apples. So is this a good time to mention that one packet of sugar substitute has absolutely zero calories? I thought so.

Serving Stew Instead of Steak

No matter how you slice it, red meat is red meat — cholesterol, saturated fats, and all. But if you stew your beef or lamb or pork rather than broiling or roasting it, you can skim off a bunch of high-calorie fat. Just make the stew and then stick it in the fridge for a couple of hours until a layer of fat hardens on top. Spoon it off: Every tablespoon of pure fat subtracts 100 calories from dinner. And, yes, you can also cut off all visible fat before preparing the meat. Same 100 calories per tablespoon of fat.

Choosing Low-Fat Desserts

Who says you have to suffer to cut calories? Not me. One half cup of Häagen-Dazs chocolate ice cream has 270 calories. One half cup of Häagen-Dazs no-fat chocolate sorbet has 140 calories. Believe me: Switching from the first to the second is no problem. If you're a true chocoholic, you'll send me valentines for this suggestion.

Peeling the Poultry

Most of the fat in poultry is in the skin. A fried chicken breast with skin has 217 calories; without the skin, it has only 160. Half a roasted duck (with skin) has a whopping 1,287 calories; without skin, it's only 444. Even if you have a fried chicken breast every night for a week (which you would never, ever do), you can save 399 calories by taking the skin off before cooking the bird. Share seven skinless half-ducks with a friend, and you each save 2,950 calories a week by removing the skin. Wow. That's practically a pound right there.

Not Oiling the Salad

True, salad can be a low-fat, low-calorie meal. Throw in some breast of chicken and a couple of no-fat croutons or cheese cubes, and it's still mostly crunch.

But the dressing can do you in. For example, two tablespoons of Wishbone Italian Dressing or one tablespoon of Hellmann's regular "real mayonnaise" have 100 calories. What to do? Ah, c'mon, you know the answer: Switch.

Two tablespoons of Wishbone Fat Free Italian dressing add just 15 — count 'em, 15! — calories. One tablespoon of Hellmann's Light cuts the calorie count in half, to 50 calories. Have salad once a day for a week, and you can save 595 calories with fat-free rather than regular salad dressing or save 525 calories with low-fat mayonnaise rather than regular. Or as University of Maine nutrition guru Alfred Bushway suggests, "Using a tablespoon of balsamic vinegar instead is even better." Neat.

Don't oil your pots and pans, either. Bake with parchment paper instead of greasing the pan. Sauté with natural juices in nonstick pans. Every tablespoon of fat you don't use means approximately 100 fewer calories in the dish.

Making One-Slice Sandwiches

Depending on the brand, one slice of bread in your daily luncheon sandwich may have anywhere from 65 to 120 calories. Eliminating one slice and serving your sandwich open-faced can cut up to 840 calories from your weekly total. And you know that making that one slice whole wheat adds dietary fiber to your menu, right? Just asking.

Eliminating the High-Fat Ingredient

A bacon, lettuce, and tomato sandwich usually comes with three strips of bacon, each one worth 100 calories. Leave off one strip and save 100 calories. Leave off two, save 200 calories. Leave off three, save 300 calories — and enjoy your lettuce and tomato sandwich with low-fat mayonnaise.

Here are some other ways to eliminate fat calories:

- ✔ Making spaghetti sauce without olive oil (100 calories a tablespoon)
- ✔ Making split pea soup without ham (55 to 90 calories an ounce)
- ✔ Making cream sauces with skim milk instead of cream (470 calories per cup for the cream; 85 to 90 calories for the skim milk)

Seasoning the Veggies instead of Drowning Them in Butter

This one's a no-brainer. Season your vegetables with herbs instead of greasing them, and you save 100 calories for every unused tablespoon of butter, margarine, or oil. Think dill on the potatoes, chives on the corn, oregano on the green beans — whatever catches your imagination.

Washing the Chopped Meat

Yes, you read that right. Heat a teapot of water. Put the chopped meat in a pan and cook it until it browns. Pour off the fat, turn the meat into a strainer, and pour a cup of hot water over it. Repeat two times. Every tablespoon of fat that melts or drains from the meat saves you 100 calories, plus cholesterol and saturated fat. Use the defatted meat in spaghetti sauce. (Check out Figure 29-1 for the visual presentation!)

Figure 29-1:
Try washing your (cooked) chopped meat to reduce fat.

Index

● *C* ●

• *Y* •

• *Z* •

Notes

SPORTS, FITNESS, PARENTING, RELIGION & SPIRITUALITY

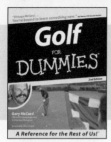

0-7645-5146-9

0-7645-5418-2

Also available:
- Adoption For Dummies
  0-7645-5488-3
- Basketball For Dummies
  0-7645-5248-1
- The Bible For Dummies
  0-7645-5296-1
- Buddhism For Dummies
  0-7645-5359-3
- Catholicism For Dummies
  0-7645-5391-7
- Hockey For Dummies
  0-7645-5228-7

- Judaism For Dummies
  0-7645-5299-6
- Martial Arts For Dummies
  0-7645-5358-5
- Pilates For Dummies
  0-7645-5397-6
- Religion For Dummies
  0-7645-5264-3
- Teaching Kids to Read For Dummies
  0-7645-4043-2
- Weight Training For Dummies
  0-7645-5168-X
- Yoga For Dummies
  0-7645-5117-5

TRAVEL

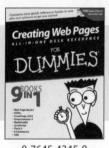

0-7645-5438-7

0-7645-5453-0

Also available:
- Alaska For Dummies
  0-7645-1761-9
- Arizona For Dummies
  0-7645-6938-4
- Cancún and the Yucatán For Dummies
  0-7645-2437-2
- Cruise Vacations For Dummies
  0-7645-6941-4
- Europe For Dummies
  0-7645-5456-5
- Ireland For Dummies
  0-7645-5455-7

- Las Vegas For Dummies
  0-7645-5448-4
- London For Dummies
  0-7645-4277-X
- New York City For Dummies
  0-7645-6945-7
- Paris For Dummies
  0-7645-5494-8
- RV Vacations For Dummies
  0-7645-5443-3
- Walt Disney World & Orlando For Dumm
  0-7645-6943-0

GRAPHICS, DESIGN & WEB DEVELOPMENT

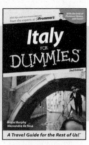

0-7645-4345-8

0-7645-5589-8

Also available:
- Adobe Acrobat 6 PDF For Dummies
  0-7645-3760-1
- Building a Web Site For Dummies
  0-7645-7144-3
- Dreamweaver MX 2004 For Dummies
  0-7645-4342-3
- FrontPage 2003 For Dummies
  0-7645-3882-9
- HTML 4 For Dummies
  0-7645-1995-6
- Illustrator CS For Dummies
  0-7645-4084-X

- Macromedia Flash MX 2004 For Dumm
  0-7645-4358-X
- Photoshop 7 All-in-One Desk
  Reference For Dummies
  0-7645-1667-1
- Photoshop CS Timesaving Technique
  For Dummies
  0-7645-6782-9
- PHP 5 For Dummies
  0-7645-4166-8
- PowerPoint 2003 For Dummies
  0-7645-3908-6
- QuarkXPress 6 For Dummies
  0-7645-2593-X

NETWORKING, SECURITY, PROGRAMMING & DATABASES

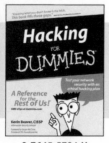

0-7645-6852-3

0-7645-5784-X

Also available:
- A+ Certification For Dummies
  0-7645-4187-0
- Access 2003 All-in-One Desk
  Reference For Dummies
  0-7645-3988-4
- Beginning Programming For Dummies
  0-7645-4997-9
- C For Dummies
  0-7645-7068-4
- Firewalls For Dummies
  0-7645-4048-3
- Home Networking For Dummies
  0-7645-42796

- Network Security For Dummies
  0-7645-1679-5
- Networking For Dummies
  0-7645-1677-9
- TCP/IP For Dummies
  0-7645-1760-0
- VBA For Dummies
  0-7645-3989-2
- Wireless All In-One Desk Reference
  For Dummies
  0-7645-7496-5
- Wireless Home Networking For Dummi
  0-7645-3910-8

Diabetes
FOR DUMMIES

0-7645-6820-5 *†

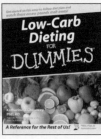

Low-Carb Dieting
FOR DUMMIES

0-7645-2566-2

Also available:
- Alzheimer's For Dummies
  0-7645-3899-3
- Asthma For Dummies
  0-7645-4233-8
- Controlling Cholesterol For Dummies
  0-7645-5440-9
- Depression For Dummies
  0-7645-3900-0
- Dieting For Dummies
  0-7645-4149-8
- Fertility For Dummies
  0-7645-2549-2

- Fibromyalgia For Dummies
  0-7645-5441-7
- Improving Your Memory For Dummies
  0-7645-5435-2
- Pregnancy For Dummies †
  0-7645-4483-7
- Quitting Smoking For Dummies
  0-7645-2629-4
- Relationships For Dummies
  0-7645-5384-4
- Thyroid For Dummies
  0-7645-5385-2

Spanish
FOR DUMMIES

0-7645-5194-9

The Origins of Tolkien's Middle-earth
FOR DUMMIES

0-7645-4186-2

Also available:
- Algebra For Dummies
  0-7645-5325-9
- British History For Dummies
  0-7645-7021-8
- Calculus For Dummies
  0-7645-2498-4
- English Grammar For Dummies
  0-7645-5322-4
- Forensics For Dummies
  0-7645-5580-4
- The GMAT For Dummies
  0-7645-5251-1
- Inglés Para Dummies
  0-7645-5427-1

- Italian For Dummies
  0-7645-5196-5
- Latin For Dummies
  0-7645-5431-X
- Lewis & Clark For Dummies
  0-7645-2545-X
- Research Papers For Dummies
  0-7645-5426-3
- The SAT I For Dummies
  0-7645-7193-1
- Science Fair Projects For Dummies
  0-7645-5460-3
- U.S. History For Dummies
  0-7645-5249-X

Get smart @ dummies.com®

- **Find a full list of Dummies titles**
- **Look into loads of FREE on-site articles**
- **Sign up for FREE eTips e-mailed to you weekly**
- **See what other products carry the Dummies name**
- **Shop directly from the Dummies bookstore**
- **Enter to win new prizes every month!**

† Separate Canadian edition also available
‡ Separate U.K. edition also available

Available wherever books are sold. For more information or to order direct: U.S. customers visit www.dummies.com or call 1-877-762-2974.
U.K. customers visit www.wileyeurope.com or call 0800 243407. Canadian customers visit www.wiley.ca or call 1-800-567-4797.